Treatment of Cornea and Ocular Surface Diseases

Treatment of Cornea and Ocular Surface Diseases

Editor

Vincenzo Scorcia

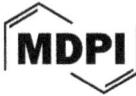 Basel • Beijing • Wuhan • Barcelona • Belgrade • Novi Sad • Cluj • Manchester

Editor
Vincenzo Scorcia
University Magna Græcia of
Catanzaro
Catanzaro, Italy

Editorial Office
MDPI
St. Alban-Anlage 66
4052 Basel, Switzerland

This is a reprint of articles from the Special Issue published online in the open access journal *Journal of Clinical Medicine* (ISSN 2077-0383) (available at: https://www.mdpi.com/journal/jcm/special_issues/Cornea_Ocular_surface).

For citation purposes, cite each article independently as indicated on the article page online and as indicated below:

Lastname, A.A.; Lastname, B.B. Article Title. *Journal Name* **Year**, *Volume Number*, Page Range.

ISBN 978-3-0365-9588-7 (Hbk)
ISBN 978-3-0365-9589-4 (PDF)
doi.org/10.3390/books978-3-0365-9589-4

© 2023 by the authors. Articles in this book are Open Access and distributed under the Creative Commons Attribution (CC BY) license. The book as a whole is distributed by MDPI under the terms and conditions of the Creative Commons Attribution-NonCommercial-NoDerivs (CC BY-NC-ND) license.

Contents

About the Editor vii

Preface ix

Karolina Urbańska, Marcin Woźniak, Piotr Więsyk, Natalia Konarska, Weronika Bartos, Mateusz Biszewski, et al.
Management and Treatment Outcomes of High-Risk Corneal Transplantations
Reprinted from: *J. Clin. Med.* **2022**, *11*, 5511, doi:10.3390/jcm11195511 1

Reiko Arita and Shima Fukuoka
Therapeutic Efficacy and Safety of Intense Pulsed Light for Refractive Multiple Recurrent Chalazia
Reprinted from: *J. Clin. Med.* **2022**, *11*, 5338, doi:10.3390/jcm11185338 17

Achim Fieß, Clara Hufschmidt-Merizian, Sandra Gißler, Ulrike Hampel, Eva Mildenberger, Michael S. Urschitz, et al.
Dry Eye Parameters and Lid Geometry in Adults Born Extremely, Very, and Moderately Preterm with and without ROP: Results from the Gutenberg Prematurity Eye Study
Reprinted from: *J. Clin. Med.* **2022**, *11*, 2702, doi:10.3390/jcm11102702 27

Giuseppe Giannaccare, Carla Ghelardini, Alessandra Mancini, Vincenzo Scorcia and Lorenzo Di Cesare Mannelli
New Perspectives in the Pathophysiology and Treatment of Pain in Patients with Dry Eye Disease
Reprinted from: *J. Clin. Med.* **2022**, *11*, 108, doi:10.3390/jcm11010108 41

Javier Martín-López, Consuelo Pérez-Rico, Selma Benito-Martínez, Bárbara Pérez-Köhler, Julia Buján and Gemma Pascual
The Role of the Stromal Extracellular Matrix in the Development of Pterygium Pathology: An Update
Reprinted from: *J. Clin. Med.* **2021**, *10*, 5930, doi:10.3390/jcm10245930 49

Miriam Idoipe, Borja de la Sen-Corcuera, Ronald M. Sánchez-Ávila, Carmen Sánchez-Pérez, María Satué, Antonio Sánchez-Pérez, et al.
Membrane of Plasma Rich in Growth Factors in Primary Pterygium Surgery Compared to Amniotic Membrane Transplantation and Conjunctival Autograft
Reprinted from: *J. Clin. Med.* **2021**, *10*, 5711, doi:10.3390/jcm10235711 71

Anna Machalińska, Agnieszka Kuligowska, Bogna Kowalska and Krzysztof Safranow
Comparative Analysis of Corneal Parameters in Swept-Source Imaging between DMEK and UT-DSAEK Eyes
Reprinted from: *J. Clin. Med.* **2021**, *10*, 5119, doi:10.3390/jcm10215119 87

Ciro Caruso, Robert Leonard Epstein, Pasquale Troiano, Francesco Napolitano, Fabio Scarinci and Ciro Costagliola
Topo-Pachimetric Accelerated Epi-On Cross-Linking Compared to the Dresden Protocol Using Riboflavin with Vitamin E TPGS: Results of a 2-Year Randomized Study
Reprinted from: *J. Clin. Med.* **2021**, *10*, 3799, doi:10.3390/jcm10173799 101

Sandra Schumann, Eva Dietrich, Charli Kruse, Salvatore Grisanti and Mahdy Ranjbar
Establishment of a Robust and Simple Corneal Organ Culture Model to Monitor Wound Healing
Reprinted from: *J. Clin. Med.* **2021**, *10*, 3486, doi:10.3390/jcm10163486 113

Javier Lacorzana, Antonio Campos, Marina Brocal-Sánchez, Juan Marín-Nieto,
Oswaldo Durán-Carrasco, Esly C. Fernández-Núñez, et al.
Visual Acuity and Number of Amniotic Membrane Layers as Indicators of Efficacy in Amniotic Membrane Transplantation for Corneal Ulcers: A Multicenter Study
Reprinted from: *J. Clin. Med.* **2021**, *10*, 3234, doi:10.3390/jcm10153234 . . . . **129**

About the Editor

Vincenzo Scorcia

Vincenzo Scorcia, MD, graduated from La Sapienza University (Roma, Italy) in 2001. He completed his residency in ophthalmology at the Eye Hospital, University "Magna Græcia" (Catanzaro, Italy), in 2006 and his clinical and surgical fellowship in Cornea and External Diseases at "Villa Serena Hospital", Eye Department, (Forlì, Italy), with Prof. Dr. M. Busin, (February 2006–January 2008). He completed an "Honorary Fellowship" with Mr. J. K. Dart, Consultant Ophthalmologist and Deputy Director of Research and Development at Moorfields Eye Hospital in 2008.

His research interests are in the fields of corneal diseases, ocular surface diseases, and corneal transplantation. He has been an invited speaker at several national and international meetings. He has served on the scientific committee of the Italian Society of Corneal Transplantation (SITRAC) and the board of several national societies. He has authored or co-authored several books and over 100 articles in peer-reviewed international journals. He is the recipient of a number of national and international prizes, and he has taken part in several multicenter trials, including PRIN (PROGETTI DI RILEVANTE INTERESSE NAZIONALE) and PON (Programma Operativo Nazionale) projects related to neurodegenerative ocular diseases, antibiotic and glaucoma therapy, the cornea, and the anterior segment.

Preface

The intricate dance of biology, pathology, and medicine finds a particularly delicate stage in the arena of ocular surface diseases. The spectrum of ocular surface diseases, as reflected upon, spans from the mild annoyance of keratoconjunctivitis sicca to the debilitating severity of conditions such as corneal ulcers which jeopardize the cornea's transparency. Such severe conditions often necessitate interventions such as keratoplasty to restore vision. However, the success of these surgical solutions hinges heavily on the preparatory steps taken to optimize the ocular surface.

Pre-surgical optimization involves crucial processes: enhancing tear function, restoring the normal lid anatomy and function, and ensuring an ample supply of limbal stem cells. Proper execution of these steps can substantially improve the outcome of subsequent surgical interventions, especially the longevity and clarity of the corneal graft.

This Special Issue entitled "Treatment of Cornea and Ocular Surface Diseases" is dedicated to showcasing the latest advancements in treatments for cornea and ocular surface diseases. The contributions herein represent the ongoing efforts of researchers to refine and develop better management strategies for these conditions.

I would like to express my gratitude to all authors for their invaluable contributions and to our readers for their interest in this crucial area of ophthalmology. Sincerely,

Vincenzo Scorcia
Editor

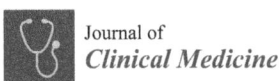

Article

Management and Treatment Outcomes of High-Risk Corneal Transplantations

Karolina Urbańska, Marcin Woźniak, Piotr Więsyk, Natalia Konarska, Weronika Bartos, Mateusz Biszewski, Michał Bielak, Tomasz Chorągiewicz * and Robert Rejdak

Chair and Department of General and Pediatric Ophthalmology, Medical University of Lublin, 20-079 Lublin, Poland
* Correspondence: tomekchor@wp.pl

Abstract: Corneal transplantation is the most effective treatment for corneal blindness. Standard planned keratoplasties have a high success rate. Conditions such as active inflammation at the time of surgery, the presence of ocular surface disease, previous graft disease, or neovascularization make them more susceptible to rejection. These are so-called high-risk corneal transplantations. In our study, we selected 52 patients with a higher risk of graft rejection. A total of 78 procedures were performed. The main indications for the first keratoplasty were infections (59.6%) and traumas (21.2%). Visual acuity (VA) significantly improved from 2.05 logMAR on the day of keratoplasty to 1.66 logMAR in the latest examination ($p = 0.003$). An analysis of the graft survival showed a 1-year survival of 54% and a 5-year survival of 19.8% of grafts. The mean observation time without complications after the first, second, and third surgery was 23, 13, and 14 months, respectively. The best results were noted among patients with infectious indications for keratoplasty ($p = 0.001$). Among them, those with bacterial infection had the best visual outcomes ($p = 0.047$).

Keywords: cornea; corneal transplantation; high-risk corneal transplantation; keratoplasty; immunosuppression in corneal transplantation; corneal immune privilege

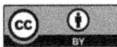

1. Introduction

Corneal disorders are the third leading cause of blindness in the human population, after cataracts and glaucoma [1]. They can be managed very effectively with keratoplasty, during which the damaged cornea is replaced with healthy tissue. Corneal grafting is the most common type of transplantation performed worldwide [1]. It is also one of the most successful ones, as it carries a low risk of graft rejection due to corneal avascularity [2]. However, in some cases, there is a higher risk of corneal transplant failure. It may be due to different factors leading to the loss of corneal immune privilege, such as ocular surface diseases or active inflammation at the time of surgery. In the case of infections unresponsive to conservative treatment or ocular traumas, the integrity of the eyeball is endangered, and the keratoplasty has to be performed urgently. The inability to examine the structures of the eyeball due to corneal opacity is another indication of urgent keratoplasty. The risk of graft failure is also higher in patients with a prior clinical history of transplant rejection or other eye surgeries, particularly glaucoma surgery [3].

Corneal transplantation is the only possible treatment in the case of extensive corneal lesions. The surgical technique depends on the size, location, cause, and depth of the corneal damage. In recent years, there have been significant advances in the treatment modalities for corneal blindness. One of the greatest breakthroughs was the introduction of endothelial keratoplasty. It provides a significantly lower risk of transplant rejection, faster visual recovery, and longer transplant survival than the traditional penetrating keratoplasty. Endothelial keratoplasty procedures include Descemet's automated endothelial keratoplasty (DSAEK) and Descemet's membrane endothelial keratoplasty (DMEK) [4].

The aim of this study was to assess the functional and structural outcomes of high-risk corneal transplantations. Specifically, we focused on different indications for keratoplasty in terms of their impact on graft rejection risk and visual outcomes. We intended to point out the potential corneal blindness etiologies whose management should be reconsidered to improve the functional and anatomical success rates of keratoplasty. In addition, we compared our results with other high-risk corneal transplantation reports found in the literature.

2. Materials and Methods

This retrospective case series involves patients of the Department of General and Pediatric Ophthalmology at the Medical University of Lublin, Poland. The study followed the tenets of the Declaration of Helsinki and was based on the data of penetrating keratoplasties performed between 2018 and 2022. In the case of patients with a prior history of keratoplasty, the surgeries performed before 2018 were also investigated. The inclusion criterion was a higher risk of graft failure. We considered the so-called hot-grafting with ongoing active inflammation (due to corneal trauma, burn, perforation, or infection) and previous graft rejection to be a high-risk setting. Previous graft rejection was qualified as a primary high-risk transplant only when the indication for the first keratoplasty was not related to a higher risk of graft failure. Patients without risk factors or with insufficient data were excluded from our research. The data extracted from the medical records included: surgical technique, history of surgical interventions prior to keratoplasty, pre- and postoperative visual acuity (VA), graft diameter, and systemic steroid therapy or immunosuppressive therapy with Mycophenolate mofetil (MMF) following the transplantation. VA was evaluated in all patients using Snellen's original test with conversions to decimal and logMAR scales for statistical analyses. Lower VAs were classified as follows: counting fingers, hand motion, light perception, or no light perception. VAs were assigned with logMAR scores of 1.9, 2.3, 2.7, and 3.0, respectively [5,6]. Bacterial and fungal infections were confirmed by the isolation and identification of the pathogens in microbiological testing. Viral infections were confirmed based on clinical presentation and slit-lamp examination. Functional success was described as an improvement in VA from the baseline to the most recent follow-up. For each analysis found in the results section, we selected those patients who met the analyzed criteria and provided enough data to include them in the specific analysis.

Statistical Analysis

Statistical analysis was performed using R programming language and RStudio: Integrated Development Environment for R language, software version number: 2022.7.1.554, author: RStudio Team (2022), Boston, MA, USA. All statistical tests were performed with 95% statistical significance. The Shapiro–Wilk test was used to examine the normality of distributions. The Chi-Squared Test of Independence was used to examine the difference in postoperative VA depending on primary etiology. Differences between pre- and postoperative VA depending on etiology and type of infection were examined with the Kruskal–Wallis test. The relationship between etiology and the time span from the first to the second keratoplasty was also examined with the Kruskal–Wallis test. The Wilcoxon test and Student's t-test were used to examine the improvement in VA. The Kaplan–Meier estimator was used to examine the survival of the first grafts. In the uncomplicated cases, we included the time between keratoplasty and the last follow-up. In the complicated cases, we used (a) the time between the first and second keratoplasty, (b) the time between keratoplasty and the discovery of an atrophic eyeball in the postoperative follow-up, (c) the time between keratoplasty and the enucleation of the eyeball. The Mantel–Haenszel test was used to examine the differences in survival probability in different groups.

3. Results

Out of the 120 patients submitted to penetrating keratoplasty, we selected 52 patients with a total of 78 keratoplasty procedures performed. The group consisted of 30 men and 22 women with an average age of 58.7 ± 18.7 years (range 22–97 years). Further analysis revealed two peaks in patients' age (Figure 1). The main indications for the first keratoplasty were infections (59.6%) and traumas (21.2%) (Figure 2). More information about the study group and indications for the first keratoplasty can be found in Table 1.

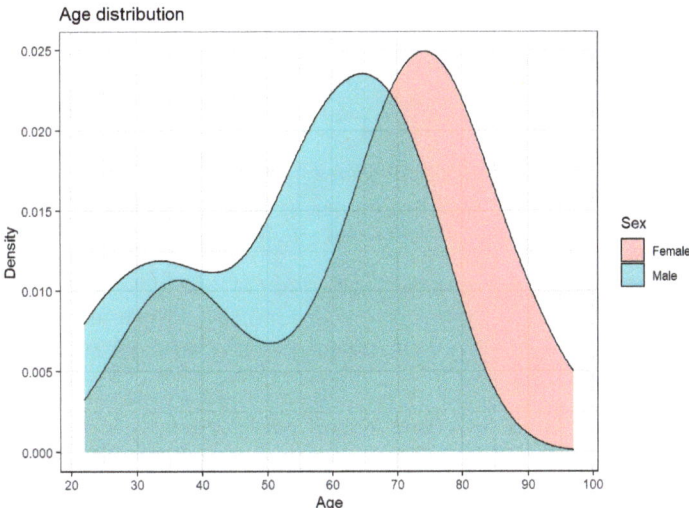

Figure 1. Age distribution with two peaks caused by traumas (first peak) and infections (second peak), being the main indications for keratoplasty in younger and older patients, respectively.

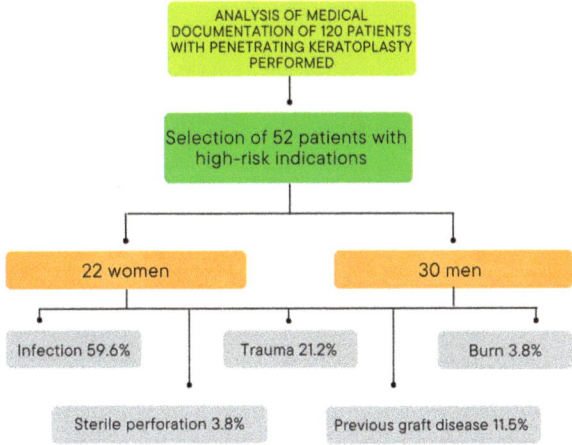

Figure 2. Structure of the study group, according to sex and the etiology of corneal blindness.

The mean observation time without complications after the first, second, and third surgery was 23, 13, and 14 months, respectively. Twenty-two patients (42.3%) required a second keratoplasty. In four cases (7.7%), a third keratoplasty was necessary. The average time between the first and second and between the second and third keratoplasty was 17 and 27 months, respectively. Thirty-two patients (61.5%) noted an improvement in VA. In nine cases (17.3%), VA remained unchanged, and in another nine cases (17.3%), it deteriorated. Two patients did not provide information about their preoperative and postoperative VA. An analysis of the average values of VA converted to logMAR indicated an improvement from 2.05 on the day of keratoplasty to 1.66 in the latest examination.

Table 1. Characteristic of the study group.

	Infection	Trauma	Previous Graft Disease	Burn	Sterile Perforation
	N = 31	N = 11	N = 6	N = 2	N = 2
	59.6%	21.2%	11.5%	3.8%	3.8%
Female	16 (51.6%)	1 (9.1%)	2 (33.3%)	1 (50.0%)	2 (100.0%)
Male	15 (48.4%)	10 (90.9%)	4 (66,7%)	1 (50.0%)	0 (0.0%)
Mean age (SD) (years)	63.4 (16.8)	42.6 (18.8)	57.3 (12.9)	57.5 (23.3)	80.0 (7.1)
Range	34.0–97.0	22.0–74.0	33.0–70.0	41.0–74.0	75.0–85.0

3.1. Preoperative VA Outcomes for Each Etiology

Fifty-one patients were included in this analysis. There were no statistically significant differences in preoperative VA depending on the etiology of corneal blindness ($p = 0.68$).

3.2. Postoperative VA Outcomes for Each Etiology

Forty-nine patients were included in this analysis. There were no statistically significant differences in postoperative VA outcomes depending on etiology ($p = 0.19$).

3.3. Differences between Pre- and Postoperative Visual Outcomes for Each Indication for Graft

Fifty patients were included in this analysis. Thirty-two patients noted an improvement in VA. In 18 cases, VA remained unchanged or became worse. There was no statistically significant relationship between VA improvement and etiology ($p = 0.12$) (Figure 3).

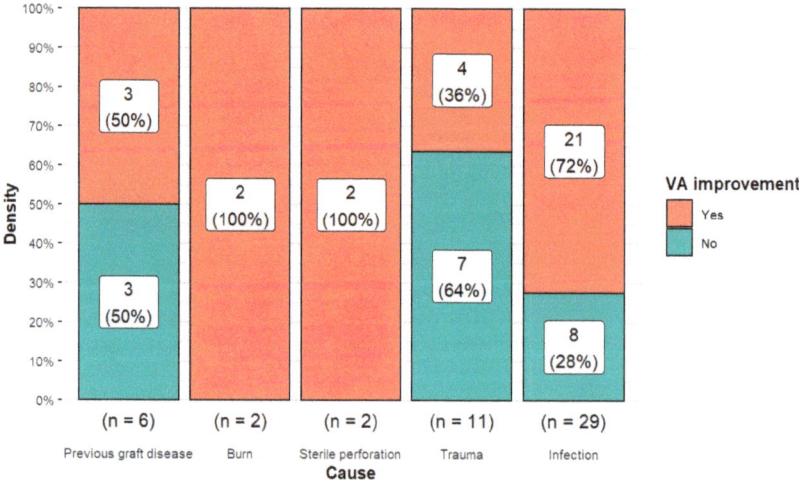

Figure 3. Relationship between VA improvement and etiology of corneal blindness.

3.4. Improvement in VA after Keratoplasty

Forty-eight patients were included in this analysis. There was a statistically significant improvement in VA in the latest follow-up ($p = 0.003$) (Figure 4).

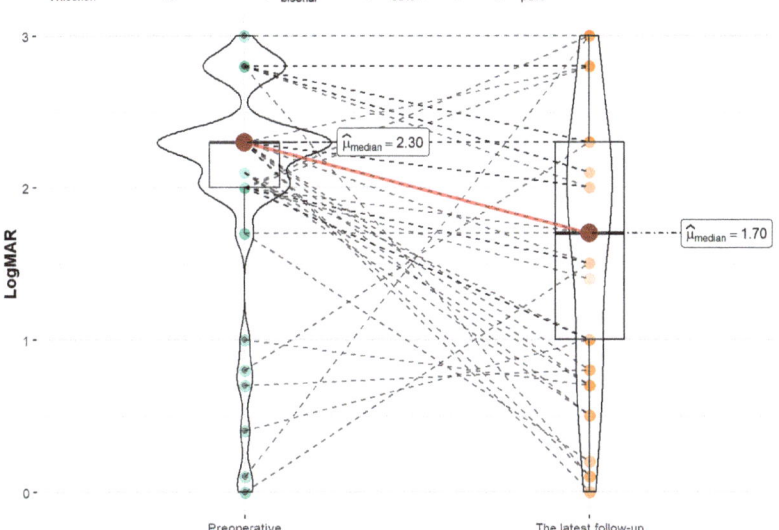

Figure 4. Visual outcomes before and after keratoplasty.

3.5. Improvement in VA for Each Indication for Graft

The improvement in VA was statistically significant only in the case of infection ($p = 0.001$) (Table 2). A summary of visual outcomes can be found in Table 3.

Table 2. Improvement in VA and etiology.

Indication for Graft	N	p-Value
Previous graft disease	6	0.387
Burn	2	0.333
Sterile perforation	2	0.167
Trauma	11	0.605
Infection	31	**0.001**

Table 3. Summary of the visual outcomes for each indication for keratoplasty.

	Previous Graft Disease	Burn	Sterile Perforation	Trauma	Infection
	(N = 6)	(N = 2)	(N = 2)	(N = 11)	(N = 31)
	11.5%	3.8%	3.8%	21.2%	59.6%
	\multicolumn{5}{c}{Preoperative logMAR}				
Mean (SD)	1.69 (0.96)	2.40 (0.57)	2.55 (0.35)	1.89 (0.98)	2.12 (0.59)
1st Quartile	1.18	2.20	2.42	1.85	2.00
Median	2.30	2.40	2.55	2.30	2.30
3rd Quartile	2.30	2.60	2.67	2.30	2.30
Min–Max	0.16–2.30	2.00–2.80	2.30–2.80	0.00–3.00	0.40–2.80
	\multicolumn{5}{c}{The last follow-up logMAR}				
Mean (SD)	1.46 (1.18)	2.00 (0.42)	1.05 (1.34)	2.19 (0.56)	1.52 (0.80)
1st Quartile	0.50	1.85	0.58	1.85	0.80
Median	1.70	2.00	01.05	2.10	1.50
3rd Quartile	2.30	2.15	1.52	2.55	2.10
Min–Max	0.00–2.80	1.70–2.30	0.10–2.00	1.40–3.00	0.10–3.00

3.6. Infections

Infection was the main indication for keratoplasty in our study group. Bacterial and fungal infections were the most common. The full characteristics of the study group can be found in Table 4.

Table 4. Characteristics of the study group with infections.

	Bacterial	Fungal	Mixed	Amebic	Viral
	(N = 10)	(N = 9)	(N = 3)	(N = 1)	(N = 3)
	38.5%	34.6%	11.5%	3.8%	11.5%
Female	5 (50.0%)	6 (66.7%)	2 (66.7%)	0 (0.0%)	2 (66.7%)
Male	5 (50.0%)	3 (33.3%)	1 (33.35)	1 (100.0%)	1 (33.3%)
Mean age (SD) (years)	60.1 (16.7)	63.0 (21.2)	63.0 (21.7)	49.0 (NA)	74.7 (6.5)
Range	35.0–75.0	34.0–97.0	38.0–77.0	49.0–49.0	68.0–81.0

3.6.1. Preoperative Visual Outcome and the Type of Infection

Twenty-five patients were included in this analysis. There were no statistically significant differences in preoperative visual outcome and the type of infection ($p = 0.59$).

3.6.2. Postoperative Visual Outcome for Different Types of Infection

Twenty-five patients were included in this analysis. There was no statistically significant difference in the postoperative VA depending on the type of infection ($p = 0.87$).

3.6.3. Improvement in Visual Outcome Depending on the Type of Infection

Twenty-four patients were included in this analysis. Eighteen patients noted an improvement in visual outcome. In six cases, visual outcomes remained unchanged or worsened. There was no statistically significant relationship between VA improvement and the type of infection ($p = 0.5$) (Figure 5).

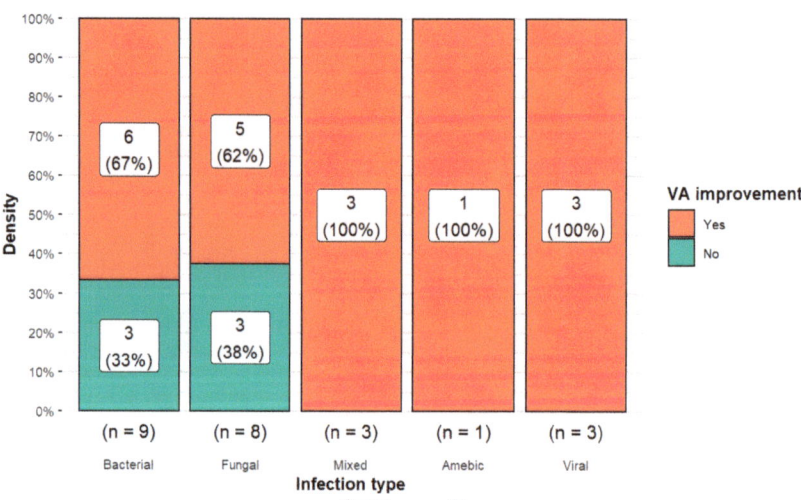

Figure 5. Improvement in VA and the type of infection.

3.6.4. Comparison of VA Improvement for Each Type of Infection

The improvement in VA was statistically significant only in the case of bacterial infection ($p = 0.047$) (Table 5). A summary of all visual outcomes can be found in Table 6.

Table 5. Improvement in VA for each type of infection.

Infection Type	Quantity	p-Value (Student's t-Test)	p-Value (Wilcoxon Test)
Bacterial	9	-	0.047
Fungal	9	-	0.072
Mixed	3	0.152	-
Amebic	1	-	0.500
Viral	3	0.109	-

Table 6. Summary of visual outcomes for each type of infection.

	Bacterial	Fungal	Mixed	Viral	Amebic
	(N = 10)	(N = 9)	(N = 3)	(N = 3)	(N = 1)
	38.5%	34.6%	11.5%	11.5%	3.8%
	Preoperative logMAR				
Mean (SD)	2.11 (0.63)	2.11 (0.76)	2.27 (0.55)	1.70 (0.61)	2.30 (NA)
1st Quartile	2.10	2.00	2.00	1.50	2.30
Median	2.30	2.30	2.30	2.00	2.30
3rd Quartile	2.30	2.42	2.55	02.05	2.30
Min–Max	0.70–2.80	0.40–2.80	1.70–2.80	1.00–2.10	2.30–2.30
	The last follow-up logMAR				
Mean (SD)	1.42 (0.89)	1.53 (0.73)	1.40 (1.08)	1.07 (0.40)	2.00 (NA)
1st Quartile	0.70	1.00	0.95	0.85	2.00
Median	1.70	1.50	1.70	1.00	2.00
3rd Quartile	2.30	2.10	2.00	1.25	2.00
Min–Max	0.10–2.30	0.70–2.80	0.20–2.30	0.70–1.50	2.00–2.00

3.7. Graft Survival

The graft survival time was defined as: (a) the time between the first and second keratoplasty; (b) the time between keratoplasty and the discovery of an atrophic eyeball in the postoperative follow-up; and (c) the time between keratoplasty and enucleation of the eyeball. In the uncomplicated cases, the graft survival time was defined as the observation time.

3.7.1. Graft survival Probability

An analysis of the graft survival showed a 1-year survival of 54% and a 5-year survival of 19.8% of grafts (Figure 6).

3.7.2. Graft Survival Probability: Influence of Primary Etiology

There was no statistically significant difference in graft survival for each etiology ($p = 0.8$) (Figure 7).

3.7.3. Graft Survival Probability: Influence of Sex

There was no statistically significant difference in graft survival between females and males ($p = 0.7$) (Figure 8).

3.7.4. Graft Survival Probability: Influence of Previous Surgical Procedures on the Eye

A history of previous surgical procedures on the eye did not have an impact on graft survival in our study group ($p = 0.5$) (Figure 9).

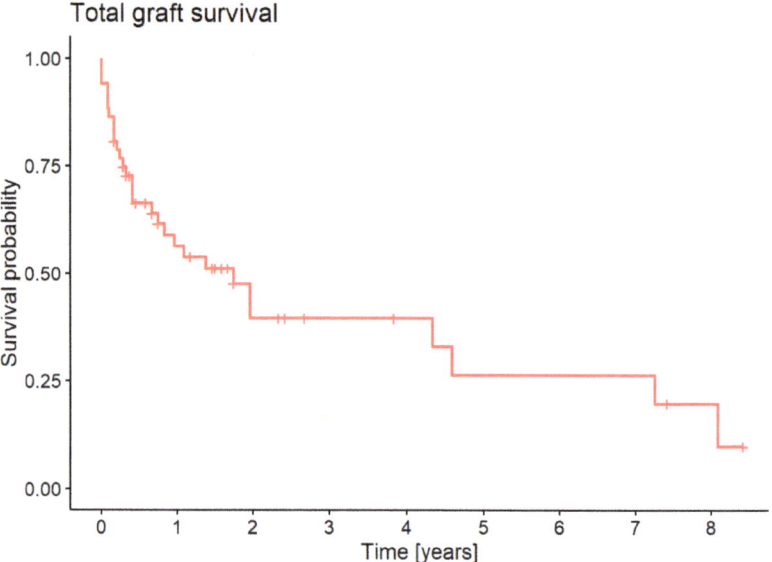

Figure 6. Overall graft survival probability.

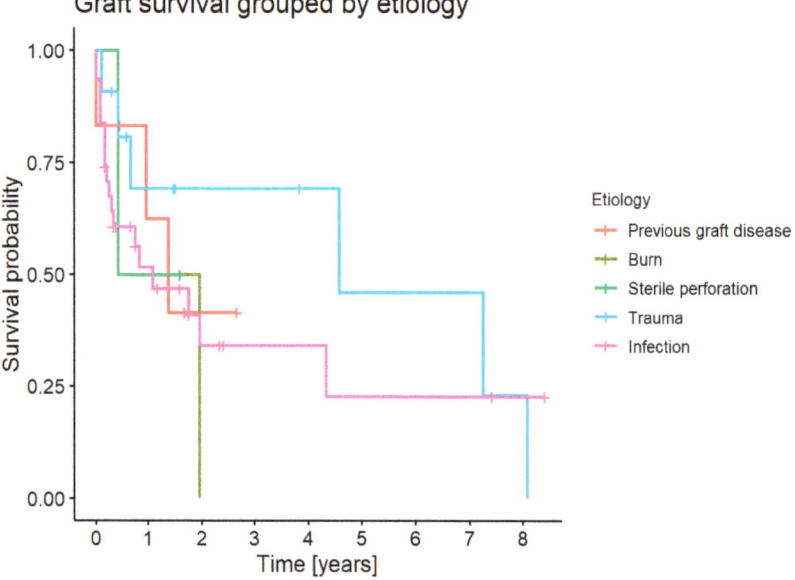

Figure 7. Survival probability for each etiology.

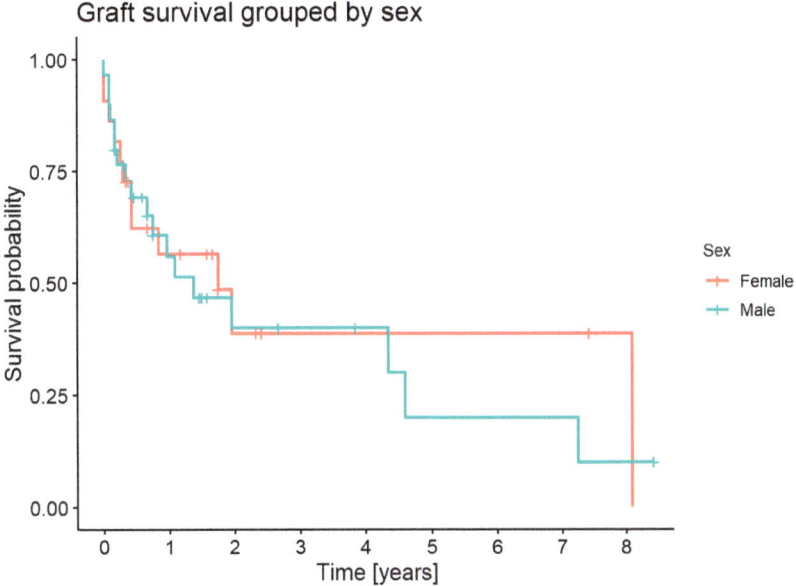

Figure 8. Survival probability for females and males.

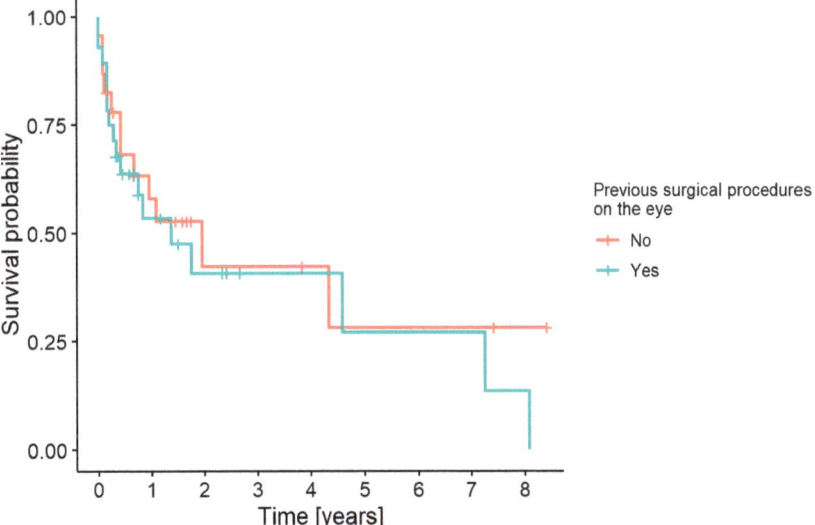

Figure 9. Survival probability and the history of previous surgical procedures.

3.7.5. Graft Survival Probability: Influence of the Recipient's Age

There was no statistically significant difference in graft survival probability depending on the recipient's age ($p = 0.7$) (Figure 10).

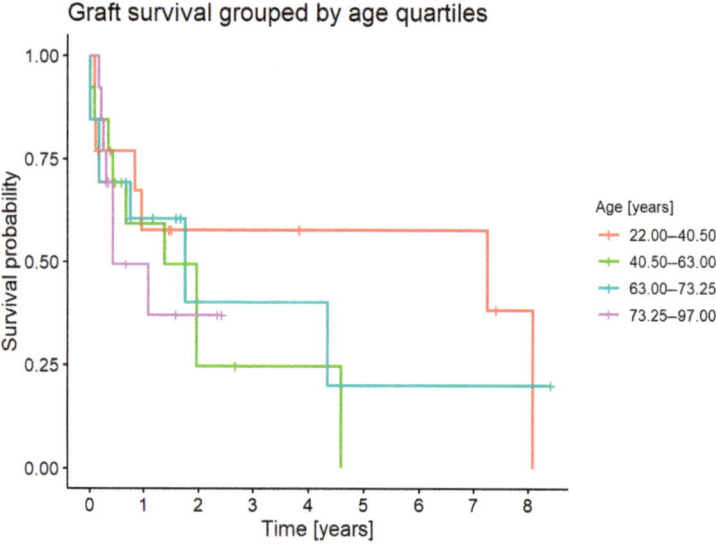

Figure 10. Graft survival grouped by age quartiles.

3.7.6. Graft Survival Probability: Influence of Additional Systemic Immunosuppression

There was no statistically significant difference in graft survival for the group with systemic immunosuppressive therapy ($p = 0.3$) (Figure 11).

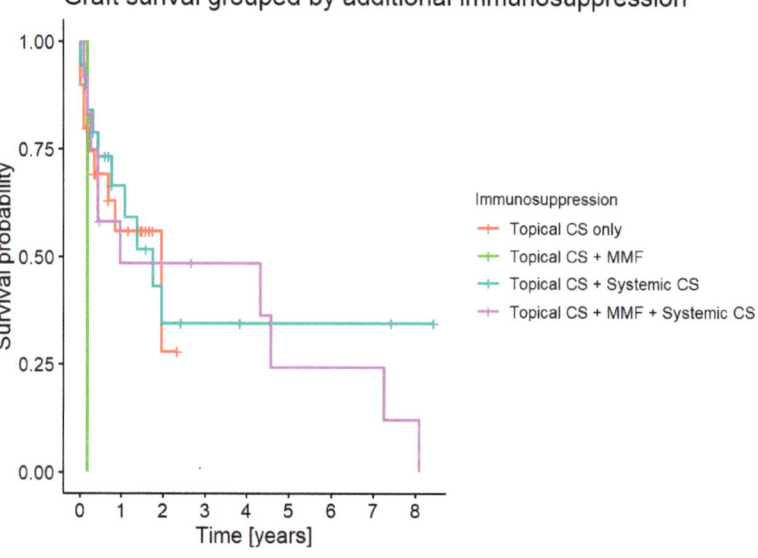

Figure 11. Graft survival grouped by the use of immunosuppression.

3.7.7. Graft Survival Probability: Influence of Graft Diameter

Graft diameter did not have an impact on graft survival ($p = 0.1$) (Figure 12).

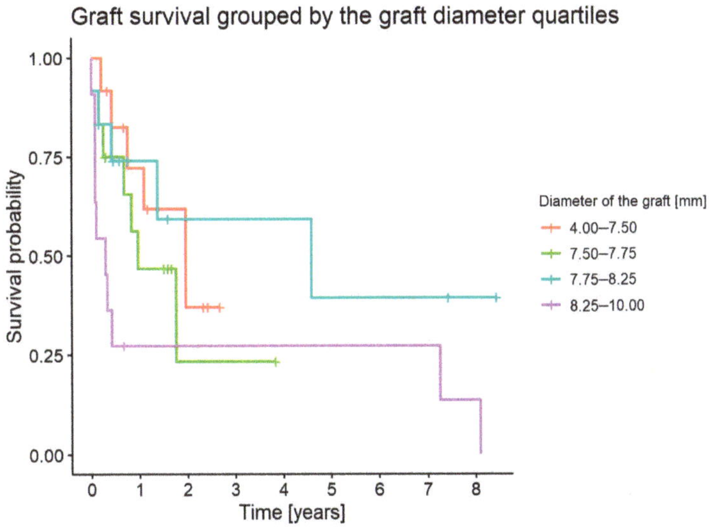

Figure 12. Graft survival grouped by the first graft diameter.

3.7.8. Graft Survival Probability: Influence of the Number of Keratoplasties

The 1-year survival was 52.8% for the first keratoplasty and 70% for the second keratoplasty. The 5-year survival was 19.9% for the first keratoplasty. None of the second keratoplasties survived 5 years (Figure 13). Previous graft disease (earlier considered as the primary high-risk etiology) was regarded as the second keratoplasty in this analysis. There was no statistically significant difference in graft survival probability for the first and second keratoplasty ($p = 0.4$).

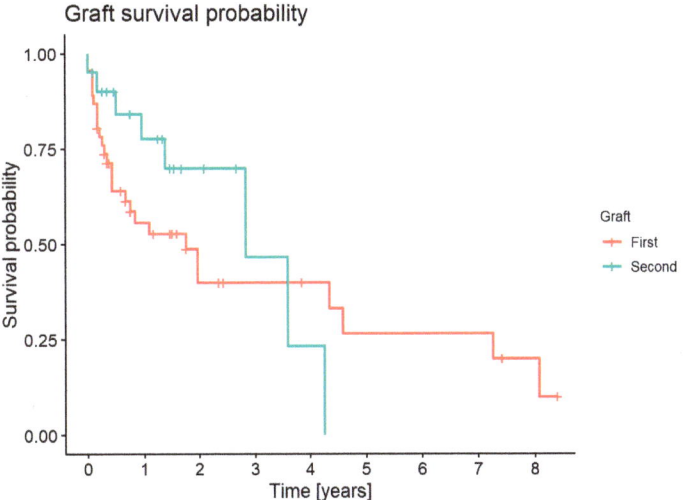

Figure 13. Graft survival probability for the first and second keratoplasty.

3.7.9. Comparison of Graft Survival Time for Each Etiology

In this analysis, we included 28 patients that required repeat keratoplasty. There were no statistically significant differences in graft survival time depending on etiology ($p = 0.44$).

3.7.10. Graft Survival Probability: Impact of Keratoplasty Combined with Vitrectomy

Within the whole study group, six patients were subjected to keratoplasty combined with vitrectomy. In four of them, vitrectomy was performed together with the first keratoplasty. The primary indications for keratoplasty in this group were trauma (3/4) and infection (1/4). Only one of the patients who had the vitrectomy combined with the first keratoplasty required a second keratoplasty (2 months after the first keratoplasty). The two other patients had a vitrectomy combined with the second keratoplasty. Their primary indications for keratoplasty were infection (1/2) and burns (1/2). The mean observation time in the group without complications was 13 months. Generally, in four patients, VA improved, in one case it remained unchanged, and in another, it deteriorated. The mean VA increased from 2.42 before to 2.08 after the operation, but this change was not statistically significant ($p = 0.17$). Despite quite a long observation time without rejection episodes, functional success was not obtained.

3.7.11. Comparison of Graft Survival Time for Different Types of Infection

In this analysis, we included 14 patients with infectious etiology that required repeat keratoplasty. There were no statistically significant differences in graft survival time depending on the type of infection ($p = 0.36$). Graft survival probability was not statistically significant ($p = 0.06$) (Figure 14).

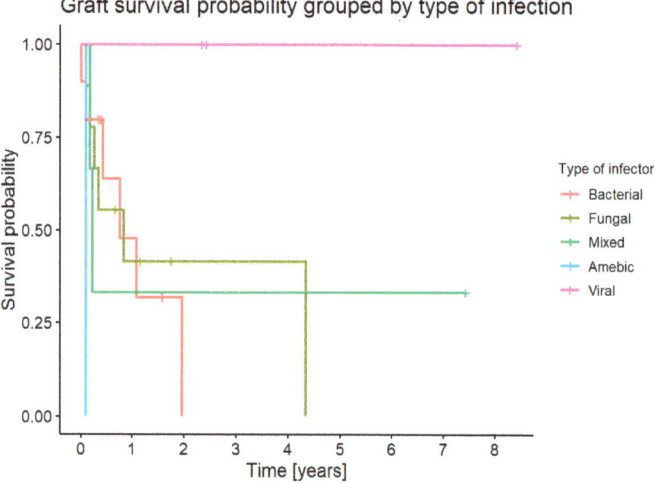

Figure 14. Graft survival probability for each type of infection.

3.8. Summary of the Results

VA in our study group significantly improved from 2.05 logMAR on the day of keratoplasty to 1.66 logMAR in the latest examination ($p = 0.003$). It proves that keratoplasty is an essential method of treatment in improving vision. An analysis of visual improvement performed separately for each etiology showed a statistically significant increase in VA only in the case of infections ($p = 0.001$). It showed poorer outcomes in patients with other etiologies, namely burns, trauma, sterile perforation, and previous graft disease. Further analysis proved patients with bacterial infections to have the best visual outcomes ($p = 0.047$). An analysis of the graft survival showed a 1-year survival of 54% and a 5-year survival of 19.8% of grafts. It proves that high-risk corneal transplants carry a greater risk of rejection than non-high-risk procedures.

4. Discussion

The immune privilege of corneal allografts is based on three fundamental processes: afferent blockade, the deviation of the immune response, and the elimination of immune effector elements. The afferent blockade of the immune response is caused by graft bed avascularity [7]. The absence of lymph vessels is also an important factor that leads to the immune privilege of the cornea [8]. Anterior chamber-associated immune deviation (ACAID) generates regulatory T cells (Tregs), which are responsible for the development and maintenance of ocular immune privilege [7,9]. Corneal allografts placed over the anterior chamber are in direct contact with anti-inflammatory and immunosuppressive cytokines from the aqueous humor [7]. In the Collaborative Corneal Transplantation Study, high risk was defined as a cornea with two or more vascularized quadrants or one in which a graft had previously been rejected [10]. High-risk corneal transplantations have lower success rates because of a higher incidence of immune-mediated graft rejection. Factors contributing to a higher risk of immunological rejection are: inflammatory, allergic, or infectious causes of corneal opacity; re-transplantation; corneal neovascularization and neo-lymphangiogenesis; glaucoma history; prior ocular surgery; blood transfusion history; larger donor cornea size; surgical complications; lens status; and male-to-female transplantation [3]. The presence of blood and lymph vessels reduces the immune privilege of corneal allografts by promoting the migration, recruitment, and infiltration of immune effector elements [8]. Immune-mediated graft rejection occurs when the main layers of the cornea are destroyed by the immune response. The rejection of the endothelium leads to irreversible endothelial cell loss and may result in permanent graft failure [11].

The probability of graft survival after penetrating keratoplasty was 86% at 1 year, 73% at 5 years, and 55% at 15 years [12]. Low-risk penetrating keratoplasty represents an even better survival rate of 90% at 5 years and 82% at 10 years [13]. High-risk recipients have a lower survival rate with a 5-year survival of 54.2% compared to 91.3% for primarily non-inflamed eyes [14]. A total of 70% of the high-risk grafts may face failure due to corneal bed vascularization or previous graft rejection [11,15]. In high-risk corneal recipients, rejection episodes occur in 40–70% of cases a year [11,16]. In our study, the 1-year survival probability for allografts was 54%, which is comparable to other studies. An increased risk of rejection was seen in young recipients [17]. However, our study did not confirm this relationship.

Repeat transplantation represented poorer outcomes [18–20]. The 5-year survival rate decreased from 72.5% in the first to 37.3–53.4% in repeat transplants [19]. Failure rates in repeat transplants were 17% at 2 years compared to 6% in first transplants [18]. In our study, the first and second keratoplasty involved a 1-year survival rate of 52.8% and 70%, respectively. This difference, however, was not statistically significant. The outcomes might have been influenced by the fact that we compared high-risk indications with repeat keratoplasty, which itself is a high-risk indication. It may suggest that all high-risk corneal transplantations have similar survival rates.

The Australian Corneal Graft Registry Report (ACGR) showed a poorer survival of grafts with a diameter of less than 7.75 mm and more than 8.5 mm [20]. Our study did not show statistically significant differences in graft survival for different graft diameters.

Some studies prove penetrating keratoplasty combined with vitrectomy to be a safe and effective procedure [21–25]. However, another study showed poorer outcomes in patients with severe ocular trauma [26]. In our study, only one out of six patients required repeat keratoplasty after this procedure, but functional success was not obtained.

Topical corticosteroids (CS) (mainly prednisolone and dexamethasone) are routinely used for the prevention and treatment of corneal graft rejection [27]. Difluprednate may be effective in penetrating keratoplasty graft rejection treatment, especially in non-high-risk grafts [28]. High-risk corneal allografts require more intensive treatment with gradually reduced doses of CS over a period of 6–12 months [17]. Besides the most common topical route, CS may also be administered by subconjunctival or systemic route [29]. However, the use of CS in corneal graft rejection treatment is limited by their ocular side effects, including infections, impaired wound healing, cataract formation, and glaucoma, as well as systemic side effects [11,17,30,31].

Cyclosporine is a calcineurin inhibitor used as an immunosuppressive agent in solid organ transplants. Topical cyclosporine was used in 48% of high-risk grafts [29]. Topical cyclosporine A (CsA) was not as effective as topical prednisolone in the prevention of graft rejection [32]. However, in another study, a combined regimen of topical CS and topical CsA was associated with a higher 1- and 2-year rejection-free graft survival rate [33]. The results of systemic CsA in the prevention of high-risk corneal transplantation rejection were inconsistent [17]. The most common adverse events of CsA therapy in high-risk corneal transplants were herpes keratitis and hypertension [34].

MMF is another systemic immunosuppressive agent used in high-risk corneal transplants. Reinhard et al. established a 1-year immune reaction-free rate of 89% in the MMF group, as compared to only 67% in the control group [35].

Other pharmacotherapeutic agents that can be used in high-risk corneal transplantation are tacrolimus and rapamycin [17].

Every patient from our study group received topical CS. Some of them were given additional systemic CS, MMF, or systemic CS + MMF. Our study showed no statistically significant difference in graft survival depending on the postoperative prophylaxis regimen.

We proved that keratoplasty was necessary and successful in restoring our patients' vision, as our study group noted a statistically significant VA improvement following keratoplasty. Considering functional success for each etiology separately, we revealed that only patients with infectious indications for keratoplasty had statistically significant VA improvement. This indicates that the management of keratoplasties after traumas, burns, previous graft diseases, and sterile perforations should be reconsidered to improve their outcomes in the future. Of all patients with an infectious etiology of corneal blindness, those with bacterial infections noted the best functional results. It is, therefore, necessary to determine the cause of worse outcomes among patients with viral, fungal, and amebic infections so as to improve their treatment.

Our study has some limitations. First of all, a greater sample size and longer observation time are required, especially in the case of less common indications for corneal transplantation, such as burns, sterile perforations, or Acanthamoeba keratitis. It is also impossible to estimate the significance of each factor accurately, as many factors can impact graft survival.

However, our study showed that similar outcomes can be reached despite the different indications for corneal transplantation. Many patients noted an improvement in VA, which proves that this treatment is essential in restoring visual functions. We proved the best functional success for bacterial infections among the infectious indications for keratoplasty. Our study showed that systemic immunosuppression with CS or MMF is necessary in many cases.

5. Conclusions

High-risk corneal transplants have poorer outcomes than routinely performed corneal transplants. Despite the lower survival rate, our study group noted statistically significant improvement in VA, which was equivalent to functional success. More studies should be performed for a better understanding of high-risk settings. It is important to establish the factors that may impact graft survival to provide better routine management that would increase the survival rate in the future.

Author Contributions: Conceptualization, T.C. and R.R.; methodology, T.C.; software, not applicable.; validation, T.C. and R.R.; formal analysis, M.W.; investigation, K.U., P.W., N.K., W.B. and M.B. (Mateusz Biszewski); resources, T.C.; data curation, K.U., M.W., P.W., N.K., W.B. and M.B. (Mateusz Biszewski); writing—original draft preparation, K.U., P.W. and M.B. (Michał Bielak); writing—review and editing, T.C., K.U. and M.B. (Michał Bielak); visualization, M.W.; supervision, T.C. and R.R.; project administration, T.C. and R.R.; funding acquisition, not applicable. All authors have read and agreed to the published version of the manuscript.

Funding: This research received no external funding.

Institutional Review Board Statement: The study was conducted in accordance with the Declaration of Helsinki.

Informed Consent Statement: Informed consent was difficult to obtain (retrospective study). Patients cannot be identified.

Data Availability Statement: Not applicable.

Conflicts of Interest: The authors declare no conflict of interest.

List of Abbreviations

VA	Visual acuity
ACAID	Anterior chamber-associated immune deviation
ACGR	Australian Corneal Graft Registry Report
CS	Corticosteroids
CsA	Cyclosporine A
MMF	Mycophenolate mofetil

References

1. Gain, P.; Jullienne, R.; He, Z.; Aldossary, M.; Acquart, S.; Cognasse, F.; Thuret, G. Global survey of corneal transplantation and eye banking. *JAMA Ophthalmol.* **2016**, *134*, 167–173. [CrossRef] [PubMed]
2. Singh, R.; Gupta, N.; Vanathi, M.; Tandon, R. Corneal transplantation in the modern era. *Indian J. Med. Res.* **2019**, *150*, 7–22. [CrossRef]
3. Armitage, W.J.; Goodchild, C.; Griffin, M.D.; Gunn, D.J.; Hjortdal, J.; Lohan, P.; Murphy, C.C.; Pleyer, U.; Ritter, T.; Tole, D.M.; et al. High-risk corneal transplantation: Recent developments and future possibilities. *Transplantation* **2019**, *103*, 2468. [CrossRef] [PubMed]
4. Ong, H.S.; Ang, M.; Mehta, J. Evolution of therapies for the Corneal Endothelium: Past, present and future approaches. *Br. J. Ophthalmol.* **2021**, *105*, 454. [CrossRef]
5. Schulze-Bonsel, K.; Feltgen, N.; Burau, H.; Hansen, L.; Bach, M. Visual acuities "hand motion" and "counting fingers" can be quantified with the Freiburg Visual Acuity Test. *Invest. Ophthalmol. Vis. Sci.* **2006**, *47*, 1236–1240. [CrossRef] [PubMed]
6. Lange, C.; Feltgen, N.; Junker, B.; Schulze-Bonsel, K.; Bach, M. Resolving the clinical acuity categories "hand motion" and "counting fingers" using the Freiburg Visual Acuity Test (FrACT). *Graefe's Arch. Clin. Exp. Ophthalmol.* **2009**, *247*, 137–142. [CrossRef] [PubMed]
7. Niederkorn, J.Y. Corneal transplantation and immune privilege. *Int. Rev. Immunol.* **2013**, *32*, 57–67. [CrossRef] [PubMed]
8. Niederkorn, J.Y. High risk corneal allografts and why they lose their immune privilege. *Curr. Opin. Allergy Clin. Immunol.* **2010**, *10*, 493. [CrossRef]
9. Keino, H.; Horie, S.; Sugita, S. Review article immune privilege and eye-derived t-regulatory cells. *J. Immunol. Res.* **2018**, *2018*, 1–12. [CrossRef]
10. The Collaborative Corneal Transplantation Studies (CCTS). Effectiveness of histocompatibility matching in high-risk corneal transplantation. *Arch. Ophthalmol.* **1992**, *110*, 1392–1403. [CrossRef]
11. Qazi, Y.; Hamrah, P. Corneal allograft rejection: Immunopathogenesis to therapeutics. *J. Clin. Cell. Immunol.* **2013**, *2013* (Suppl. 9), 006. [CrossRef]
12. Williams, K.A.; Esterman, A.J.; Bartlett, C.; Holland, H.; Hornsby, N.B.; Coster, D.J. How effective is penetrating corneal transplantation? Factors influencing long-term outcome in multivariate analysis. *Transplantation* **2006**, *81*, 896–901. [CrossRef] [PubMed]
13. Thompson, R.W.; Price, M.O.; Bowers, P.J.; Price, F.W. Long-term graft survival after penetrating keratoplasty. *Ophthalmology* **2003**, *110*, 1396–1402. [CrossRef]
14. Yu, T.; Rajendran, V.; Griffith, M.; Forrester, J.V.; Kuffová, L. High-risk corneal allografts: A therapeutic challenge. *World J. Transplant.* **2016**, *6*, 10. [CrossRef]
15. Maguire, M.G.; Stark, W.J.; Gottsch, J.D.; Stulting, R.D.; Sugar, A.; Fink, N.E.; Schwartz, A. Risk factors for corneal graft failure and Rejection in the Collaborative Corneal Transplantation Studies. Collaborative Corneal Transplantation Studies Research group. *Ophthalmology* **1994**, *101*, 1536–1547. [CrossRef]
16. Major, J.; Foroncewicz, B.; Szaflik, J.P.; Mucha, K. Immunology and donor-specific antibodies in corneal transplantation. *Arch. Immunol. Ther. Exp.* **2021**, *69*, 32. [CrossRef]

17. Di Zazzo, A.; Kheirkhah, A.; Abud, T.B.; Goyal, S.; Dana, R. Management of high-risk corneal transplantation. *Surv. Ophthalmol.* **2017**, *62*, 816. [CrossRef]
18. Claesson, M.; Armitage, W.J. Clinical outcome of repeat penetrating keratoplasty. *Cornea* **2013**, *32*, 1026–1030. [CrossRef]
19. Aboshiha, J.; Jones, M.N.A.; Hopkinson, C.L.; Larkin, D.F.P. Differential survival of penetrating and lamellar transplants in management of failed corneal grafts. *JAMA Ophthalmol.* **2018**, *136*, 859–865. [CrossRef]
20. Williams, K.A.; Keane, M.C.; Galettis, R.A.; Jones, V.J.; Mills, R.; Coster, D.J. *The Australian Corneal Graft Registry 2015 Report*; South Australian Health and Medical Research Institute: Adelaide, Australia, 2015.
21. Bové Álvarez, M.; Arumí, C.G.; Distéfano, L.; Güell, J.L.; Gris, Ó.; Mateo, C.; Corcóstegui, B.; García-Arumí, J. Comparative study of penetrating keratoplasty and vitreoretinal surgery with Eckardt temporary keratoprosthesis in ocular trauma versus non-trauma patients. *Graefes Arch. Clin. Exp. Ophthalmol.* **2019**, *257*, 2547–2558. [CrossRef]
22. Dave, A.; Acharaya, M.; Agarwal, M.; Dave, P.A.; Singh, M.; Mathur, U. Outcomes of combined keratoplasty and pars plana vitrectomy for endophthalmitis with compromised corneal clarity. *Clin. Experiment. Ophthalmol.* **2019**, *47*, 49–56. [CrossRef] [PubMed]
23. Dave, V.; Pappuru, R.; Khader, M.; Basu, S.; Tyagi, M.; Pathengay, A. Endophthalmitis with opaque cornea managed with primary endoscopic vitrectomy and secondary keratoplasty: Presentations and outcomes. *Indian J. Ophthalmol.* **2020**, *68*, 1587–1592. [CrossRef] [PubMed]
24. Hayashi, T.; Yasutsugu, I.; Shimizu, T.; Kuroki, T.; Kobashigawa, Y.; Iijima, Y.; Yuda, K. Pars plana vitrectomy combined with penetrating keratoplasty and transscleral-sutured intraocular lens implantation in complex eyes: A case series. *BMC Ophthalmol.* **2020**, *20*, 369. [CrossRef] [PubMed]
25. Yokogawa, H.; Kobayashi, A.; Okuda, T.; Mori, N.; Masaki, T.; Sugiyama, K. Combined keratoplasty, pars plana vitrectomy, and flanged intrascleral intraocular lens fixation to restore vision in complex eyes with coexisting anterior and posterior segment problems. *Cornea* **2018**, *37* (Suppl. 1), S78–S85. [CrossRef]
26. Nowomiejska, K.; Haszcz, D.; Forlini, C.; Forlini, M.; Moneta-Wielgos, J.; Maciejewski, R.; Zarnowski, T.; Juenemann, A.G.; Rejdak, R. Wide-field landers temporary keratoprosthesis in severe ocular trauma: Functional and anatomical results after one year. *J. Ophthalmol.* **2015**, *2015*, 1–6. [CrossRef]
27. Randleman, J.B.; Stulting, R.D. Prevention and treatment of corneal graft rejection: Current practice patterns (2004). *Cornea* **2006**, *25*, 286–290. [CrossRef]
28. Sorkin, N.; Yang, Y.; Mednick, Z.; Einan-Lifshitz, A.; Trinh, T.; Santaella, G.; Telli, A.; Chan, C.C.; Slomovic, A.R.; Rootman, D.S. Outcomes of difluprednate treatment for corneal graft rejection. *Can. J. Ophthalmol.* **2020**, *55*, 82–86. [CrossRef]
29. Kharod-Dholakia, B.; Randleman, J.B.; Bromley, J.G.; Stulting, R.D. Prevention and treatment of corneal graft rejection: Current practice patterns of the cornea society (2011). *Cornea* **2015**, *34*, 609–614. [CrossRef]
30. Abud, T.B.; Di Zazzo, A.; Kheirkhah, A.; Dana, R. Systemic immunomodulatory strategies in high-risk corneal transplantation. *J. Ophthalmic Vis. Res.* **2017**, *12*, 81. [CrossRef]
31. Uchiyama, E.; Papaliodis, G.N.; Lobo, A.M.; Sobrin, L. Side-effects of anti-inflammatory therapy in Uveitis. *Semin. Ophthalmol.* **2014**, *29*, 456–467. [CrossRef]
32. Price, M.O.; Price, F.W. Efficacy of topical cyclosporine 0.05% for Prevention of Cornea Transplant Rejection Episodes. *Ophthalmology* **2006**, *113*, 1785–1790. [CrossRef] [PubMed]
33. Marques, R.E.; Leal, I.; Guerra, P.S.; Barão, R.C.; Quintas, A.M.; Rodrigues, W. Topical corticosteroids with topical cyclosporine A versus topical corticosteroids alone for immunological corneal graft rejection. *Eur. J. Ophthalmol.* **2022**, *32*, 1469–1481. [CrossRef] [PubMed]
34. Lee, J.J.; Kim, M.K.; Wee, W.R. Adverse effects of low-dose systemic cyclosporine therapy in high-risk penetrating keratoplasty. *Graefes Arch. Clin. Exp. Ophthalmol.* **2015**, *253*, 1111–1119. [CrossRef] [PubMed]
35. Reinhard, T.; Mayweg, S.; Sokolovska, Y.; Seitz, B.; Mittelviefhaus, H.; Engelmann, K.; Voiculescu, A.; Godehardt, E.; Sundmacher, R. Systemic mycophenolate mofetil avoids immune reactions in penetrating high-risk keratoplasty: Preliminary results of an ongoing prospectively randomized multicentre study. *Transpl. Int.* **2005**, *18*, 703–708. [CrossRef]

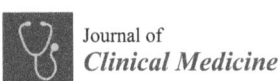

Article

Therapeutic Efficacy and Safety of Intense Pulsed Light for Refractive Multiple Recurrent Chalazia

Reiko Arita [1,2,*] and Shima Fukuoka [2,3]

1. Itoh Clinic, Saitama 3370042, Japan
2. Lid and Meibomian Gland Working Group, Saitama 3370042, Japan
3. Omiya Hamada Eye Clinic, Omiya, Saitama 3300854, Japan
* Correspondence: ritoh@za2.so-net.ne.jp; Tel.: +81-48-686-5588

Abstract: To evaluate the efficacy and safety of intense pulsed light (IPL) combined with meibomian gland expression (MGX) for the treatment of refractory multiple and recurrent chalazia without surgery or curettage. This was a retrospective controlled study. Patients with multiple and recurrent chalazia, who had performed the conventional treatment at least 2 months without any surgery or curettage, were enrolled in this study. Twenty-nine consecutive multiple recurrent chalazia (12 patients) were assigned to receive either the combination of IPL and MGX or MGX alone as a control. Each eye underwent one to four treatment sessions with 2-week intervals. Parameters were evaluated before and 1 month after the final treatment session. Clinical assessments included symptom, size of each chalazion, lid margin abnormalities, corneal and conjunctival fluorescein staining, meibum grade, the number of Demodex mites, the Schirmer value and meiboscore. All parameters except meiboscore and the Schirmer value were significantly improved with IPL-MGX therapy, whereas only meibum grade was significantly improved with MGX alone. There were no adverse events which occurred in either group. IPL-MGX was safe and effective for multiple and recurrent chalazia without surgery or curettage by reducing the size of chalazion and improving lid margin abnormalities and meibum grade.

Keywords: chalazion; intense pulsed light; meibomian gland; meibomian gland dysfunction; blepharitis

Citation: Arita, R.; Fukuoka, S. Therapeutic Efficacy and Safety of Intense Pulsed Light for Refractive Multiple Recurrent Chalazia. *J. Clin. Med.* **2022**, *11*, 5338. https://doi.org/10.3390/jcm11185338

Academic Editor: Vincenzo Scorcia

Received: 27 July 2022
Accepted: 7 September 2022
Published: 11 September 2022

Publisher's Note: MDPI stays neutral with regard to jurisdictional claims in published maps and institutional affiliations.

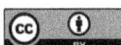

Copyright: © 2022 by the authors. Licensee MDPI, Basel, Switzerland. This article is an open access article distributed under the terms and conditions of the Creative Commons Attribution (CC BY) license (https://creativecommons.org/licenses/by/4.0/).

1. Introduction

Chalazion is a non-infectious chronic granulomatous inflammation of the lipids of the meibomian glands [1,2]. Blepharitis [3] and ocular demodicosis [4] are risk factors for chalazia. Patients with demodicosis tend to demonstrate recurrence [4,5]. MGD, blepharitis and marginal keratitis are significantly associated with a higher rate of developing multiple chalazia in pediatric patients [6]. Traditionally, the "cutting" treatment of chalazion by incision and curettage has been the mainstay of treatment [7], but "non-surgical" treatment of chalazion is attracting attention in order to protect the morphology and function of the meibomian glands [1,2]. Non-surgical common therapies for patients with chalazion include various topical medications such as steroidal injection [8,9], oral and/or topical antibiotics (eyedrops and/or ointment) [10], and topical steroids (eyedrops and/or ointment) [10] as well as warming eyelids and/or lid hygiene [1,10]. While some cases are cured spontaneously with the non-surgical conventional therapies above, some cases are refractory with multiple or recurrent episodes. Chalazion is considered a pathognomonic localized form of meibomian gland dysfunction (MGD) [11]. Chalazion is a risk factor of meibomian gland loss [12]. Indeed, many cases with multiple or recurrent episodes present with MGD, which show lid margin abnormalities such as plugging and vascularity of orifices and large loss of meibomian glands. Adding surgical resection to multiple recurrent chalazion tumors not only carries the risk of recurrence, but also the concern of losing even more of the meibomian gland area, resulting in dry eye in the future [13].

Intense pulsed light (IPL) therapy based on the delivery of intense pulses of non-coherent light with wavelengths of 500 to 1200 nm has been applied in dermatology to treat various conditions, including benign cavernous hemangiomas or venous malformations, telangiectasia, port wine stains, and other pigmented lesions [14]. IPL has been published internationally for the treatment of MGD and is listed as a Step 2 treatment in the International Guidelines for Dry Eye [15]. More than seventy papers and 14 randomized controlled trials have been conducted on MGD to date [16] and the treatment has been proven to be useful. IPL is a treatment that can be a fundamental treatment for MGD. A systematic review found that IPL is an effective and well-tolerated treatment option for a range of dermatologic conditions, having been shown to result in a reduction in the extent of telangiectasia and the severity of facial erythema [17]. Side effects of IPL ophthalmic treatment include redness, swelling, hair removal [18], and although rare, pupillary constriction, anterior uveitis, and pupillary defect have been reported [19]. The efficacy of IPL therapy for patients with dry eye due to MGD was discovered during IPL treatment of facial rosacea [20]. Subsequent studies found that IPL, with or without concomitant meibomian gland expression (MGX), is effective for improvement of subjective symptoms and objective findings in patients with mild to moderate MGD or dry eye [21–32]. The combination of IPL and MGX was also shown to be effective in patients with refractory MGD [32,33].

Recently, the efficacy of IPL has been reported for recurrent chalazion after excisional surgery in a single-arm study [34]. Still, there are no reports on the treatment of multiple and recurrent chalazia using IPL without surgery, with a control group.

Although the usefulness of IPL for chalazion has been investigated, there is still no international consensus on specific indications and protocols. Based on this study, we would like to propose a protocol for IPL for multiple and recurrent chalazia. We have, therefore, performed a retrospective controlled study to evaluate the efficacy of IPL combined with MGX in patients with refractory multiple recurrent chalazia who have been treated with non-surgical conventional therapies for at least 2 months. In addition, we analyzed the factors associated with the number of IPL treatment sessions until improvement.

2. Materials and Methods

2.1. Patients

This retrospective cohort study was approved by the Institutional Review Boards of Itoh Clinic (IRIN-202109), and it adhered to the tenets of the Declaration of Helsinki. Patients with refractory multiple recurrent chalazia who were treated with IPL and MGX or MGX alone between April and December 2021 at Itoh Clinic in Japan were assigned in the study. Informed consent was obtained from all subjects involved in the study. Inclusion criteria included: (1) an age of at least 18 years; (2) a diagnosis of multiple and recurrent chalazia which occurred within 6 months in more than 2 chalazions; (3) refractoriness of chalazion as defined by the failure to respond over a period of ≥ 2 months to at least three types of conventional therapy prescribed in Japan, including warming eyelids, lid hygiene, topical antibiotics eyedrops and/or ointment, topical steroid eyedrops and/or ointment, and/or systemic antibiotics oral medication; and (4) a Fitzpatrick skin type of 1 to 4 based on sun sensitivity and appearance [35]. Exclusion criteria included the presence of active skin lesions, skin cancer, or other specific skin pathology or of active ocular infection or ocular inflammatory disease.

2.2. Experimental Design

Patients treated with IPL-MGX underwent a series of one to four IPL-MGX treatment sessions at 2-week intervals and patients with MGX alone received treatment four times at 2-week intervals. Both groups were subjected to clinical assessment as described below both before treatment as well as 4 weeks after the final treatment session. Six months later, recurrence and safety were confirmed (Figure 1). Since this was an exploratory study, the number of IPL sessions was not determined, and the IPL was terminated when the size of the chalazion was reduced by 80–100% and the Standard Patient Evaluation of Eye Dryness (SPEED) score was less than 6 [36]. All of the patients were asked to continue warming eyelids and lid hygiene as well as not to initiate therapy with a new topical or systemic agent during the treatment course.

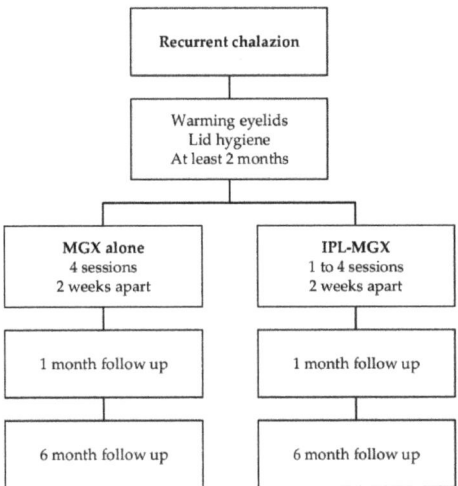

Figure 1. The Clinical Flow of this study.

2.3. Clinical Assessment

The diameter (mm) of each chalazion was measured with a ruler and we took a photograph with a slit lamp. Lid margin abnormalities (plugging of meibomian gland orifices and vascularity of lid margins) [37], corneal and conjunctival fluorescein staining (CFS) [38], and meibum grade [39] were evaluated with a slit lamp microscope. Morphological changes of meibomian glands were assessed on the basis of the meiboscore [40] as determined by noninvasive meibography. Tear fluid production was measured by Schirmer's test without anesthesia [41]. The number of Demodex mite was counted using a light microscope after pulling out three lashes. Symptoms were assessed with the SPEED validated questionnaire (scale of 0 to 28) for both eyes [36,42] and with visual analogue scale (VAS) scores of 0 (no symptom) to 100 (maximum conceivable symptom) of ocular discomfort and foreign body sensation for each eye separately. Visual acuity, intraocular pressure, lens opacity as well as fundus examination were also examined before and at 1 month after the final treatment session. We checked for recurrence of chalazion up to 6 months.

2.4. IPL-MGX Procedure

Before the first treatment, each patient underwent Fitzpatrick skin typing [35] and the IPL machine (AQUA CEL; Jeysis, Seoul, South Korea) was adjusted to the appropriate setting (upper eyelid; 15 J/cm^2, lower eyelid; 20 J/cm^2). At each treatment session, both eyes of the patient were closed and sealed with disposable eye shields (AQUA CEL HYDROGEL EYE CARE PATCH, KBM Inc., Seoul, Korea). After generous application of ultrasonic gel to the targeted skin area, each patient received ~13 pulses of light (with slightly overlapping applications) from the right preauricular area, across the cheeks and nose, to the left preauricular area, reaching up to the inferior boundary of the eye shields. Then, IPL was applied to the upper orbit along the bottom of the eyebrow from the temple to the base of the nose. These procedures were then repeated in a second pass. Immediately after the IPL treatment, MGX was performed on both upper and lower eyelids of each eye with an Arita Meibomian Gland Expressor (M-2073, Inami, Tokyo, Japan). Pain was minimized during MGX by the application of 0.4% oxybuprocaine hydrochloride to each eye.

2.5. Statistical Analysis

Data were found to be nonnormally distributed with the Shapiro–Wilk test ($p < 0.05$), and nonparametric testing was therefore applied. Wilcoxon rank sum test was used to compare the background characteristics of patients between the IPL-MGX and the MGX alone groups. Numerical data were compared between before and after treatment with the use of the Wilcoxon signed-rank test. Wilcoxon rank sum test was applied to compare the parameters between the IPL-MGX and the MGX alone groups. The number of IPLs required to improve the chalazion was investigated with background characteristics of the patients and each parameter using the Spearman's rank correlation coefficient.

We performed a statistical power analysis for both size of chalazion and the SPEED score. For the size of chalazion, the mean difference between before and four weeks after the final treatment was 4.3, with a corresponding standard deviation (SD) of 5.0; for the SPEED score, the mean difference was 5.4 with an SD of 6.3. For the size of chalazion, the mean difference between the IPL-MGX and the MGX groups after treatment was 9.2, with a corresponding SD of 1.9; for the SPEED score, the mean difference was 12.1 with an SD of 1.4. These changes were calculated from the results of all 12 eyes in the current study. The number of eyes in each group for the power analysis was assumed as 6. The power ($1 - \beta$) was >0.9 at the level of $\alpha = 0.05$ for both size of chalazion and SPEED score, and the sample size was sufficient.

Statistical analysis was performed with JMP Pro version 16 software (SAS, Cary, NC, USA). Data are shown as means $\pm$ SDs. All statistical tests were two-sided, and a p value of <0.05 was considered statistically significant.

3. Results

Patient demographics are shown in Table 1. Twenty-nine chalazia of 24 eyelids of 12 patients (14 chalazia of 14 eyelids of 6 patients in the MGX alone group and 15 chalazia of 14 eyelids of 6 patients in the IPL-MGX group) were enrolled in the study. No significant differences in parameters were detected between the two groups before treatment (Table 1).

Table 1. Demographics of the patients with chalazion in Intense pulsed light (IPL)–meibomian gland expression (MGX) ($n = 6$) and MGX alone ($n = 6$) groups.

	IPL-MGX		MGX Alone		p Value
	Mean $\pm$ SD	(Range)	Mean $\pm$ SD	(Range)	
Age (years)	36.8 $\pm$ 12.1	(19–51)	37.7 $\pm$ 13.1	(22–54)	1.00
Number of chalazia	2.5 $\pm$ 0.8	(2–4)	2.3 $\pm$ 0.5	(2–3)	0.92
Number of eyelids with chalazia	2.3 $\pm$ 0.5	(2–3)	2.3 $\pm$ 0.5	(2–3)	1.00
Duration of pre-lid-warming (months)	30.9 $\pm$ 41.2	(0.5–104)	2.0 $\pm$ 2.1	(0.5–6)	0.29
Size of the largest chalazion (mm)	12.2 $\pm$ 5.6	(5–18)	10.5 $\pm$ 2.0	(7–12)	0.81

p values were obtained using Wilcoxon rank sum test.

3.1. Efficacy of IPL-MGX

The characteristics of the eyes in the IPL-MGX group and the control group before as well as 4 weeks after the final treatment are shown in Table 2. The size of chalazia and VAS score were significantly decreased (Figure 2, Table 2). Significant decreases in irregularity ($p = 0.031$), plugging, vascularity, CFS, meibum grade, the number of Demodex, diameter of chalazion, and VAS score ($p < 0.001$, respectively) were apparent at 4 weeks after the final treatment in the IPL-MGX group (Table 2). Meiboscore and Schirmer test value at 4 weeks after the final treatment did not differ significantly in the IPL-MGX group ($p = 1.00$, 0.76, respectively) (Table 2). The SPEED score was significantly reduced at 4 weeks after the final treatment in the IPL-MGX group ($p = 0.031$) (Table 3).

All of the parameters except meibum grading in the MGX alone group remained unchanged (Table 2). Comparing the IPL-MGX and MGX alone groups, the size of chalazia, VAS, plugging, vascularity, CFS, meibum grade, and number of Demodex were significantly improved ($p < 0.001$, respectively) (Table 2).

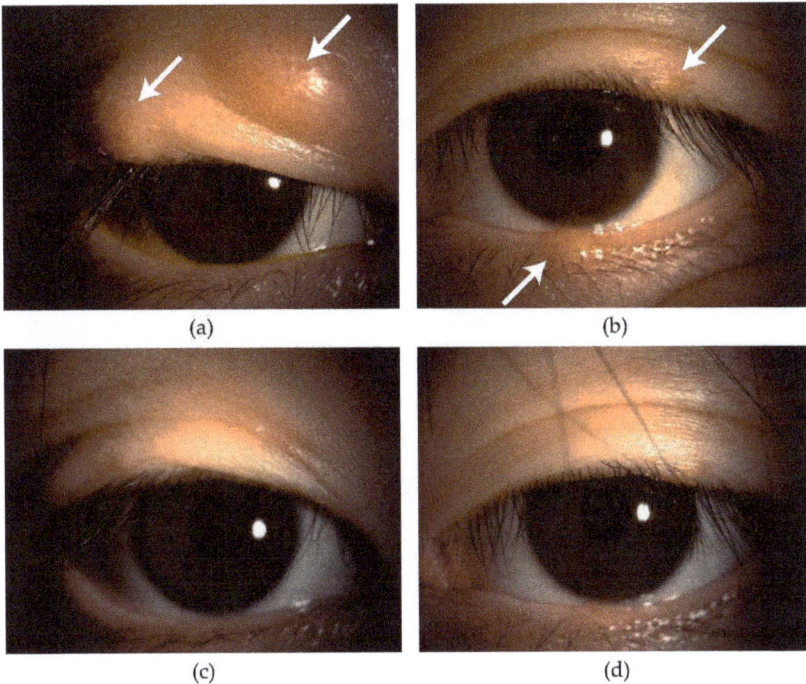

Figure 2. A 19-year-old female. Changes in chalazion in upper and lower eyelids before and after IPL. (**a**) Upper right eye. 18mm of chalazia (right white arrow) and 7 mm of chalazia (left white arrow) recurrenced. (**b**) Upper left eye. 4 mm of chalazia (upper white arrow) and 6 mm of chalazia (lower white arrow) recurrenced. (**c**) Two upper chalazia much improved. (**d**) Tow upper and lower chalazia much improved.

Table 2. Characteristics of the patients with chalazion in intense pulsed light (IPL)–meibomian gland expression (MGX) (treatment group) (n = 12) and MGX alone (control group) (n = 12) groups before and four weeks after the final treatment session.

Characteristics		Baseline Mean ± SD	(Range)	p Value for IPL-MGX vs. MGX Alone	Post-Treatment Mean ± SD	(Range)	p Value vs. Baseline	p Value for IPL-MGX vs. MGX Alone
Number of IPL for improvement	MGX alone							
	IPL-MGX				2.8 ± 1.3	(1–4)		
Plugging (0–3)	MGX alone	2.7 ± 0.5	(2–3)	0.92	2.1 ± 0.9	(1–3)	0.063	<0.001 **
	IPL-MGX	2.6 ± 0.7	(1–3)		0.2 ± 0.4	(0–1)	<0.001 **	
Vascularity (0–3)	MGX alone	2.3 ± 0.8	(1–3)	0.77	2.3 ± 0.8	(1–3)	1.00	<0.001 **
	IPL-MGX	2.4 ± 0.8	(1–3)		0 ± 0	(0–0)	<0.001 **	
Irregularity (0–2)	MGX alone	0.9 ± 0.9	(0–2)	0.83	0.9 ± 0.9	(0–2)	1.00	0.27
	IPL-MGX	1.0 ± 0.9	(0–2)		0.5 ± 0.5	(0–1)	0.031 *	
CFS (0–9)	MGX alone	2.0 ± 0.7	(1–3)	0.54	1.7 ± 0.7	(1–3)	0.125	<0.001 **
	IPL-MGX	2.1 ± 1.5	(1–5)		0.2 ± 0.4	(0–1)	<0.001 **	
Meibum grade (0–3)	MGX alone	2.5 ± 0.5	(2–3)	0.57	1.9 ± 0.8	(1–3)	0.016 *	<0.001 **
	IPL-MGX	2.6 ± 0.7	(1–3)		0.3 ± 0.5	(0–1)	<0.001 **	
Meiboscore (0–6)	MGX alone	3.2 ± 0.9	(2–4)	0.88	3.2 ± 0.9	(2–4)	1.00	0.88
	IPL-MGX	3.4 ± 1.5	(2–6)		3.4 ± 1.5	(2–6)	1.00	
Number of *Demodex*	MGX alone	3.1 ± 0.9	(2–4)	0.52	3.3 ± 0.8	(2–4)	0.50	<0.001 **
	IPL-MGX	2.8 ± 0.9	(2–4)		0 ± 0	(0–0)	<0.001 **	
Schirmer test value (mm)	MGX alone	11.7 ± 4.7	(5–20)	0.50	11.0 ± 4.2	(6–20)	0.30	0.75
	IPL-MGX	11.5 ± 7.5	(4–26)		11.5 ± 5.5	(6–20)	0.76	
Size (diameter) of chalazion (mm)	MGX alone	8.8 ± 2.4	(6–12)	0.47	9.2 ± 2.6	(6–12)	0.38	<0.001 **
	IPL-MGX	9.0 ± 5.2	(3–18)		0 ± 0	(0–0)	<0.001 **	
VAS score (0–100)	MGX alone	61.2 ± 22	(23–90)	1.00	67.3 ± 21.2	(30–90)	0.063	<0.001 **
	IPL-MGX	61.7 ± 23.8	(23–90)		0 ± 0	(0–0)	<0.001 **	

CFS, corneal and conjunctival fluorescein staining; VAS score, visual analogue scale score of ocular discomfort and foreign body sensation. p values were determined with Wilcoxon signed-rank test or Wilcoxon rank sum test (* $p < 0.05$, ** $p < 0.001$).

Table 3. Standard Patient Evaluation of Eye Dryness (SPEED) validated questionnaire score (0–28) of the patients with chalazion in intense pulsed light (IPL)–meibomian gland expression (MGX) ($n = 6$) and MGX alone ($n = 6$) groups before and four weeks after the final treatment session.

	Baseline Mean ± SD	(Range)	p Value for IPL-MGX vs. MGX Alone	Post-Treatment Mean ± SD	(Range)	p Value vs. Baseline	p Value for IPL-MGX vs. MGX Alone
MGX alone	11.8 ± 2.0	(9–15)	0.94	12.3 ± 2.2	(9–15)	1.00	0.003 *
IPL-MGX	11.2 ± 4.3	(4–15)		0 ± 0	(0–0)	0.031 *	

p values were determined with Wilcoxon signed-rank test or Wilcoxon rank sum test (* $p < 0.05$).

3.2. The Number of IPLs Required to Improve the Chalazion

Among the background factors, only the size of the chalazion correlated with the number of IPL-MGX sessions for treatment. (Table 4). Among the parameters related to the meibomian gland and tear film, plugging, CFS score, meibum grade, the number of *Demodex*, and Schirmer value were positively correlated with the number of IPL-MGX sessions for the treatment of chalazia (Table 5).

Table 4. Spearman's correlation coefficient (ρ) and p values for the relation between baseline characteristics and the number of treatment sessions in the intense pulsed light (IPL)–meibomian gland expression (MGX) group ($n = 6$).

Characteristics	ρ	p Value
Age	0.12	0.82
Number of chalazia	0.66	0.16
Number of eyelids with chalazia	0.67	0.15
Duration of pre-lid-warming	0.62	0.19
Size of the largest chalazion	0.94	0.005 *
SPEED score at baseline	−0.03	0.95

* $p < 0.05$. SPEED score, Standard Patient Evaluation of Eye Dryness validated questionnaire score.

Table 5. Spearman's correlation coefficient (ρ) and p values for the relation between baseline parameters and the number for treatment in the intense pulsed light (IPL)–meibomian gland expression (MGX) group ($n = 12$ eyes).

Baseline Parameters	ρ	p Value
Plugging	0.74	0.006 *
Vascularity	0.56	0.059
Irregularity	0.52	0.086
CFS	0.89	<0.001 **
Meibum grade	0.74	0.006 *
Meiboscore	0.57	0.051
Number of Demodex	0.73	0.007 *
Schirmer test value	0.61	0.034 *
VAS score	−0.24	0.45

* $p < 0.05$, ** $p < 0.001$. CFS, corneal and conjunctival fluorescein staining; VAS score, visual analogue scale score of ocular discomfort and foreign body sensation.

3.3. Safety of IPL-MGX

There were no significant differences in visual acuity and intraocular pressure before and 4 weeks after the final treatment in either treatment group (Table 6). Lens opacity and fundus condition showed no change between before and 4 weeks after the final treatment in either treatment group.

Table 6. Visual acuity and intraocular pressure of the patients with chalazion in intense pulsed light (IPL)–meibomian gland expression (MGX) ($n = 12$) and MGX alone ($n = 12$) groups before and four weeks after the final treatment session.

Characteristics		Baseline Mean ± SD	(Range)	p Value for IPL-MGX vs. MGX Alone	Post-Treatment Mean ± SD	(Range)	p Value for IPL-MGX vs. MGX Alone	p Value vs. Baseline
LogMAR visual acuity	MGX alone	−0.06 ± 0.07	(−0.18–0.00)	0.37	−0.07 ± 0.06	(−0.18–0.00)	0.38	0.50
	IPL-MGX	−0.07 ± 0.03	(−0.08–0.00)		−0.08 ± 0	(−0.08–0.08)		0.50
IOP (mmHg)	MGX alone	16.7 ± 1.4	(15–19)	0.93	16.6 ± 1.1	(14–19)	0.98	0.77
	IPL-MGX	16.8 ± 1.5	(15–19)		16.6 ± 1.7	(15–18)		1.00

LogMAR, logarithm of minimum angle of resolution; IOP, intraocular pressure. p values were determined with Wilcoxon signed-rank test or Wilcoxon rank sum test.

4. Discussion

The safety and effectiveness of IPL combined with MGX: Although chalazion is a non-infectious granuloma that often resolves spontaneously without special treatment, it can recur frequently, resulting in refractory chalazion. In this study, we treated multiple recurrent chalazia in the IPL-MGX and the MGX alone groups without surgery or incision, and found that the IPL-MGX treatment significantly reduced the size of the chalazion and increased patient satisfaction. This is the first study to examine the usefulness of IPL-MGX without surgical treatment and to compare its efficacy with MGX alone. The results showed that the IPL-MGX group significantly improved the size of chalazion, subjective symptoms, MGD-related parameters, and number of Demodex compared to the control group. The treatment was safe and effective with no side effects.

The mechanism by which IPL was effective for chalazion may be due to the anti-inflammatory effect of IPL and the mechanism of chalazion by temperature rise [29], since chalazion is an inflammatory granuloma. In addition, the IPL-MGX group was able to suppress recurrence for 6 months, suggesting that the environment of the ocular surface, including the eyelid, improved and the recurrence of the chalazion itself was suppressed by the treatment with IPL not only in the meibomian glands affected by the chalazion but also in the entire eyelid. The larger the size of chalazion at baseline was, and the poorer the function and morphology of the meibomian gland was, the higher the number of IPL cycles which was required to cure the chalazion in our study. An average of 2.8 (maximum 4) IPL cycles were required for the treatment of recurrent chalazion, which is similar to the number of IPL cycles required for the treatment of MGD.

4.1. Risk Factors for Chalazion

Blepharitis is the most common risk factor for chalazion. The probability of having a chalazion in the presence of blepharitis is 4.7 times greater than in the absence of blepharitis [3]. Posterior blepharitis describes inflammatory condition of the posterior lid margin, of which MGD is one possible cause [43]. Moreover, the previous report showed that MGD, dry eye, and blepharitis were the risk factors for recurrent chalazion [6,44]. Recently, the relationship between Demodex and chalazion has become a controversial topic. The rate of Demodex positivity is very high, ranging from approximately 70% to 90% in eyes affected by chalazion [4,45]. Demodex positivity is also associated with a high recurrence rate of chalazion [45]. Therefore, we investigated the meibomian-gland-related parameters, tear-film-related parameters and the presence of Demodex to determine the effect of IPL on multiple recurrent chalazia.

4.2. Compared to the Previous Results

In this study, three cases (50%) cured within 1 month; three (50%) cured after 1.5 months. In addition, all six cases had no recurrence 6 months after the end of the IPL treatment. A prospective randomized clinical trial reported that complete resolution rates in the surgical treatment and the triamcinolone acetonide injection groups were 79% and 81% [46]. The average time to resolution in the surgical treatment and the triamcinolone acetonide injection groups was 4 days and 5 days [46]. A single-center prospective randomized clinical study reported that the resolution rates in the surgical treatment, one triamcinolone acetonide injection, and hot compress groups were 87%, 84%, and 46% at the 3-week follow-up [47]. Patients with more than one chalazion on the same eyelid were excluded from the study. A prospective randomized multicenter treatment study reported that the resolution rates of single or multiple chalazia in the hot compresses alone, the hot compresses plus tobramycin, and hot compresses plus tobramycin/dexamethasone groups were 21%, 16%, and 18%, respectively, for 4–6 weeks of treatment [10].

4.3. Compared to the Conventional Therapies

Conventional treatments for chalazion include surgery, incision, warm compresses, lid hygiene, and topical steroid injection [1]. Non-ablative treatment takes longer (about 6 months on average) than surgery and incision. According to the previous literature, a meta-analysis on the recurrence rate of primary chalazion showed that the recurrence rate for curettage for chalazia was 0–16.7% and 0–27.3% for intralesional steroid injections [48]. Demodex blepharitis, MGD, and dry eye are also reported to be risks for multiple recurrent chalazia [34,44], and repeated surgery may further damage the meibomian glands, leading to decreased visual function [13] and eventual dry eye. In particular, the younger generation can be damaged cosmetically, mentally, and visually by multiple recurrences. Therefore, it is preferable to treat multiple recurrent chalazia without surgery and to treat subclinical/clinical MGD to prevent recurrence. We believe that proactive treatment for MGD, in addition to the local treatment of chalazion, can prevent future recurrence of chalazion and contribute to the patient's quality of life and quality of vision.

4.4. Limitations

There are several limitations in this study. First, this was a retrospective study. Second, the sample size was small, although the number of cases was sufficient for the power analysis. Third, the number of IPL sessions was not identical from case to case due to the search for the optimal IPL protocol for chalazion. Fourth, no automatic procedure was used to determine effectiveness. Finally, the decision point is relatively subjective, as patient satisfaction with improvement is clinically important for chalazion. Further addition of cases and multicenter studies are desirable with a randomized controlled prospective study. Further studies for the investigation of IPL protocols for recurrent multiple chalazia based on MGD treatment are needed.

5. Conclusions

In conclusion, our study demonstrated that an average of 2.5 ± 0.8 chalazia per patient, 9.0 ± 5.2 mm in size, were improved with an average of 2.8 ± 1.3 IPLs, with no recurrence for 6 months. IPL was safe and effective as non-surgical treatment of multiple recurrent chalazia. IPL is probably the best treatment option for multiple recurrent chalazia in terms of prevention of recurrence in order to minimize loss of the meibomian glands.

Author Contributions: Conceptualization, R.A.; methodology, R.A. and S.F.; software, S.F.; validation, R.A. and S.F.; formal analysis, S.F.; investigation, R.A.; resources, R.A.; data curation, R.A.; writing—original draft preparation, R.A.; writing—review and editing, S.F.; visualization, R.A.; supervision, R.A.; project administration, R.A. All authors have read and agreed to the published version of the manuscript.

Funding: This research received no external funding.

Institutional Review Board Statement: The study was conducted in accordance with the Declaration of Helsinki and approved by the Institutional Review Board (or Ethics Committee) of Itoh Clinic (protocol code: IRIN-202109 and date of approval: 15 March 2021).

Informed Consent Statement: Informed consent was obtained from all subjects involved in the study.

Data Availability Statement: The datasets generated during and analyzed in the current study are available from the corresponding author on request.

Conflicts of Interest: The authors declare no conflict of interest.

References

1. Perry, H.D.; Serniuk, R.A. Conservative treatment of chalazia. *Ophthalmology* **1980**, *87*, 218–221. [CrossRef]
2. Gary, A.; Jordan, K.B. *Chalazion*; StatPearls Publishing: San Francisco, CA, USA, 2022.
3. Nemet, A.Y.; Vinker, S.; Kaiserman, I. Associated morbidity of blepharitis. *Ophthalmology* **2011**, *118*, 1062–1068. [CrossRef] [PubMed]
4. Liang, L.; Ding, X.; Tseng, S.C. High prevalence of demodex brevis infestation in chalazia. *Am. J. Ophthalmol.* **2014**, *157*, 342–348.e341. [CrossRef] [PubMed]
5. Yam, J.C.; Tang, B.S.; Chan, T.M.; Cheng, A.C. Ocular demodicidosis as a risk factor of adult recurrent chalazion. *Eur. J. Ophthalmol.* **2014**, *24*, 159–163. [CrossRef]
6. Evans, J.; Vo, K.B.H.; Schmitt, M. Chalazion: Racial risk factors for formation, recurrence, and surgical intervention. *Can. J. Ophthalmol.* **2021**, *57*, 242–246. [CrossRef]
7. Duarte, A.F.; Moreira, E.; Nogueira, A.; Santos, P.; Azevedo, F. Chalazion surgery: Advantages of a subconjunctival approach. *J. Cosmet. Laser Ther.* **2009**, *11*, 154–156. [CrossRef]
8. Wong, M.Y.; Yau, G.S.; Lee, J.W.; Yuen, C.Y. Intralesional triamcinolone acetonide injection for the treatment of primary chalazions. *Int. Ophthalmol.* **2014**, *34*, 1049–1053. [CrossRef]
9. Lee, J.W.; Yau, G.S.; Wong, M.Y.; Yuen, C.Y. A comparison of intralesional triamcinolone acetonide injection for primary chalazion in children and adults. *Sci. World J.* **2014**, *2014*, 413729. [CrossRef]
10. Wu, A.Y.; Gervasio, K.A.; Gergoudis, K.N.; Wei, C.; Oestreicher, J.H.; Harvey, J.T. Conservative therapy for chalazia: Is it really effective? *Acta Ophthalmol.* **2018**, *96*, e503–e509. [CrossRef]
11. Nelson, J.D.; Shimazaki, J.; Benitez-del-Castillo, J.M.; Craig, J.P.; McCulley, J.P.; Den, S.; Foulks, G.N. The international workshop on meibomian gland dysfunction: Report of the definition and classification subcommittee. *Investig. Ophthalmol. Vis. Sci.* **2011**, *52*, 1930–1937. [CrossRef]
12. Machalinska, A.; Zakrzewska, A.; Safranow, K.; Wiszniewska, B.; Machalinski, B. Risk Factors and Symptoms of Meibomian Gland Loss in a Healthy Population. *J. Ophthalmol.* **2016**, *2016*, 7526120. [CrossRef]
13. Fukuoka, S.; Arita, R.; Shirakawa, R.; Morishige, N. Changes in meibomian gland morphology and ocular higher-order aberrations in eyes with chalazion. *Clin. Ophthalmol.* **2017**, *11*, 1031–1038. [CrossRef]
14. Raulin, C.; Greve, B.; Grema, H. IPL technology: A review. *Lasers Surg. Med.* **2003**, *32*, 78–87. [CrossRef]
15. Jones, L.; Downie, L.E.; Korb, D.; Benitez-Del-Castillo, J.M.; Dana, R.; Deng, S.X.; Dong, P.N.; Geerling, G.; Hida, R.Y.; Liu, Y.; et al. TFOS DEWS II Management and Therapy Report. *Ocul. Surf.* **2017**, *15*, 575–628. [CrossRef]
16. Tashbayev, B.; Yazdani, M.; Arita, R.; Fineide, F.; Utheim, T.P. Intense pulsed light treatment in meibomian gland dysfunction: A concise review. *Ocul. Surf.* **2020**, *18*, 583–594. [CrossRef]
17. Wat, H.; Wu, D.C.; Rao, J.; Goldman, M.P. Application of intense pulsed light in the treatment of dermatologic disease: A systematic review. *Dermatol. Surg.* **2014**, *40*, 359–377. [CrossRef]
18. Moreno-Arias, G.A.; Castelo-Branco, C.; Ferrando, J. Side-effects after IPL photodepilation. *Dermatol. Surg.* **2002**, *28*, 1131–1134.
19. Lee, W.W.; Murdock, J.; Albini, T.A.; O'Brien, T.P.; Levine, M.L. Ocular damage secondary to intense pulse light therapy to the face. *Ophthalmic Plast Reconstr. Surg.* **2011**, *27*, 263–265. [CrossRef]
20. Toyos, R.; McGill, W.; Briscoe, D. Intense pulsed light treatment for dry eye disease due to meibomian gland dysfunction; a 3-year retrospective study. *Photomed. Laser Surg.* **2015**, *33*, 41–46. [CrossRef]
21. Craig, J.P.; Chen, Y.H.; Turnbull, P.R. Prospective trial of intense pulsed light for the treatment of meibomian gland dysfunction. *Investig. Ophthalmol. Vis. Sci.* **2015**, *56*, 1965–1970. [CrossRef]
22. Vora, G.K.; Gupta, P.K. Intense pulsed light therapy for the treatment of evaporative dry eye disease. *Curr. Opin. Ophthalmol.* **2015**, *26*, 314–318. [CrossRef] [PubMed]
23. Gupta, P.K.; Vora, G.K.; Matossian, C.; Kim, M.; Stinnett, S. Outcomes of intense pulsed light therapy for treatment of evaporative dry eye disease. *Can. J. Ophthalmol.* **2016**, *51*, 249–253. [CrossRef] [PubMed]
24. Vegunta, S.; Patel, D.; Shen, J.F. Combination Therapy of Intense Pulsed Light Therapy and Meibomian Gland Expression (IPL/MGX) Can Improve Dry Eye Symptoms and Meibomian Gland Function in Patients with Refractory Dry Eye: A Retrospective Analysis. *Cornea* **2016**, *35*, 318–322. [CrossRef] [PubMed]
25. Jiang, X.; Lv, H.; Song, H.; Zhang, M.; Liu, Y.; Hu, X.; Li, X.; Wang, W. Evaluation of the Safety and Effectiveness of Intense Pulsed Light in the Treatment of Meibomian Gland Dysfunction. *J. Ophthalmol.* **2016**, *2016*, 1910694. [CrossRef]
26. Dell, S.J. Intense pulsed light for evaporative dry eye disease. *Clin. Ophthalmol.* **2017**, *11*, 1167–1173. [CrossRef]
27. Dell, S.J.; Gaster, R.N.; Barbarino, S.C.; Cunningham, D.N. Prospective evaluation of intense pulsed light and meibomian gland expression efficacy on relieving signs and symptoms of dry eye disease due to meibomian gland dysfunction. *Clin. Ophthalmol.* **2017**, *11*, 817–827. [CrossRef]

28. Rong, B.; Tu, P.; Tang, Y.; Liu, R.X.; Song, W.J.; Yan, X.M. [Evaluation of short-term effect of intense pulsed light combined with meibomian gland expression in the treatment of meibomian gland dysfunction]. *Zhonghua Yan Ke Za Zhi* **2017**, *53*, 675–681.
29. Liu, R.; Rong, B.; Tu, P.; Tang, Y.; Song, W.; Toyos, R.; Toyos, M.; Yan, X. Analysis of Cytokine Levels in Tears and Clinical Correlations After Intense Pulsed Light Treating Meibomian Gland Dysfunction. *Am. J. Ophthalmol.* **2017**, *183*, 81–90. [CrossRef]
30. Guilloto Caballero, S.; Garcia Madrona, J.L.; Colmenero Reina, E. Effect of pulsed laser light in patients with dry eye syndrome. *Arch. Soc. Esp. Oftalmol.* **2017**, *92*, 509–515. [CrossRef]
31. Yin, Y.; Liu, N.; Gong, L.; Song, N. Changes in the Meibomian Gland After Exposure to Intense Pulsed Light in Meibomian Gland Dysfunction (MGD) Patients. *Curr. Eye Res.* **2017**, *43*, 308–313. [CrossRef]
32. Albietz, J.M.; Schmid, K.L. Intense pulsed light treatment and meibomian gland expression for moderate to advanced meibomian gland dysfunction. *Clin. Exp. Optom.* **2018**, *101*, 23–33. [CrossRef]
33. Arita, R.; Fukuoka, S.; Morishige, N. Therapeutic efficacy of intense pulsed light in patients with refractory meibomian gland dysfunction. *Ocul. Surf.* **2019**, *17*, 104–110. [CrossRef]
34. Zhu, Y.; Huang, X.; Lin, L.; Di, M.; Chen, R.; Dong, J.; Jin, X. Efficacy of Intense Pulsed Light in the Treatment of Recurrent Chalaziosis. *Front. Med.* **2022**, *9*, 839908. [CrossRef]
35. Fitzpatrick, T.B. The validity and practicality of sun-reactive skin types I through VI. *Arch Dermatol.* **1988**, *124*, 869–871. [CrossRef]
36. Ngo, W.; Situ, P.; Keir, N.; Korb, D.; Blackie, C.; Simpson, T. Psychometric properties and validation of the Standard Patient Evaluation of Eye Dryness questionnaire. *Cornea* **2013**, *32*, 1204–1210. [CrossRef]
37. Arita, R.; Minoura, I.; Morishige, N.; Shirakawa, R.; Fukuoka, S.; Asai, K.; Goto, T.; Imanaka, T.; Nakamura, M. Development of Definitive and Reliable Grading Scales for Meibomian Gland Dysfunction. *Am. J. Ophthalmol.* **2016**, *169*, 125–137. [CrossRef]
38. van Bijsterveld, O.P. Diagnostic tests in the Sicca syndrome. *Arch. Ophthalmol.* **1969**, *82*, 10–14. [CrossRef]
39. Shimazaki, J.; Sakata, M.; Tsubota, K. Ocular surface changes and discomfort in patients with meibomian gland dysfunction. *Arch. Ophthalmol.* **1995**, *113*, 1266–1270. [CrossRef]
40. Arita, R.; Itoh, K.; Inoue, K.; Amano, S. Noncontact infrared meibography to document age-related changes of the meibomian glands in a normal population. *Ophthalmology* **2008**, *115*, 911–915. [CrossRef]
41. Shirmer, O. Studiun zur Physiologie und Pathologie der Tranenabsonderung und Tranenabfuhr. *Albrecht von Graefes Arch. für Ophthalmol.* **1903**, *56*, 197–291. [CrossRef]
42. Korb, D.R.; Blackie, C.A.; McNally, E.N. Evidence suggesting that the keratinized portions of the upper and lower lid margins do not make complete contact during deliberate blinking. *Cornea* **2013**, *32*, 491–495. [CrossRef]
43. Knop, E.; Knop, N.; Millar, T.; Obata, H.; Sullivan, D.A. The international workshop on meibomian gland dysfunction: Report of the subcommittee on anatomy, physiology, and pathophysiology of the meibomian gland. *Investig. Ophthalmol. Vis. Sci.* **2011**, *52*, 1938–1978. [CrossRef]
44. Patel, S.; Tohme, N.; Gorrin, E.; Kumar, N.; Goldhagen, B.; Galor, A. Prevalence and risk factors for chalazion in an older veteran population. *Br. J. Ophthalmol.* **2021**, *106*, 1200–1205. [CrossRef]
45. Tarkowski, W.; Owczynska, M.; Blaszczyk-Tyszka, A.; Mlocicki, D. Demodex mites as potential etiological factor in chalazion—A study in Poland. *Acta Parasitol.* **2015**, *60*, 777–783. [CrossRef]
46. Ben Simon, G.J.; Rosen, N.; Rosner, M.; Spierer, A. Intralesional triamcinolone acetonide injection versus incision and curettage for primary chalazia: A prospective, randomized study. *Am. J. Ophthalmol.* **2011**, *151*, 714–718 e711. [CrossRef]
47. Goawalla, A.; Lee, V. A prospective randomized treatment study comparing three treatment options for chalazia: Triamcinolone acetonide injections, incision and curettage and treatment with hot compresses. *Clin. Exp. Ophthalmol.* **2007**, *35*, 706–712. [CrossRef]
48. Aycinena, A.R.; Achiron, A.; Paul, M.; Burgansky-Eliash, Z. Incision and Curettage Versus Steroid Injection for the Treatment of Chalazia: A Meta-Analysis. *Ophthalmic Plast Reconstr. Surg.* **2016**, *32*, 220–224. [CrossRef]

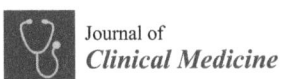

Article

Dry Eye Parameters and Lid Geometry in Adults Born Extremely, Very, and Moderately Preterm with and without ROP: Results from the Gutenberg Prematurity Eye Study

Achim Fieß [1,*], Clara Hufschmidt-Merizian [1], Sandra Gißler [1], Ulrike Hampel [2], Eva Mildenberger [3], Michael S. Urschitz [4], Fred Zepp [3], Bernhard Stoffelns [1], Norbert Pfeiffer [1] and Alexander K. Schuster [1]

1. Department of Ophthalmology, University Medical Center of the Johannes Gutenberg University Mainz, 55131 Mainz, Germany; clara.hufschmidt-merizian@gast.unimedizin-mainz.de (C.H.-M.); sandra.gissler@unimedizin-mainz.de (S.G.); bernhard.stoffelns@unimedizin-mainz.de (B.S.); norbert.pfeiffer@unimedizin-mainz.de (N.P.); alexander.schuster@unimedizin-mainz.de (A.K.S.)
2. Department of Ophthalmology, University Hospital Leipzig, 04103 Leipzig, Germany; uli.hampel@medizin.uni-leipzig.de
3. Division of Neonatology, Department of Pediatrics, University Medical Center of the Johannes Gutenberg University Mainz, 55131 Mainz, Germany; eva.mildenberger@unimedizin-mainz.de (E.M.); zepp@uni-mainz.de (F.Z.)
4. Division of Pediatric Epidemiology, Institute for Medical Biostatistics, Epidemiology and Informatics, University Medical Center of the Johannes Gutenberg University Mainz, 55131 Mainz, Germany; urschitz@uni-mainz.de
* Correspondence: achim.fiess@gmail.com; Tel.: +49-(0)6131-17-5150; Fax: +49-(0)6131-17-8495

Citation: Fieß, A.; Hufschmidt-Merizian, C.; Gißler, S.; Hampel, U.; Mildenberger, E.; Urschitz, M.S.; Zepp, F.; Stoffelns, B.; Pfeiffer, N.; Schuster, A.K. Dry Eye Parameters and Lid Geometry in Adults Born Extremely, Very, and Moderately Preterm with and without ROP: Results from the Gutenberg Prematurity Eye Study. *J. Clin. Med.* 2022, *11*, 2702. https://doi.org/10.3390/jcm11102702

Academic Editor: Vincenzo Scorcia

Received: 15 March 2022
Accepted: 3 May 2022
Published: 11 May 2022

Publisher's Note: MDPI stays neutral with regard to jurisdictional claims in published maps and institutional affiliations.

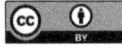

Copyright: © 2022 by the authors. Licensee MDPI, Basel, Switzerland. This article is an open access article distributed under the terms and conditions of the Creative Commons Attribution (CC BY) license (https:// creativecommons.org/licenses/by/ 4.0/).

Abstract: Background/Aims: This study aimed to analyze the effects of perinatal history on tear film properties and lid geometry in adults born preterm. Methods: The Gutenberg Prematurity Eye Study (GPES) is a German prospective examination of adults born preterm and term aged 18 to 52 years with Keratograph® 5M and Schirmer test I. Main outcome measures were first non-invasive tear film break-up time (F-NITBUT), bulbar redness (BR), Schirmer test, and nasal palpebral angle measurement. The associations with gestational age (GA), birth weight (BW), and BW percentile, retinopathy of prematurity (ROP), ROP treatment, and other perinatal factors were evaluated using regression analyses. Results: 489 eyes of 255 preterm and 277 eyes of 139 full-term individuals (aged 28.6 +/− 8.8 years, 220 females) were included. Of these, 33 participants (56 eyes) had a history of spontaneously regressed ROP and 9 participants (16 eyes) had a history of ROP treatment. After adjustment for age and sex, lower F-NITBUT (<20 s) was associated with ROP treatment (OR = 4.42; $p = 0.025$). Lower GA correlated with increased bulbar redness (B = −0.02; $p = 0.011$) and increased length of wetting in the Schirmer test (B = −0.69; $p = 0.003$). Furthermore, low GA was associated with narrowing of the nasal palpebral angle (B = 0.22; $p = 0.011$) adjusted for age and sex, but not when considering ROP in the multivariable model. Conclusion: Our analyses indicate that perinatal history affects ocular surface properties, tear production and lid geometry in adults born term and preterm. This might indicate that affected persons have a predisposition to diseases of the corneal surface such as the dry eye disease.

Keywords: Schirmer test; dry eye; sicca; prematurity; retinopathy of prematurity; epidemiology

1. Introduction

Preterm delivery leads to an abrupt change in the surrounding fetal environment and may result in ocular changes, especially in those with immediate exposure to the environment such as the ocular surface. Indeed, children born preterm have altered ocular morphology, including a steeper corneal geometry [1], a smaller anterior chamber depth [2], thicker lens [2], shorter axial length [1,2], and altered posterior pole [3–5]. Similar results were reported in adults indicating that low birth weight (<2500 g) as a surrogate marker for prematurity is associated with steeper corneas and shorter axial lengths [6]. These results show that the effects of prematurity on ocular shape persist throughout life. Furthermore, extreme preterm newborns are at increased risk for the postnatal development of retinopathy of prematurity (ROP) which is a vasoproliferative disease of the retina caused by high oxygen levels and the major cause for reduced visual acuity in childhood [7,8]. Several reports observed that ROP is an additional parameter affecting corneal shape in children [1]. Additionally, the corneal surface is less regular as indicated by increased corneal aberrations measured in preterm children [9] and adults [10]. This is of particular importance because every year about 15 million newborns are born preterm globally and the prevalence of ROP has still been increasing for several decades worldwide [7,11].

There are different hypotheses and models explaining the effects of an altered corneal geometry. For example, Fielder et al. hypothesized that the lower extrauterine temperature leads to a decreased flattening of the cornea after preterm birth [12], whereas other researchers supposed that a shorter time in the intrauterine milieu and different periods of opened eyes [13] may result in ultrastructural corneal remodeling processes including collagen fiber layers. Impaired prenatal growth also leads to altered organ morphology and functioning [14], as well as increased inflammation in a hyper-responsive innate immune system [15]. Until now, it is unclear whether this pro-inflammatory tendency after premature birth and different environmental exposure may also influence the ocular surface in which subacute inflammation is a risk factor for homeostasis and may lead to dry eye disease. Previous reports demonstrated that dry eye disease has many features in common with autoimmune disease [16], which may lead to an increased risk of dry eye disease in preterm individuals.

Dry eye disease is a multifactorial disease of the tears and ocular surface leading to discomfort, an unstable tear film, and visual disturbance [17], with up to every third person worldwide suffering from dry eye disease [18]. In recent decades, many studies investigated triggers of dry eye disease such as environmental factors, endogenous stress, antigens, infections, and genetic factors [16,19]. Another risk factor may be the perinatal history, potentially leading to life-long alterations of the ocular surface. As prematurity is linked to altered ocular geometry, there is the possibility that perinatal history may also affect eyelid formation and ocular surface characteristics. Hence, this investigation assessed the status of the ocular surface by measuring the tear film break-up time, bulbar redness, length of wetting the Schirmer test I, and nasal palpebral angle of subjects born preterm at different gestational ages (GA) with and without ROP compared to full-term controls now aged between 18 to 52 years.

Precis: This study investigated the long-term effects of prematurity on dry eye disease parameters and lid geometry in adulthood. The results indicate that the more preterm individuals are born, the more frequently alterations of ocular surface occur.

Key messages of the article:
- What is already known on this topic? Prematurity is associated with altered ocular morphology and functioning in childhood and adulthood, so we investigated whether perinatal factors have long-term effects on the ocular surface and lid configuration in adulthood.
- What does this study add? ROP treatment is linked to reduced tear film break-up time later in life. Furthermore, low gestational age is associated with increased bulbar redness, longer Schirmer strip measurement, and a narrower nasal lid angle.
- How might this study affect research or practice? Perinatal history affects the ocular surface, tear production, and lid geometry in adults born term and preterm, which might predispose affected persons to diseases of the corneal surface and dry eye disease in later life.

2. Materials and Methods

2.1. Study Population

The Gutenberg Prematurity Eye Study (GPES) is a single-center cohort study at the University Medical Center of the Johannes Gutenberg University Mainz in Germany (UMCM) that recruits individuals that (i) have been born preterm or at term between 1969 and 2002 and (ii) were between 18 and 52 years of age at study enrolment. According to these design elements, the study is a retrospective cohort study with a prospective acquisition of follow-up data. For the GPES, every preterm newborn with a GA $\leq$ 32 weeks and every second randomly chosen preterm newborn with GA 33–36 weeks was contacted and invited to participate. From each month from 1969 to 2002, 6 (3 males and 3 females) randomly selected full-term subjects with a birth weight between the 10th and 90th percentile were also invited to serve as controls as reported earlier [20–24].

The study examinations were performed between 2019 and 2021. The flow chart for eligibility and recruitment efficacy proportion is shown in Figure S1. Every participant underwent a detailed ophthalmological examination including measurement with a Keratograph® 5M (Oculus, Wetzlar, Germany) and a medical history interview. Furthermore, their medical records documenting the perinatal and postnatal history were assessed.

Written informed consent was obtained from all participants before their entry into the study and the GPES complies with Good Clinical Practice (GCP), Good Epidemiological Practice (GEP), and the ethical principles of the Declaration of Helsinki. The study protocol and documents were approved by the local ethics committee of the Medical Chamber of Rhineland-Palatinate, Germany (reference no. 2019-14161; original vote: 29 May 2019, latest update: 2 April 2020).

2.2. Assessment of Pre-, Peri- and Postnatal Medical History

The medical histories were assessed from medical records stored at the UMCM. Data were collected regarding GA (weeks), birth weight (kg), presence of ROP, stage of ROP, ROP treatment, placental insufficiency, preeclampsia, maternal smoking during pregnancy and breastfeeding. Birth weight percentiles were also calculated according to Voigt et al. [25].

2.3. Categorization

For descriptive analysis, participants were allocated to group 1: full-term participants (GA $\geq$ 37 weeks), group 2: preterm participants with GA between 33–36 weeks without ROP, group 3: preterm participants with GA between 29–32 weeks without ROP, group 4: preterm participants with GA $\leq$ 28 weeks without ROP, group 5: preterm participants with GA $\leq$ 32 weeks with postnatal ROP without ROP treatment and group 6: preterm participants with GA $\leq$ 32 weeks with postnatal ROP and ROP treatment as reported earlier [21,22]. In the case that only one eye of a participant had ROP, the other non-ROP eye was excluded from the analysis.

2.4. Ophthalmological Examination

Each participant was examined with a Keratograph® 5M (Oculus, Wetzlar, Germany) to measure the non-invasive tear film break-up time (first: F-NITBUT) and grade of break-up time. Furthermore, the software of the Keratograph® 5M measures the nasal and temporal conjunctival areas, detects conjunctival blood vessels and calculates redness grade. Values for the mean global bulbar redness consist of values from temporal and nasal bulbar redness. The limbal nasal and limbal temporal redness values are subcategories of the nasal and temporal bulbar redness, respectively. Lid geometry was determined by analyzing photographs of the anterior segment and measuring the palpebral fissure and the nasal palpebral angle. Each parameter was controlled for outliers.

Tear production was measured by the Schirmer test. In every participant, the distance of the tears to travel along the length of a paper test strip was measured [1] without anesthesia of the ocular surface (Schirmer test I). Furthermore, the study participants completed the ocular surface and disease questionnaire, and the Ocular Surface Disease Index (OSDI) was calculated [26].

2.5. Covariates

Covariates were factors that may have affected the main outcome measures such as sex (female), age (years), GA (weeks), birth weight (gram), birth weight percentile, ROP (yes), ROP treatment (yes), placental insufficiency (yes), preeclampsia (yes), breastfeeding (yes), and maternal smoking during pregnancy (yes).

2.6. Inclusion/Exclusion Criteria

Only participants with successful measurement of the tear film break-up time were included. Each measurement was checked for correctness and centration and excluded if considered invalid. Participants with a history of corneal or cataract surgery were excluded as this may have contributed to an altered ocular surface.

2.7. Statistical Analysis

The main outcome measures were non-invasive tear film break-up time, bulbar redness, length of wetting in the Schirmer test I, and nasal palpebral angle. Descriptive statistics were computed for these measures stratified by clinical group. Absolute and relative frequencies were calculated for dichotomous parameters; the mean and standard deviation were calculated for approximately normally distributed variables, otherwise median and interquartile range. Categorical data were compared with the chi-square test, with not-normally distributed continuous parameters compared with the Mann–Whitney U-test. Linear regression models in the case of normal distribution with general estimating equations (GEE) were used to assess associations and account for correlations between corresponding eyes. For non-normally distributed parameters, quantile regression was performed including only right eyes (Schirmer I test). Binary logistic regression analyses were conducted for reduced F-NITBUT (<20 s). First, univariate analyses of the main outcome measures and sex (female), age (years), GA (weeks), birth weight (kg), birth weight percentile, ROP (yes), ROP treatment (yes), placental insufficiency (yes), preeclampsia (yes), breastfeeding (yes) and maternal smoking during pregnancy (yes) were computed. Then, only parameters associated in the univariate analyses were included in model #1 with additional adjustment for sex and age. In a further model, the potential effect of ROP occurrence (yes) and/or ROP treatment (yes) were analyzed. Birth weight was excluded in the multivariable models to avoid collinearity which was strong between GA and birth weight. This was an explorative study, so there was no adjustment for multiple testing. Calculations were performed using commercial software (IBM SPSS 20.0; SPSS, Inc., Chicago, IL, USA; R version 4.0.0 (24 April 2020), R Core Team (2020), R: A language and environment for statistical computing and R Foundation for Statistical Computing, Vienna, Austria. URL https://www.R-project.org/; package "quantreg" (accessed 10 January 2022).

3. Results

3.1. Participant Characteristics

The present analysis included 489 eyes of 255 preterm and 277 eyes of 139 full-term individuals (age 28.6 +/− 8.8 years, 220 females). Overall, there were 277 eyes of 139 participants with GA ≥ 37 weeks (group 1), 256 eyes of 129 participants with a GA between 33–36 weeks without ROP (group 2), 133 eyes of 70 participants with a GA between 29–32 weeks without ROP (group 3), 28 eyes of 14 participants with a GA ≤ 28 weeks without ROP (group 4), 56 eyes of 33 participants with a GA between 24–32 weeks with ROP without treatment (group 5), and 16 eyes of 9 participants with a GA between 24–32 and with postnatal treatment for ROP (group 6). Of the ROP-treated group, five (nine eyes) participants underwent laser coagulation, while four (seven eyes) participants had cryocoagulation. The recruitment efficacy proportion for each group is presented in Supplementary Figure S1. Overall, 7 participants were excluded because of previous corneal refractive surgery, cataract surgery, or ocular trauma, and further 40 participants were excluded because measurement with a keratograph was invalid or not possible. In total, eight eyes without ROP were excluded in which the fellow eye had postnatal ROP. The participants' characteristics are presented in Table 1.

Table 1. Characteristics of the sample of the Gutenberg Prematurity Eye Study stratified by study groups.

Gestational Age [Weeks]	Group 1 GA ≥ 37	Group 2 GA 33–36 no ROP	Group 3 GA 29–32 no ROP	Group 4 GA ≤ 28 no ROP	Group 5 GA ≤ 32 ROP	Group 6 GA ≤ 32 ROP with Treatment
Participants/eyes (n)	139/277	129/256	70/133	14/28	33/56	9/16
Sex (Women) (%)	81 (58.3%)	77 (59.7%)	37 (52.9%)	8 (57.1%)	15 (45.5%)	2 (22.2%)
Age (y)	29.9 ± 9.2	29.3 ± 9.2	27.8 ± 8.1	23.9 ± 8.2	24.5 ± 5.3	27.9 ± 6.3
Birth weight (g)	3420 ± 393	2064 ± 473	1587 ± 347	930 ± 218	1120 ± 392	862 ± 304
Birth weight < 1500 g (yes)	0 (0%)	13 (10.1%)	28 (40%)	14 (100%)	28 (84.8%)	9 (100%)
Birth weight < 1000 g (yes)	0 (0%)	0 (0%)	4 (5.7%)	7 (50%)	12 (36.4%)	6 (66.7%)
Birth weight percentile	48.7 ± 21.4	25.2 ± 24.5	45.2 ± 23.8	41.1 ± 24.6	37.7 ± 29.4	24.2 ± 27.1
Gestational age (wks)	39.3 ± 1.3	34.3 ± 1.0	30.7 ± 1.1	26.8 ± 1.6	28.4 ± 1.9	27.4 ± 2.7
(min–max)	(37–43)	(33–36)	(29–32)	(23–28)	(24–32)	(24–32)
ROP stage (1/2/3/4/5)	0/0/0/0/0	0/0/0/0/0	0/0/0/0/0	0/0/0/0/0	25/25/5/0/1	0/2/14/0/0
Preeclampsia (yes)	11 (7.9%)	23 (17.8%)	8 (11.4%)	2 (14.3%)	7 (21.2%)	2 (22.2%)
Placental insufficiency (yes)	2 (1.4%)	16 (12.4%)	1 (1.4%)	1 (7.1%)	2 (6.1%)	0 (0%)
HELLP-syndrome	0 (0%)	6 (4.7%)	0 (0%)	0 (0%)	4 (12.1%)	0 (0%)
Maternal smoking (yes)	7 (5%)	7 (5.4%)	5 (7.1%)	1 (7.1%)	3 (9.1%)	1 (11.1%)
Gestational diabetes (yes)	1 (0.7%)	6 (4.7%)	1 (1.4%)	0 (0%)	1 (3%)	0 (0%)
Breastfeeding (yes)	78 (56.1%)	69 (53.5%)	37 (52.9%)	7 (50%)	16 (48.5%)	5 (55.6%)
Ocular parameters						
Visual acuity (logMAR) OD	0.0 (0.0; 0.0)	0.0 (0.0; 0.0)	0.0 (0.0; 0.0)	0.0 (0.0; 0.0)	0.0 (0.0; 0.1)	0.0 (0.0; 0.3)
Visual acuity (logMAR) OS	0.0 (0.0; 0.0)	0.0 (0.0; 0.0)	0.0 (0.0; 0.0)	0.0 (0.0; 0.0)	0.0 (0.0; 0.0)	0.1 (0.0; 0.7)
Spherical equivalent (diopter) OD	−0.98 ± 2.2	−1.10 ± 2.20	−0.59 ± 2.19	−0.9 ± 2.53	−1.52 ± 3.39	−5.12 ± 7.51
Spherical equivalent (diopter) OS	−0.97 ± 2.09	−1.16 ± 2.18	−0.63 ± 2.19	−0.45 ± 2.19	−1.75 ± 3.41	−4.26 ± 10.98
Intraocular pressure (mmHg) OD	15.3 ± 2.8	14.7 ± 2.9	14.6 ± 3.3	16.1 ± 3.0	15.8 ± 3.5	16.0 ± 4.1
Intraocular pressure (mmHg) OS	15.2 ± 2.8	14.5 ± 3.0	14.5 ± 3.1	14.7 ± 3.0	16.3 ± 3.7	17.0 ± 4.4

g—gram; mm—millimeter; ROP—retinopathy of prematurity; dpt—diopter; OD—right eye; OS—left eye.

3.2. Descriptive Anterior Surface Parameters

Participants treated for ROP showed a lower F-NITBUT ($p = 0.032$; Table 2) (Figure 1). Bulbar redness was increased in the preterm group with a GA 33–36 weeks ($p = 0.034$; group 2) and the group with untreated ROP participants ($p = 0.024$; group 5) and in the ROP treated participants ($p = 0.048$; group 6) compared to the full-term control group (group 1) (Table 2). Furthermore, the measurement in the Schirmer test was significantly increased in the preterm groups with a GA 33–36 weeks ($p = 0.001$; group 2), GA 29–32 weeks without ROP ($p = 0.001$; group 3), and GA ≤ 28 weeks without ROP ($p < 0.001$; group 4), and descriptively increased in participants with GA ≤ 32 weeks with ROP without treatment ($p = 0.092$; group 5) and with ROP treatment ($p = 0.054$; group 6) compared to the full-term control group (group 1) (Table 2; Figure 2). Parameters for palpebral fissure and angle are displayed in Table 3 and Figure 3.

Table 2. Anterior segment parameters of the study groups.

Gestational Age [Weeks]	Group 1 GA ≥ 37	Group 2 GA 33–36 no ROP	Group 3 GA 29–32 no ROP	Group 4 GA ≤ 28 no ROP	Group 5 GA ≤ 32 ROP	Group 6 GA ≤ 32 ROP with Treatment
Participants/eyes (n)	139/277	129/256	70/133	14/28	33/56	9/16
Break-up time						
First BUT OD	20.7 ± 5.8	20.7 ± 6.2	20.2 ± 6.8	21.4 ± 5.4	19.6 ± 6.2	14.9 ± 7.8 #
First BUT OS	21.6 ± 5.2	19.6 ± 6.8 #	20.9 ± 5.9	20.3 ± 5.1	20.3 ± 5.1	12.2 ± 7.6 #
BUT ≤ 20 s OD + OS	89 (33.0%)	90 (36.0%)	41 (32.3%)	10 (37.0%)	21 (42.0%)	10 (71.4%) #
BUT ≤ 10 s OD + OS	21 (7.8%)	29 (11.6%)	14 (11.0%)	1 (3.7%)	3 (6.0%)	6 (42.9%) #
BUT ≤ 5 s OD + OS	0 (0%)	6 (2.4%) #	0 (0%)	0 (0%)	0 (0%)	1 (7.1%) #
BUT grade OD	13.9 ± 6.1	14.7 ± 5.9	13.9 ± 6.6	16.0 ± 5.0	14.0 ± 6.4	10.4 ± 5.3
BUT grade OS	15.4 ± 5.3	13.6 ± 5.9 #	15.6 ± 6.0	14.4 ± 4.8	14.6 ± 4.6	8.5 ± 5.6 #
OSDI score	4.73 ± 7.79	4.73 ± 7.47	3.58 ± 5.69	2.79 ± 6.09	4.14 ± 5.64	5.13 ± 10.16
Available measurements OD/OS	130/129	117/116	61/61	13/13	22/23	6/6
Schirmer test OD (mm/5 min)	17.6 ± 12.1	20.8 ± 11.8 #	21.2 ± 12	26.9 ± 9.5 #	19.3 ± 13	24.5 ± 12.1
Schirmer test OS (mm/5 min)	16.2 ± 11.3	20.1 ± 11.7 #	20.7 ± 11.7 #	28.5 ± 9.6 #	21.1 ± 12.5	23.5 ± 12.1
Schirmer test ≤ 10 mm/5 min OD + OS	102 (39.2%)	64 (27.2%) #	31 (24.8%) #	1 (3.8%) #	12 (26.7%) #	2 (18.2%)
Schirmer test ≤ 5 mm/5 min OD + OS	52 (20%)	29 (12.3%) #	15 (12%) #	0 (0%) **	7 (15.6%)	2 (18.2%)
Bulbar redness						
Valid measurements participants OD/OS	81/76	71/69	42/39	9/6	16/13	6/3
Global bulbar redness OD	0.82 ± 0.32	0.87 ± 0.4	0.87 ± 0.61	0.92 ± 0.32	1.15 ± 0.53 #	1.08 ± 0.43
Global bulbar redness OS	0.72 ± 0.31	0.96 ± 0.56 #	0.81 ± 0.59	0.97 ± 0.56	1.08 ± 0.89	0.9 ± 0.2
Bulbar temporal OD	0.7 ± 0.33	0.78 ± 0.35	0.75 ± 0.43	0.86 ± 0.32	0.92 ± 0.38 #	1.0 ± 0.4
Bulbar temporal OS	0.66 ± 0.28	0.79 ± 0.38 #	0.69 ± 0.34	0.78 ± 0.38	0.78 ± 0.34	1.03 ± 0.15 #
Bulbar nasal OD	1.01 ± 0.4	0.96 ± 0.4	0.88 ± 0.48	1.12 ± 0.39	1.52 ± 0.78 #	1.17 ± 0.52
Bulbar nasal OS	0.91 ± 0.45	1.05 ± 0.52	0.92 ± 0.49	1.42 ± 0.7	1.27 ± 0.82	1.13 ± 0.32
Limbal temporal OD	0.37 ± 0.28	0.43 ± 0.23	0.39 ± 0.28	0.62 ± 0.45	0.53 ± 0.3 #	0.52 ± 0.34
Limbal temporal OS	0.39 ± 0.22	0.5 ± 0.31 #	0.44 ± 0.29	0.5 ± 0.35	0.47 ± 0.29	0.53 ± 0.23
Limbal nasal OD	0.53 ± 0.3	0.5 ± 0.27	0.5 ± 0.35	0.61 ± 0.28	0.79 ± 0.48	0.67 ± 0.33
Limbal nasal OS	0.47 ± 0.31	0.58 ± 0.38	0.49 ± 0.39	0.9 ± 0.81	0.68 ± 0.53	0.87 ± 0.55

GA—gestational age; ROP—retinopathy of prematurity; mm—millimeter; OD—right eye; OS—left eye; BUT—Break-up time. Linear regression analysis was applied for normally distributed parameters to compare the different groups with the full-term control group (reference). When parameters were not normally distributed, Mann–Whitney U-test was conducted to compare the different preterm groups with the full-term control group (reference group). # statistical difference ($p < 0.05$) compared to the control group. ** statistical difference ($p < 0.001$) compared to the control group.

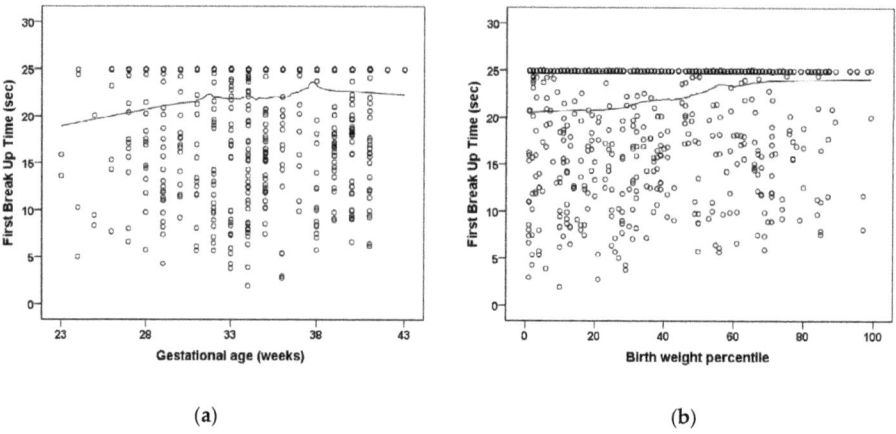

(a) (b)

Figure 1. Relationship of (a) gestational age and (b) birth weight percentile to the first break-up time (sec.) in the Gutenberg Prematurity Eye Study. Figure legend 1: There is no significant association between low gestational age and low birth weight percentile with first break-up time. The line presents the Loess (Locally Weighted Scatterplot Smoothing) curve.

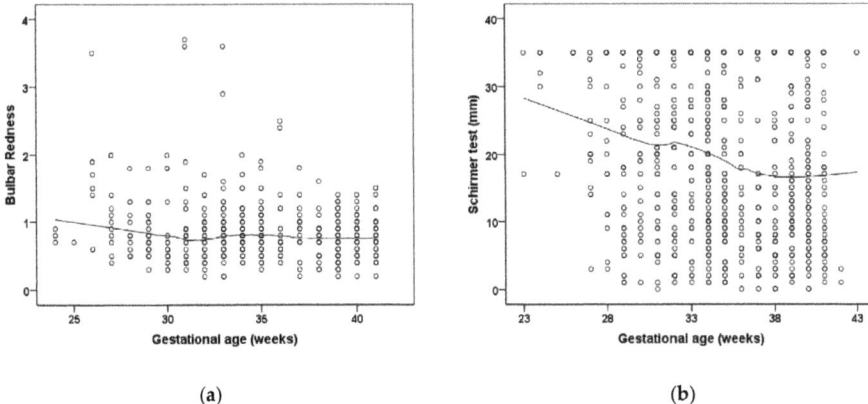

Figure 2. The relationship of gestational age to (**a**) bulbar redness, and (**b**) wetting in the Schirmer test in the Gutenberg Prematurity Eye Study. Figure legend 2: Individuals born preterm with low gestational age show an increased bulbar redness and a higher Schirmer test result. The line presents the Loess (Locally Weighted Scatterplot Smoothing) curve.

Table 3. Lid parameters of the study groups.

Gestational Age [Weeks]	Group 1 GA ≥ 37	Group 2 GA 33–36 no ROP	Group 3 GA 29–32 no ROP	Group 4 GA ≤ 28 no ROP	Group 5 GA ≤ 32 ROP	Group 6 GA ≤ 32 Treated ROP
Available lid measurements Participants/eyes (n)	134/268	125/245	64/125	14/28	29/50	8/15
Palpebral fissure (mm) OD	9.52 ± 1.11	9.41 ± 1.43	9.39 ± 1.19	9.25 ± 1.03	9.5 ± 1.17	8.85 ± 1.97
Palpebral fissure (mm) OS	9.17 ± 1.19	8.98 ± 1.56	9.11 ± 1.27	8.61 ± 1.41	9.36 ± 2.35	8.39 ± 2.34
Nasal palpebral angle (degree) OD	53.86 ± 6.83	52.46 ± 7.62	52.92 ± 8.78	51.43 ± 8.48	51.8 ± 6.41	47.88 ± 10.52
Nasal palpebral angle (degree) OS	53.47 ± 7.42	51.72 ± 7.6	52.49 ± 8.6	50.79 ± 6.93	47.68 ± 5.39	46.86 ± 13.23
Bulbar area OD	11.3 ± 4.3	10.9 ± 5.0	11.1 ± 4.9	10.4 ± 3.1	9.6 ± 2.5 #	8.8 ± 3.6
Bulbar area OS	11.2 ± 4.6	9.8 ± 5.2	10.3 ± 5.2	9.7 ± 4.1	9.4 ± 4.4	8.1 ± 2.3 #

GA—gestational age; ROP—retinopathy of prematurity; mm—millimeter; OD—right eye; OS—left eye. Linear regression analysis was applied to compare the different groups with the full-term control group (reference). Categorical data were compared using the chi-square test with the full-term group as reference. # statistical difference ($p < 0.05$) compared to the control group.

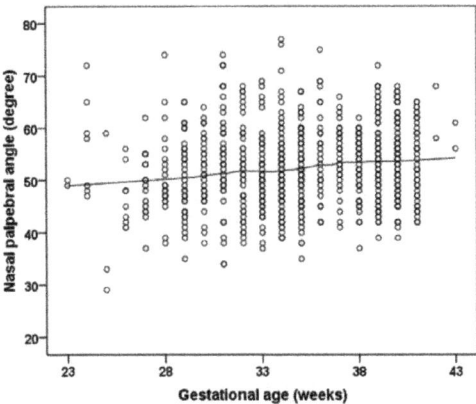

Figure 3. The relationship of gestational age to the nasal palpebral angle. Figure legend 3: Participants with lower gestational age reveal a smaller nasal palpebral angle. The line presents the Loess (Locally Weighted Scatterplot Smoothing) curve.

3.3. Uni- and Multivariable Analyses

In the association analyses, first univariable analyses were performed. Associated parameters were then included in model #1 without the inclusion of ROP occurrence and ROP treatment. In a second multivariable model, ROP occurrence and treatment were additionally included if they were associated in the univariable model. Models #1 and #2 were additionally adjusted for sex and age. First tear film break-up time (<20 s) correlated in univariable analyses with ROP occurrence (p = 0.024) and ROP treatment (p = 0.009). After adjustment for sex and age and the additional inclusion of ROP occurrence and treatment, ROP treatment (OR = 4.42 [95% CI: 1.20; 16.28]; p = 0.025) but not ROP occurrence was associated with F-NITBUT < 20 s. In the univariable analyses, Bulbar redness was associated with GA (p = 0.004), birth weight (p = 0.003), and ROP occurrence (p = 0.05). After adjustment for sex and age in model #1, GA (p < 0.001) was still associated with bulbar redness. In model #2, a low GA revealed an association (B = −0.015 [95% CI: −0.027; −0.003]; p = 0.011) with bulbar redness but not ROP occurrence.

The measurement in the Schirmer test was associated with GA (p < 0.001), birth weight (<0.001), and placental insufficiency (p = 0.029) in univariable analyses. In multivariable model #1, the Schirmer test results were still associated with gestational age (B = −0.692 [95% CI: −1.158; −0.226] mm; p = 0.003) and placental insufficiency (B = 8.596 [95% CI: 4.643; 12.55] mm; p < 0.001).

Nasal palpebral angle correlated with GA (p = 0.002), birth weight (p < 0.002), ROP occurrence (p = 0.002), and preeclampsia (p = 0.040). After adjustment for sex and age, GA (p = 0.011) and preeclampsia (p = 0.034) showed both associations. In model #2, GA and ROP treatment showed no association, while preeclampsia was associated (B = 2.492 [95% CI: 0.320; 4.664] mm; p = 0.025) (Table 4).

Table 4. Linear associations of anterior segment parameters with different perinatal parameters for the sample of the Gutenberg Prematurity Eye Study.

First Break-Up Time < 20 s (yes)	Univariate OR [95% CI]	p	Model 1 B [95% CI]	p	Model 2 B [95% CI]	p
Gestational age (weeks)	0.981 (0.947; 1.017)	0.29	-	-	-	-
Birth weight (kg)	0.878 (0.750; 1.028)	0.88	*	*	*	*
Birth weight percentile	0.994 (0.988; 1.000)	0.057	-	-	-	-
ROP (yes)	1.813 (1.083; 3.036)	0.024	-	-	1.425 (0.783; 2.591)	0.25
ROP treatment (yes)	4.711 (1.463; 15.17)	0.009	-	-	4.421 (1.200; 16.28)	0.025
Placental insufficiency (yes)	1.204 (0.617; 2.349)	0.59	-	-	-	-
Preeclampsia (yes)	1.389 (0.896; 2.153)	0.14	-	-	-	-
Breastfeeding (yes)	0.962 (0.711; 1.301)	0.80	-	-	-	-
Smoking pregnancy (yes)	1.144 (0.623; 2.103)	0.66	-	-	-	-
Bulbar redness	**B [95% CI]**	***p***	**B [95% CI]**	***p***	**B [95% CI]**	***p***
Gestational age (weeks)	−0.018 (−0.03; −0.006)	0.004	−0.019 (−0.030; −0.008)	<0.001	−0.015 (−0.027; −0.003)	0.011
Birth weight (kg)	−0.076 (−0.127; −0.026)	0.003	*	*	*	*
Birth weight percentile	−0.002 (−0.003; 0)	0.098	-	-	-	-
ROP (yes)	0.202 (−0.001; 0.405)	0.05	-	-	0.108 (−0.102; 0.319)	0.31
ROP treatment (yes)	0.147 (−0.097; 0.390)	0.24	-	-	-	-
Placental insufficiency (yes)	−0.067 (−0.255; 0.121)	0.49	-	-	-	-
Preeclampsia (yes)	0.055 (−0.098; 0.207)	0.48	-	-	-	-
Breastfeeding (yes)	−0.087 (−0.193; 0.018)	0.10	-	-	-	-
Smoking pregnancy (yes)	−0.135 (−0.328; 0.058)	0.17	-	-	-	-
Wetting Schirmer test (mm)	**B [95% CI]**	***p***	**B [95% CI]**	***p***	**B [95% CI]**	***p***
Gestational age (weeks)	−1.067 (−1.638; −0.496)	<0.001	−0.692 (−1.158; −0.226)	0.003		
Birth weight (kg)	−4.918 (−7.330; −2.506)	0.001	*	*		
Birth weight percentile	0.048 (−0.068; 0.163)	0.41	-	-		
ROP (yes)	3.0 (−3.137; 9.137)	0.34	-	-		
ROP treatment (yes)	3.0 (−13.203; 19.203)	0.22	-	-		
Placental insufficiency (yes)	12.0 (1.259; 22.74)	0.029	8.596 (4.643; 12.55)	<0.001		
Preeclampsia (yes)	0.0 (−10.73; 10.73)	1.0	-	-		
Breastfeeding (yes)	3.0 (−2.514; 8.515)	0.29	-	-		
Smoking pregnancy (yes)	8.0 (−1.875; 17.87)	0.11	-	-		

Table 4. *Cont.*

	Univariate		Model 1		Model 2	
Nasal palpebral angle (degree)	B [95% CI]	p	B [95% CI]	p	B [95% CI]	p
Gestational age (weeks)	0.266 (0.098; 0.435)	0.002	0.220 (0.050; 0.390)	0.011	0.142 (0.039; 0.323)	0.125
Birth weight (kg)	1.159 (0.418; 1.9)	0.002	*	*	*	*
Birth weight percentile	0.019 (−0.009; 0.048)	0.19	-	-	-	-
ROP (yes)	−3.643 (−5.998; −1.288)	0.002	-	-	−2.384 (−4.986; 0.219)	0.073
ROP treatment (yes)	−5.175 (−11.934; 1.584)	0.13	-	-	-	-
Placental insufficiency (yes)	−0.555 (−4.721; 3.611)	0.79	-	-	-	-
Preeclampsia (yes)	2.31 (0.107; 4.513)	0.040	2.360 (0.177; 4.544)	0.034	2.492 (0.320; 4.664)	0.025
Breastfeeding (yes)	−0.668 (−2.098; 0.762)	0.36	-	-	-	-
Smoking pregnancy (yes)	0.622 (−2.422; 3.667)	0.69	-	-	-	-

B—Beta; CI—confidence interval; mm—millimeter. Linear regression analysis using generalized estimating equations to control for correlations between right and left eyes for normally distributed parameters. Binary logistic regression analyses were used for the parameter BUT < 20 s and quantile regression analyses for wetting of the Schirmer test (mm). Model 1 included sex (female), age (years), and univariate associated factors ≤ 0.05 but not ROP occurrence and treatment. * Birth weight (kg) was not included in this model due to the high correlation with gestational age. Model 2 included sex (female), age (years), gestational age (weeks), and univariate associated factors ≤ 0.05 and ROP occurrence and ROP treatment (if associated in univariate analyses).

4. Discussion

The present study provides new data describing the long-term effects of prematurity, ROP, and perinatal factors on ocular surface health in adults born preterm. Our study shows that prematurity correlated with an increase in bulbar redness, increased length of wetting in the Schirmer test, and a narrower nasal palpebral angle. Furthermore, ROP treatment was associated with a tear film break-up time lower than 20 s. Overall, this data indicates that adults born preterm may have altered ocular surface homeostasis.

This study provided new insights regarding the long-term effects of perinatal history on ocular surface characteristics. It is well known that preterm birth and the postnatal occurrence of ROP are linked to an altered organ morphology in childhood, adolescence, and adulthood. The Wiesbaden Prematurity Study observed that prematurity was linked with a steeper corneal curvature, while postnatal ROP occurrence and treatment were linked to a shorter anterior chamber depth [1]. In congruence, a population-based report analyzing adolescents showed an association between lower birth weight as a proxy for prematurity and steeper corneal curvature [27]. Recent reports indicate that these alterations persist throughout life, as results from the Gutenberg Health Study showed that low birth weight (<2500 g) was associated with a steeper corneal radius, smaller corneal diameter [6], and altered posterior pole [28–31]. Furthermore, other studies reported a less regular corneal surface in subjects born preterm with low birth weight, as indicated by increased corneal aberrations in childhood and adulthood [9,10]. The present results indicate that prematurity affects not only ocular geometry but also other ocular surface properties such as tear film quantity and stability.

While Raffa and colleagues [32] observed no association between the eyelid aperture in individuals born preterm and term aged 4 to 15 years, the present study found a narrower nasal palpebral angle in individuals born preterm. One may speculate that this is an unknown risk factor potentially influencing ocular refractive and geometric development in individuals born preterm, as previous reports observed that palpebral angles and lid aperture are risk factors for spherical refractive error development [33,34].

Individuals affected by dry eye diseases suffer from ocular discomfort, burning, instable tear film, and visual disturbance that can lead to inflammatory damage of the ocular surface [17]. They may also have reduced quality of life [35] and lower vision-related quality of life [36] with a prevalence up to one in three in the general population [37] with a high economic impact [38]. There are different recognized risk factors, such as environmental factors, endogenous stress, antigens, infections, genetic factors, and autoimmune disorders [16], which only partially explain the occurrence of dry eye disease, so other risk factors may be involved. Our data are the first to suggest that prematurity and associated factors may predispose to dry eye disease later in life. Dry eye disease can be classified as decreased tear secretion or increased tear evaporation. Since the preterm participants revealed significantly increased Schirmer test measures, one may speculate that preterm birth leads to tear overproduction accompanied by a less stable tear film. However, the pathophysiological mechanisms remain unclear, and it remains to be determined whether the increased tear evaporation is caused by dysfunction of the Meibomian glands or by reduced mucin from the goblet cells. Other pathophysiological mechanisms causing long-term effects on the corneal surface might be the lower extrauterine temperature after preterm birth compared to the intrauterine environment [12] and a shorter time in the intrauterine milieu, or different periods of opened eyes in the interval until reaching full GA [13]. There is evidence that dry eye disease is caused, among other reasons, by subacute inflammation and has many features in common with autoimmune disease [16]. Prematurity is linked to a hyper-responsive innate immune system [15]; thus, one may speculate that this pro-inflammatory tendency also influences the ocular surface. In addition, participants being treated for postnatal ROP revealed a shorter tear film break-up time also potentially indicating that absorbed energy during treatment leads to life-long alterations of corneal hemostasis. It is well known that prematurity is a risk factor for psychosomatic diseases, such as depression, which is also a risk factor for dry eye disease [39]. However, the clinical significance of our findings remains unclear because we observed no difference in the OSDI score between the different study groups. It is possible that the observed ocular changes are of subclinical importance and might predispose to dry eye diseases in later life.

5. Strengths and Limitations

One limitation of the present study is the single-center hospital-based study design. Furthermore, other lid parameters were not investigated, such as frequency of blinking in different environments, horizontal lid aperture, and temporal lid aperture. Invalid or missing keratograph examinations may further limit the present data. Moreover, the number of individuals with a history of ROP and ROP treatment was low, which must be considered during the data interpretation. A further limitation is the missing data about tissue status and function of the meibomian gland in the present study which should be examined in future studies.

The strengths are that this study was one of the largest cohorts of adults born preterm at different GA with and without ROP. Detailed assessment of perinatal history from medical records enabled a comprehensive data analysis of the perinatal effects on the ocular surface, with all measurements and validation steps blinded with respect to GA and other perinatal factors.

6. Conclusions

In conclusion, our analyses indicate that perinatal history affects the ocular surface later in life. Preterm birth was associated with increased bulbar redness, increased length of wetting in the Schirmer test, and a narrower palpebral angle, while ROP treatment was associated with a reduced tear film break-up time of less than 20 s, suggesting that affected persons may be predisposed to diseases of the corneal surface in later life, such as dry eye disease.

Supplementary Materials: The following supporting information can be downloaded at: https://www.mdpi.com/article/10.3390/jcm11102702/s1, Figure S1: Gutenberg Prematurity Eye Study design.

Author Contributions: Conceived and designed the study: A.F. and A.K.S. analyzed the data, A.F., C.H.-M., S.G., U.H., E.M., M.S.U. and A.K.S. wrote the paper, A.F. critically revised the manuscript, A.F., C.H.-M., S.G., U.H., E.M., M.S.U., F.Z., B.S., N.P. and A.K.S. read and approved the final manuscript. This study contains parts of the thesis of Clara Hufschmidt-Merizian. All authors have read and agreed to the published version of the manuscript.

Funding: Fieß is supported by the Intramural Research Funding (Stufe I) of the University Medical Center of Johannes Gutenberg University Mainz. The present study was supported by the Ernst- und Berta-Grimmke Stiftung and the Else Kröner-Fresenius-Stiftung. The funders had no role in the study design, data collection and analysis, decision to publish, or preparation of the manuscript. Schuster AK holds the professorship for ophthalmic healthcare research endowed by "Stiftung Auge" and financed by "Deutsche Ophthalmologische Gesellschaft" and "Berufsverband der Augenärzte Deutschlands e.V." Pfeiffer N receives financial support and grants from Novartis, Ivantis, Santen, Thea, Boehringer Ingelheim Deutschland GmbH & Co. KG, Alcon, and Sanoculis. Schuster AK receives research support from Allergan, Bayer, Heidelberg Engineering, PlusOptix and Norvartis.

Institutional Review Board Statement: The Gutenberg Prematurity Eye Study (GPES) complies with Good Clinical Practice (GCP), Good Epidemiological Practice (GEP), and the ethical principles of the Declaration of Helsinki. The study protocol and documents were approved by the local ethics committee of the Medical Chamber of Rhineland-Palatinate, Germany (reference no. 2019-14161; original vote: 29 May 2019, latest update: 2 April 2020).

Informed Consent Statement: Written informed consent was obtained from all participants before their entry into the study.

Data Availability Statement: A.F. had full access to all study data and takes responsibility for the integrity of the data and the accuracy of the data analysis. Statistical analyses were performed by A.F. The analysis presents clinical data of a cohort. This project constitutes a major scientific effort with high methodological standards and detailed guidelines for analysis and publication to ensure scientific analyses are on the highest level; therefore, data are not made available for the scientific community outside the established and controlled workflows and algorithms. To meet the general idea of verification and reproducibility of scientific findings, we offer access to data at the local database upon request at any time. Interested researchers may make their requests to the coordinating PI of the GPES (Achim Fieß; achim.fiess@unimedizin-mainz.de). More detailed contact information is available at the homepages of the UM (www.unimedizin-mainz.de).

Acknowledgments: The study team thanks all participants who took part in this study and the GPES, which involved an enthusiastic team to explore perinatal factors on long-term eye development.

Conflicts of Interest: The authors declare no conflict of interest.

Abbreviations

GA	Gestational age
GCP	Good Clinical Practice
GEE	General estimating equations
GEP	Good Epidemiological Practice
GPES	The Gutenberg Prematurity Eye Study
OSDI	Ocular Surface Disease Index
ROP	Retinopathy of prematurity
UMCM	University Medical Center of the Johannes Gutenberg University Mainz in Germany

References

1. Fieß, A.; Kolb-Keerl, R.; Knuf, M.; Kirchhof, B.; Blecha, C.; Oberacher-Velten, I.; Muether, P.S.; Bauer, J. Axial Length and Anterior Segment Alterations in Former Preterm Infants and Full-Term Neonates Analyzed With Scheimpflug Imaging. *Cornea* **2017**, *36*, 821–827. [CrossRef] [PubMed]
2. Wu, W.C.; Lin, R.I.; Shih, C.P.; Wang, N.K.; Chen, Y.P.; Chao, A.N.; Chen, K.J.; Chen, T.L.; Hwang, Y.S.; Lai, C.C.; et al. Visual acuity, optical components, and macular abnormalities in patients with a history of retinopathy of prematurity. *Ophthalmology* **2012**, *119*, 1907–1916. [CrossRef] [PubMed]
3. Fieß, A.; Christian, L.; Kolb-Keerl, R.; Knuf, M.; Kirchhof, B.; Muether, P.S.; Bauer, J. Peripapillary Choroidal Thickness in Former Preterm and Full-Term Infants Aged From 4 to 10 Years. *Investig. Ophthalmol. Vis. Sci.* **2016**, *57*, 6548–6553. [CrossRef] [PubMed]
4. Fieß, A.; Christian, L.; Janz, J.; Kolb-Keerl, R.; Knuf, M.; Kirchhof, B.; Muether, P.S.; Bauer, J. Functional analysis and associated factors of the peripapillary retinal nerve fibre layer in former preterm and full-term infants. *Br. J. Ophthalmol.* **2017**, *101*, 1405–1411. [CrossRef] [PubMed]

5. Fieß, A.; Janz, J.; Schuster, A.K.; Kolb-Keerl, R.; Knuf, M.; Kirchhof, B.; Muether, P.S.; Bauer, J. Macular morphology in former preterm and full-term infants aged 4 to 10 years. *Graefe's Arch. Clin. Exp. Ophthalmol. Albrecht Graefes Arch. Klin. Exp. Ophthalmol.* **2017**, *255*, 1433–1442. [CrossRef] [PubMed]
6. Fieß, A.; Schuster, A.K.; Nickels, S.; Urschitz, M.S.; Elflein, H.M.; Schulz, A.; Munzel, T.; Wild, P.S.; Beutel, M.E.; Schmidtmann, I.; et al. Association of Low Birth Weight With Altered Corneal Geometry and Axial Length in Adulthood in the German Gutenberg Health Study. *JAMA Ophthalmol.* **2019**, *137*, 507–514. [CrossRef]
7. Darlow, B.A.; Gilbert, C. Retinopathy of prematurity—A world update. *Semin. Perinatol.* **2019**, *43*, 315–316. [CrossRef]
8. Hartnett, M.E.; Penn, J.S. Mechanisms and management of retinopathy of prematurity. *N. Engl. J. Med.* **2012**, *367*, 2515–2526. [CrossRef]
9. Fieß, A.; Schuster, A.K.; Kolb-Keerl, R.; Knuf, M.; Kirchhof, B.; Muether, P.S.; Bauer, J. Corneal Aberrations in Former Preterm Infants: Results From The Wiesbaden Prematurity Study. *Investig. Ophthalmol. Vis. Sci.* **2017**, *58*, 6374–6378. [CrossRef]
10. Fieß, A.; Uschitz, M.; Nagler, M.; Mickels, S. Association of birth weight with corneal aberrations in adulthood—Results from a population-based study. *J. Optom.* **2021**.
11. Howson, C.P.; Kinney, M.V.; Lawn, J.E. Born Too Soon: The Global Action Report on Preterm Birth. March of Dimes, PMNCH, Save the Children, World Health Organization. Geneva. 2012. Available online: https://assets.publishing.service.gov.uk/media/57a08a76e5274a27b20005e3/201204_borntoosoon-report.pdf (accessed on 8 February 2019).
12. Fielder, A.R.; Levene, M.I.; Russell-Eggitt, I.M.; Weale, R.A. Temperature—A factor in ocular development? *Dev. Med. Child Neurol.* **1986**, *28*, 279–284. [CrossRef] [PubMed]
13. Fieß, A.; Urschitz, M.S.; Marx-Groß, S.; Nagler, M.; Wild, P.S.; Münzel, T.; Beutel, M.E.; Lackner, K.J.; Pfeiffer, N.; Schuster, A.K. Association of Birth Weight with Central and Peripheral Corneal Thickness in Adulthood-Results from the Population-Based German Gutenberg Health Study. *Children* **2021**, *8*, 1006. [CrossRef] [PubMed]
14. Barker, D.J. The developmental origins of adult disease. *J. Am. Coll. Nutr.* **2004**, *23*, 588s–595s. [CrossRef] [PubMed]
15. Pellanda, L.C.; Duncan, B.B.; Vigo, A.; Rose, K.; Folsom, A.R.; Erlinger, T.P. Low birth weight and markers of inflammation and endothelial activation in adulthood: The ARIC study. *Int. J. Cardiol.* **2009**, *134*, 371–377. [CrossRef]
16. Stern, M.E.; Schaumburg, C.S.; Pflugfelder, S.C. Dry eye as a mucosal autoimmune disease. *Int. Rev. Immunol.* **2013**, *32*, 19–41. [CrossRef]
17. The definition and classification of dry eye disease: *Report of the Definition and Classification Subcommittee of the International Dry Eye WorkShop (2007)*. *Ocul. Surf.* **2007**, *5*, 75–92. [CrossRef]
18. Chia, E.M.; Mitchell, P.; Rochtchina, E.; Lee, A.J.; Maroun, R.; Wang, J.J. Prevalence and associations of dry eye syndrome in an older population: The Blue Mountains Eye Study. *Clin. Exp. Ophthalmol.* **2003**, *31*, 229–232. [CrossRef]
19. Stapleton, F.; Alves, M.; Bunya, V.Y.; Jalbert, I.; Lekhanont, K.; Malet, F.; Na, K.S.; Schaumberg, D.; Uchino, M.; Vehof, J.; et al. TFOS DEWS II Epidemiology Report. *Ocul. Surf.* **2017**, *15*, 334–365. [CrossRef]
20. Fieß, A.; Gißler, S.; Mildenberger, E.; Urschitz, M.S.; Zepp, F.; Hoffmann, E.M.; Brockmann, M.A.; Stoffelns, B.; Pfeiffer, N.; Schuster, A.K. Optic nerve head morphology in adults born extreme, very and moderate preterm with and without retinopathy of prematurity: Results from the Gutenberg Prematurity Eye Study. *Am. J. Ophthalmol.* **2022**. [CrossRef]
21. Fieß, A.; Gißler, S.; Mildenberger, E.; Urschitz, M.S.; Fauer, A.; Elflein, H.M.; Zepp, F.; Stoffelns, B.; Pfeiffer, N.; Schuster, A.K. Anterior Chamber Angle in Adults Born Extremely, Very, and Moderately Preterm with and without Retinopathy of Prematurity-Results of the Gutenberg Prematurity Eye Study. *Children* **2022**, *9*, 281. [CrossRef]
22. Fieß, A.; Nauen, H.; Mildenberger, E.; Zepp, F.; Urschitz, M.S.; Pfeiffer, N.; Schuster, A.K.-G. Ocular geometry in adults born extremely, very and moderately preterm with and without retinopathy of prematurity: Results from the Gutenberg Prematurity Eye Study. *Br. J. Ophthalmol.* **2022**. [CrossRef] [PubMed]
23. Fieß, A.; Fauer, A.; Mildenberger, E.; Urschitz, M.S.; Elflein, H.M.; Zepp, F.; Stoffelns, B.; Pfeiffer, N.; Schuster, A.K. Refractive error, accommodation and lens opacification in adults born preterm and full-term: Results from the Gutenberg Prematurity Eye Study (GPES). *Acta Ophthalmol.* **2022**. [CrossRef] [PubMed]
24. Fieß, A.; Gißler, S.; Fauer, A.; Riedl, J.C.; Mildenberger, E.; Urschitz, M.S.; Zepp, F.; Stoffelns, B.; Pfeiffer, N.; Schuster, A.K. Short report on retinal vessel metrics and arterial blood pressure in adult individuals born preterm with and without retinopathy of prematurity: Results from the Gutenberg Prematurity Eye Study. *Acta Ophthalmol.* **2022**. [CrossRef] [PubMed]
25. Voigt, M.; Fusch, C.; Olbertz, D. Analyse des Neugeborenenkollektivs der Bundesrepublik Deutschland 12. Mitteilung: Vorstellung engmaschiger Perzentilwerte (-kurven) für die Körpermaße Neugeborener. *Geburtsh Frauenheilk* **2006**, *66*, 956–970. [CrossRef]
26. Schiffman, R.M.; Christianson, M.D.; Jacobsen, G.; Hirsch, J.D.; Reis, B.L. Reliability and validity of the Ocular Surface Disease Index. *Arch. Ophthalmol.* **2000**, *118*, 615–621. [CrossRef]
27. Fieß, A.; Schuster, A.K.; Pfeiffer, N.; Nickels, S. Association of birth weight with corneal power in early adolescence: Results from the National Health and Nutrition Examination Survey (NHANES) 1999–2008. *PLoS ONE* **2017**, *12*, e0186723. [CrossRef]
28. Fieß, A.; Nickels, S.; Urschitz, M.S.; Münzel, T.; Wild, P.S.; Beutel, M.E.; Lackner, K.J.; Hoffmann, E.M.; Pfeiffer, N.; Schuster, A.K. Association of Birth Weight with Peripapillary Retinal Nerve Fiber Layer Thickness in Adulthood—Results from a Population-Based Study. *Investig. Ophthalmol. Vis. Sci.* **2020**, *61*, 4. [CrossRef]
29. Fieß, A.; Ponto, K.A.; Urschitz, M.S.; Nickels, S.; Schulz, A.; Münzel, T.; Wild, P.S.; Beutel, M.E.; Lackner, K.J.; Pfeiffer, N.; et al. Birthweight and its association with retinal vessel equivalents—Results from the population-based German Gutenberg Health Study. *Acta Ophthalmol.* **2020**, *99*, e773–e774. [CrossRef]

30. Fieß, A.; Stingl, J.; Urschitz, M.S.; Hoffmann, E.M.; Münzel, T.; Wild, P.S.; Beutel, M.E.; Lackner, K.J.; Pfeiffer, N.; Schuster, A.K. Birth weight and its association with optic nerve head morphology—Results from the population-based German Gutenberg Health Study. *Acta Ophthalmol.* **2021**.
31. Fieß, A.; Wagner, F.M.; Urschitz, M.S.; Nagler, M.; Stoffelns, B.; Wild, P.S.; Münzel, T.; Beutel, M.E.; Lackner, K.J.; Pfeiffer, N.; et al. Association of Birth Weight With Foveolar Thickness in Adulthood: Results From a Population-Based Study. *Investig. Ophthalmol. Vis. Sci.* **2021**, *62*, 9. [CrossRef]
32. Raffa, L.H.; Hellstrom, A.; Aring, E.; Andersson, S.; Gronlund, M.A. Ocular dimensions in relation to auxological data in a sample of Swedish children aged 4–15 years. *Acta Ophthalmol.* **2014**, *92*, 682–688. [CrossRef]
33. Grey, C.; Yap, M. Influence of lid position on astigmatism. *Am. J. Optom. Physiol. Opt.* **1986**, *63*, 966–969. [CrossRef] [PubMed]
34. Read, S.A.; Collins, M.J.; Carney, L.G. The influence of eyelid morphology on normal corneal shape. *Investig. Ophthalmol. Vis. Sci.* **2007**, *48*, 112–119. [CrossRef] [PubMed]
35. Rajagopalan, K.; Abetz, L.; Mertzanis, P.; Espindle, D.; Begley, C.; Chalmers, R.; Caffery, B.; Snyder, C.; Nelson, J.D.; Simpson, T.; et al. Comparing the discriminative validity of two generic and one disease-specific health-related quality of life measures in a sample of patients with dry eye. *Value Health J. Int. Soc. Pharm. Outcomes Res.* **2005**, *8*, 168–174. [CrossRef] [PubMed]
36. Li, M.; Gong, L.; Chapin, W.J.; Zhu, M. Assessment of vision-related quality of life in dry eye patients. *Investig. Ophthalmol. Vis. Sci.* **2012**, *53*, 5722–5727. [CrossRef] [PubMed]
37. Tian, Y.J.; Liu, Y.; Zou, H.D.; Jiang, Y.J.; Liang, X.Q.; Sheng, M.J.; Li, B.; Xu, X. Epidemiologic study of dry eye in populations equal or over 20 years old in Jiangning District of Shanghai. *[Zhonghua Yan Ke Za Zhi] Chin. J. Ophthalmol.* **2009**, *45*, 486–491.
38. Bielory, L.; Syed, B.A. Pharmacoeconomics of anterior ocular inflammatory disease. *Curr. Opin. Allergy Clin. Immunol.* **2013**, *13*, 537–542. [CrossRef]
39. Upadhyaya, S.; Sourander, A.; Luntamo, T.; Matinolli, H.M.; Chudal, R.; Hinkka-Yli-Salomäki, S.; Filatova, S.; Cheslack-Postava, K.; Sucksdorff, M.; Gissler, M.; et al. Preterm Birth Is Associated With Depression From Childhood to Early Adulthood. *J. Am. Acad. Child Adolesc. Psychiatry* **2021**, *60*, 1127–1136. [CrossRef]

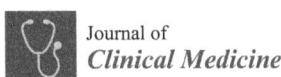

Review

New Perspectives in the Pathophysiology and Treatment of Pain in Patients with Dry Eye Disease

Giuseppe Giannaccare [1,*,†], Carla Ghelardini [2,†], Alessandra Mancini [1], Vincenzo Scorcia [1] and Lorenzo Di Cesare Mannelli [2]

1. Department of Ophthalmology, University Magna Graecia of Catanzaro, 88100 Catanzaro, Italy; alessandra.mancini@studenti.unicz.it (A.M.); vscorcia@unicz.it (V.S.)
2. Department of Neuroscience, Psychology, Drug Research and Child Health–NEUROFARBA–Pharmacology and Toxicology Section, University of Florence, 50139 Florence, Italy; carla.ghelardini@unifi.it (C.G.); lorenzo.mannelli@unifi.it (L.D.C.M.)
* Correspondence: giuseppe.giannaccare@unicz.it
† These authors contributed equally to this work.

Abstract: Ocular discomfort and eye pain are frequently reported by patients with dry eye disease (DED), and their management remains a real therapeutic challenge for the Ophthalmologist. In DED patients, injury at the level of each structure of the ocular surface can determine variable symptoms, ranging from mild ocular discomfort up to an intolerable pain evoked by innocuous stimuli. In refractory cases, the persistence of this harmful signal is able to evoke a mechanism of maladaptive plasticity of the nervous system that leads to increased pain responsiveness. Peripheral and, subsequently, central sensitization cause nociceptor hyperexcitability and persistent pain perception that can culminate in the paradoxical situation of perceiving eye pain even in the absence of ocular surface abnormalities. Effective therapeutic strategies of these cases are challenging, and new options are desirable. Recently, a theoretical novel therapeutic approach concerns enkephalins thanks to the evidence that eye pain sensations are modulated by endogenous opioid peptides (enkephalins, endorphins and dynorphins). In this regard, new topical agents open up a new theoretical scenario in the treatment of ocular discomfort and eye pain in the setting of DED, such as, for example, a multimolecular complex based on proteins and glycosaminoglycans also containing opiorphin that may assist the physiological pain-relieving mechanism of the eye.

Keywords: dry eye disease; pain; neuropathic pain; opiorphin; glicopro

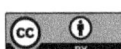

1. Introduction

Dry eye disease (DED) is a multifactorial condition occurring due to reduced tear production (hyposecretive DED), excessive tear evaporation (evaporative DED) or both (mixed DED). This disorder is characterized by a loss of homeostasis of the tear film in which instability and hyperosmolarity of the tear film itself, inflammation, as well as neurosensory abnormalities play an important role in the development and the maintenance of the disease [1]. DED is characterized by symptoms such as burning, photophobia, blurred vision, and eye discomfort or pain; it is divided into primary or secondary DED, depending on whether it is present in an isolated form or in association with other diseases, mostly autoimmune, such as systemic lupus erythematosus, rheumatoid arthritis, scleroderma, or Sjögren's syndrome [2]. The pathophysiological mechanism that determines the onset of DED is a change in the quantity and/or composition of tears, which become richer in solutes (tear hyperosmolarity) due to reduced production of the aqueous component secreted by the main lacrimal gland, or its excessive evaporation. The increase in osmolarity, in turn, causes damage to the epithelial cells of the conjunctiva and cornea, as well as to the goblet cells that produce the normal mucous component of tears, and induces an inflammatory reaction at the level of the entire ocular surface [3]. These alterations trigger a vicious circle that aggravates the condition of DED, and determines the chronicization of the process, with damage of the nerve fibers that conduct the stimuli to the main lacrimal gland for the production of the tear film [3]. Recently, the non-invasive imaging of corneal nerves has become possible thanks to the introduction of in vivo confocal microscopy that revealed profound alterations in patients with DED compared to control subjects (Figure 1) [4,5].

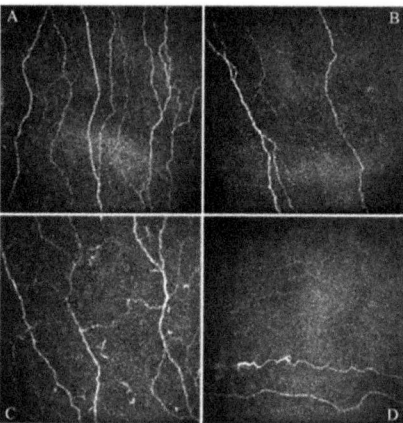

Figure 1. In vivo confocal microscopy scans of the corneal sub-basal nerve plexus obtained in a healthy patient (**A**) and in different patients affected by dry eye disease (**B–D**). All images are in the scale of 400 × 400 µm. Part (**A**) shows a normal nerve plexus, part (**B**) shows a nerve plexus with reduced density, part (**C**) shows a nerve plexus with increased tortuosity, part (**D**) shows an altered nerve plexus characterized by the presence of neuroma.

In the context of DED, it is of particular importance not only to improve the clinical signs of the disease (e.g., corneal epithelial damage) but also to control symptoms that, in some cases, represent a very invalidating complication for the patient. In fact, a study on health-related quality of life (HR-QoL) of patients with DED has shown that severe forms of the disease affect HR-QoL in a manner comparable to hospital dialysis and severe forms of angina [6]. Furthermore, a more recent study stated that worse mental HR-QoL is present in severe DED patients not having received a clear diagnosis [7].

The management of DED symptoms still remains a great unmet therapeutic need in Ophthalmology and new advances in this field are desirable. The recent advent of a new lubricating ophthalmic solution containing GlicoPro® (Lacricomplex®, FB Vision Spa, Ascoli Piceno, Italy) opens up a new theoretical scenario in the treatment of ocular discomfort and eye pain occurring in the setting of DED. GlicoPro® is a multimolecular complex extracted from Helix aspersa snail mucus and based on proteins and sulfured and unsulfured glycosaminoglycans (GAGs), which is carried by a mucin base consisting of hydroxypropyl methylcellulose. GAGs have been shown to be essential for maintaining corneal homeostasis, epithelial cell differentiation, and wound healing. In addition, more recently, a role has been suggested for the extracellular matrix in regulating limbal stem cells, corneal innervation, corneal inflammation, and corneal angiogenesis and lymphangiogenesis. The simple GAGs confer to the GlicoPro® solution a lubricating, moisturizing, antioxidant, and protective action, by reintegrating the mucinic component of the tear film [8]. Sulfur GAGs are thiomers that form covalent bonds (disulfide bridges) with the cysteine residues of mucin. This property makes the GlicoPro® solution highly mucoadhesive and capable of forming the glycocalyx structure in a prolonged manner [9]. Therefore, GlicoPro® has a triple mucomimetic component important for the lubrication of the ocular surface, the stabilization of the tear film, and the prolonged pre-corneal stay. In the protein kit of GlicoPro® there is opiorphin, which assists the physiological pain-relieving mechanism of the eye.

The aim of this review is to summarize the emerging role of opiorphin in the control of ocular discomfort and eye pain.

2. Ocular Discomfort and Eye Pain

Symptoms of ocular discomfort or eye pain referred by patients with DED are sustained by various phenomena, such as ocular surface epithelial damage, inflammation, and neurosensory abnormalities. The consequence is the presence of variable symptoms for each single patient, ranging from a mild sensation of ocular discomfort (often reported by the patient as a "foreign body sensation") to an intolerable pain evoked by innocuous stimuli under normal conditions (allodynia following light, wind, etc.) [10]. The procrastination of this harmful signal is able to evoke a mechanism of maladaptive plasticity of the nervous system that leads to increased pain responsiveness. Peripheral and, subsequently, central sensitization cause nociceptor hyperexcitability and persistent pain perception that can culminate in the paradoxical situation of eye pain, even in the absence of frank ocular surface abnormalities [11,12].

The rupture of the tear film during the blink interval, the hyperosmolarity of the tears, the rubbing between the eyelid and the ocular globe in the presence of decreased tear volume or reduced expression of mucins on the ocular surface, as well as the presence of inflammatory mediators participate in the activation of corneal sensitive fibers capable of triggering nociceptive mechanisms. In fact, the cornea is among the most densely innervated tissues of the body, possessing exclusively C and Ad fibers, comprising mechanonociceptors, polymodal nociceptors (activated by mechanical, chemical, and thermal stimuli), and nociceptors activated by cold stimuli that carry the information to the respective cell bodies located in the trigeminal ganglion projecting to the brainstem nuclei [13,14]. Corneal neurosensory alterations play a fundamental role in both the development and the maintenance of DED. From the initial inflammatory phase, it is possible to evolve toward a neurogenic inflammation that is the basis of real nerve damage with a reduction in the density and branching of nerve fibers up to the formation of neuromas [15]. These phenomena can lead to the onset of a neuropathic type of pain, different in clinical manifestations, amplified in intensity, and persistent over time. The dynamic response of the altered nervous tissue evokes mechanisms of peripheral and central sensitization with increased electrical activity of neurons, excitatory dysregulation of the neurotransmitter milieu, and activation of glial cells that actively participate in synaptic signaling. Neuroplasticity makes this pain central (although originating in the periphery), coupled with a disinhibition of descending pathways, resulting in the loss of the mechanisms that physiologically underlie pain reduction [16]. As the neuropathic component increases, the description of hot, burning, stinging, or granular eye sensation increases as well. Failure of common treatments used for DED is a further indicator of the neuropathic component; patients with little or no relief after the use of conventional treatment based on tear substitutes are often the same ones who report high levels of burning, pain, and wind sensitivity, as well as a decreased threshold for systemic pain [17]. Therapeutic strategies of this challenging condition include: (i) intense lubrication of the ocular surface with tear substitutes in order to, among others, decrease the hyperosmolarity of tears and the consequent stimulation of corneal nociceptors [18]; (ii) contact lens bandaging; (iii) anti-inflammatory agents, such as corticosteroids or immunomodulators, such as cyclosporine or lifitegrast, that can reduce inflammation and increase tear stability; (iv) serum and platelet derivatives, which are rich in growth factors and can promote epithelial wound healing and nerve regeneration [19,20]; and (v) analgesics or anti-neuropathic drugs, such as antiepileptics or antidepressants, for systemic use [17]. This type of persistent pain cannot be controlled by chronically using topical anesthetics because, as reported by Harnish et al., these drugs induce damage to corneal cell metabolism with rarefaction of microvilli and increased cytoplasmic degeneration [21].

Recently, a possible novel therapeutic approach to eye pain concerns enkephalins thanks to the evidence that this symptom is modulated by endogenous opioid peptides (enkephalins, endorphins, and dynorphins) through binding to mu, delta, and kappa opioid receptors widely distributed in the nervous system [22]. The endogenous peptides Met- and Leu-enkephalin, released in the presence of an insult or due to the presence of an inflammatory state by the ocular and corneal nerves, as well as by immune cells (lymphocytes, dendritic cells, and monocytes) recruited at the inflamed site, bind to both mu and delta opioid receptors expressed at the level of the eye [22]. However, enkephalins evoke short-lived local analgesic effects due to their rapid degradation by the concomitant action of two enzymes: neprilysin neutral endopeptidase (NEP) and aminopeptidase N (APN) [23]. On the basis of these aspects, just to overcome the fact that the analgesic action induced by enkephalins is transient, it has been proposed to enhance the effect using compounds that can inhibit the degradation by blocking both enzymes involved (Figure 2).

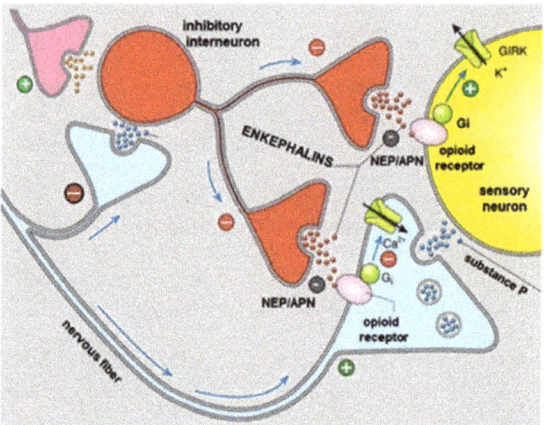

Figure 2. Enkephalin signaling in the pain pathway. Enkephalins are released by inhibitory interneurons activated as a result of the balance between positive (anti-nociceptive) and negative (pain) inputs. Enkephalins are able to activate opioid receptors evoking analgesic signaling; their efficacy is limited by the catabolic enzymes NEP and APN. GIRK = G protein-coupled inwardly rectifying potassium, NEP = neutral endopeptidase, APN = Aminopeptidase N, Gi = Gi protein. Modified from an image available on: www.slideplayer.it. (Accessed on 23 July 2021).

Reaux-Le Goazigo et al. reported that topical administration of the compound PL265 (a dual inhibitor of the enkephalin-degrading enzymes NEP and APN) appeared to be significantly effective in mouse models of corneal pain [23]. Repeated instillations of this product significantly reduced mechanical and chemical hypersensitivity of the cornea with an action completely antagonized by the opioid antagonist naloxone, highlighting that it was mediated by peripheral corneal opioid receptors. In addition, flow cytometry (quantification of CD11b1 cells) and confocal microscopy analysis revealed that PL265 instillations significantly reduced the active inflammatory process in a model of corneal inflammatory pain by decreasing macrophage infiltrate and expression of the neuronal injury marker ATF3 (Activating Transcription Factor 3) in the ipsilateral trigeminal ganglion. These results, therefore, suggest that the activation of opioid receptors in the eye, through the strategy of raising the concentration of endogenous enkephalins by inhibiting their physiological degradation, could be an effective approach to reduce not only the hyper-nociceptive responses observed in the setting of DED but also the ones following toxic, traumatic, and inflammatory corneal injuries. Molecular and histological studies conducted at the corneal level after repeated instillations of PL265 in a healthy eye have shown that the compound has no detrimental effects on corneal integrity [23]. Furthermore, a recent study suggested that Leu-enkephalin (derived from the same precursor as pro-enkephalin, Met-enkephalin, and prodynorphin) is also able to promote corneal wound repair through the regulation of matrix metalloproteases (MMP-2 and MMP-9) [24]. Finally, regarding the studies about the role of APN/LTA4 (Leukotriene A4) hydrolases (LTA4H) aminopeptidases in extracellular matrix degradation 13, it has been reported that the inhibition of APN/LTA4H activity could prevent the action of extracellular matrix proteases (such as heparanase and MMP-9), thereby slowing down the extracellular matrix degradation process [25]. The prediction of the usefulness of enkephalinase degradation blockers as a new class of topical analgesics, devoid of the side effects of exogenous opioids, is based on the assumption that they merely increase the extracellular physiological concentrations of enkephalins released following stimulus-evoked depolarization. Unlike exogenous opioids that directly stimulate all available opioid receptors, enkephalinase inhibitors act specifically where endogenous enkephalins are released in response to stimulus. On this basis, ocular pain relief by selectively increasing local enkephalin concentrations is likely to be safer than using exogenous opioids in the presence of significant efficacy. A further advantage derives from the absence of an anesthetic effect which, on the contrary, could be harmful for various reasons. On the one hand, corneal anesthesia could conceal the patient's symptoms in the event of any corneal complications (e.g., erosions, ulcers, etc.), which, although rare, can complicate the course of DED [26]. Moreover, a reduction in corneal sensitivity has already been described in the majority of patients with DED compared to healthy patients of the same age [27]. On the other hand, topical anesthetics, when administered to patients with DED, and the consequent disruption of the corneal epithelium, can lead to an obstacle to the repair of the epithelial defect, alteration of lacrimation, increased corneal permeability with edema and opacification, and, finally, alteration of the elements of the cytoskeleton of the corneal epithelium with alteration of cell motility [28]. These phenomena can lead to chronicity of the corneal epithelial defect and stromal colliquation (melting) up to corneal perforation in the most severe cases [29].

3. Opiorphin

Human opiorphin is an endogenous pentapeptide with modulatory capabilities of opioid signaling pathways. It has been identified in human saliva and has potent analgesic properties due to its ability to enhance endogenous opioid signaling by protecting enkephalins from degradation by human NEP and APN [30–32]. The opiorphin molecule does not cross the blood–brain barrier due to its intrinsic ability to form bonds with plasma proteins, degree of ionization, and lipid/water partition coefficient. Opiorphin is present in blood, urine, and other body fluids, but because the PROL1 gene, which codes for the opiorphin precursor, is found primarily in human lacrimal and salivary glands, the amount of opiorphin in tears and saliva is higher compared to that one present in other body fluids. Opiorphin is synthesized more in pathological conditions with pain symptomatology [30–32]. Salaric et al. reported an increase in salivary opiorphin in patients with burning mouth syndrome [33], while, more recently, Ozdogan et al. described an increase in salivary opiorphin in patients with dental pain caused by pulp inflammation [34]. Opiorphin levels were reported to be increased in the tears of patients with ocular pain caused by a corneal foreign body [35]. This suggests that opiorphin may play a role in the modulation of orofacial and eye pain [8,35]. Opiorphin reduces pain caused by different origins in a manner comparable, if not greater, to morphine in terms of both efficacy and potency [30,36]. Opiorphin exhibits anti-nociceptive effects toward pain induced by thermal stimuli with an opioid receptor-dependent mechanism, and thus the action is lost in the presence of the antagonist naloxone [36–38]. In addition, its antihyperalgesic efficacy has been demonstrated in models of alteration of the pain threshold even with neuropathic components, such as following treatment with the neurotoxic substance formalin. Moreover, in this case, the effect of opiorphin is mediated by opioid receptors since the raising of the threshold is antagonized by naloxone [38]. The same authors demonstrated that the effect is selectively µ-receptor dependent as it is blocked by the µ-selective antagonist CTAP, while it is not modified by the K-selective receptor antagonist nor by the δ-selective antagonist naltrindole [38]. Opiorphin has a lower ability to induce constipation, tolerance, and dependence compared to the direct opioid agonist morphine [37,38]. Evidence suggests that after 7 days of treatment, the analgesic effect of opiorphin exceeds the one induced by morphine (at a similar dose), offering a demonstration of the progressive loss of efficacy of the latter and, on the contrary, the maintenance of the effect over time of the former [38]. The greater balance between analgesia and side effects guaranteed by opiorphin is undoubtedly due to its ability to activate opioid pathways by inhibiting the destruction of endogenous enkephalins released in response to a painful stimulus [30,38]. This action has been confirmed by preclinical experiments that reported the achievement of a roof effect (a concentration reached beyond which the effectiveness does not change) [37], highlighting how the action of opiorphin depends on the concentration of enkephalins released following a painful stimulus rather than a direct receptor action independent of physiological regulation and, therefore, easily encroaching on adverse effects [23]. Several studies have shown that other dual NEP and APN enkephalinase inhibitors, such as kelatorphan and thiorphan [39], also induce potent dose-dependent pain suppression in various animal models of pain. However, none of them have been able to produce analgesic effects comparable to those of opiorphin, a greater effectiveness explained by a higher inhibitory capacity of the catabolism of enkephalins [30]. These effects allow a physiological modulation of opioid receptors compared to direct agonists, reducing their side effects (such as respiratory depression, sedation, constipation, physical and psychic dependence, and tolerance). Subchronic treatments with opiorphin do not induce a significant predisposition to abuse, and no dependence phenomena or anti-peristaltic effects have been observed [40]. These aspects represent a crucial aspect as DED has a chronic course characterized by acute episodes of worsening of the symptoms ("poussé") alternating with periods of partial control, so its treatment is necessarily of long duration.

4. Conclusions

DED is a common ocular condition whose symptoms may range from ocular discomfort up to eye pain. To date, the management of chronic ocular pain remains a real therapeutic challenge in Ophthalmology as no specific treatments are effective. GlicoPro® may open up a new theoretical scenario in the treatment of ocular discomfort and eye pain occurring in the setting of DED thanks to its ability to activate opioid pathways by inhibiting the destruction of endogenous enkephalins released in response to a painful stimulus. A recent study has demonstrated the in vitro anti-inflammatory action, the optimal mucoadhesive and regenerative properties, as well as the potential analgesic role of this ocular formulation [41].

However, it should be pointed out that, although the theoretical therapeutic effects in the management of eye pain owing to DED have been described in this paper, in vivo studies on humans are still ongoing and positive results are required in order to support the role of GlicoPro® in the armamentarium of DED therapies.

Author Contributions: Conceptualization, G.G., C.G., L.D.C.M.; methodology, G.G., C.G., A.M., L.D.C.M.; validation, G.G., C.G., A.M., V.S., L.D.C.M.; writing—original draft preparation, G.G., C.G., L.D.C.M.; writing—review and editing, G.G., C.G., V.S., L.D.C.M.; funding acquisition, G.G., C.G., V.S., L.D.C.M. All authors have read and agreed to the published version of the manuscript.

Funding: This research received no external funding.

Institutional Review Board Statement: Not applicable.

Informed Consent Statement: The data presented in this study are available on request from the corresponding author.

Conflicts of Interest: The authors declare no conflict of interest.

References

1. Craig, J.P.; Nichols, K.K.; Akpek, E.K.; Caffery, B.; Dua, H.S.; Joo, C.-K.; Liu, Z.; Nelson, J.; Nichols, J.J.; Tsubota, K.; et al. TFOS DEWS II Definition and Classification Report. *Ocul. Surf.* **2017**, *15*, 276–283. [CrossRef] [PubMed]

2. Versura, P.; Giannaccare, G.; Vukatana, G.; Mulè, R.; Malavolta, N.; Campos, E.C. Predictive role of tear protein expression in the early diagnosis of Sjögren's syndrome. *Ann. Clin. Biochem. Int. J. Lab. Med.* **2018**, *55*, 561–570. [CrossRef] [PubMed]
3. Zhang, X.; Qu, Y.; He, X.; Ou, S.; Bu, J.; Jia, C.; Wang, J.; Wu, H.; Liu, Z.; Li, W. Dry Eye Management: Targeting the Ocular Surface Microenvironment. *Int. J. Mol. Sci.* **2017**, *18*, 1398. [CrossRef] [PubMed]
4. Giannaccare, G.; Pellegrini, M.; Sebastiani, S.; Moscardelli, F.; Versura, P.; Campos, E.C. In vivo confocal microscopy morphometric analysis of corneal subbasal nerve plexus in dry eye disease using newly developed fully automated system. *Graefes Arch. Clin. Exp. Ophthalmol.* **2019**, *257*, 583–589. [CrossRef]
5. Giannaccare, G.; Pellegrini, M.; Bernabei, F.; Moscardelli, F.; Buzzi, M.; Versura, P.; Campos, E.C. In Vivo Confocal Microscopy Automated Morphometric Analysis of Corneal Subbasal Nerve Plexus in Patients with Dry Eye Treated With Different Sources of Homologous Serum Eye Drops. *Cornea* **2019**, *38*, 1412–1417. [CrossRef] [PubMed]
6. Buchholz, P.; Steeds, C.S.; Stern, L.S.; Wiederkehr, D.P.; Doyle, J.J.; Katz, L.M.; Figueiredo, F.C. Utility assessment to measure the impact of dry eye disease. *Ocul. Surf.* **2006**, *4*, 155–161. [CrossRef]
7. Morthen, M.K.; Magno, M.S.; Utheim, T.P.; Snieder, H.; Hammond, C.J.; Vehof, J. The physical and mental burden of dry eye dis-ease: A large population-based study investigating the relationship with health-related quality of life and its determinants. *Ocul. Surf.* **2021**, *21*, 107–117. [CrossRef] [PubMed]
8. Dufour, E.; Villard-Saussine, S.; Mellon, V.; Leandri, R.; Jouannet, P.; Ungeheuer, M.N.; Rougeot, C. Opiorphin secretion pattern in healthy volunteers: Gender difference and organ specificity. *Biochem. Anal. Biochem.* **2013**, *2*, 2–11.
9. Puri, S.; Coulson-Thomas, Y.M.; Gesteira, T.F.; Coulson-Thomas, V.J. Distribution and function of glycosaminoglycans and proteoglycans in the development, homeostasis and pathology of the ocular surface. *Front. Cell Dev. Biol.* **2020**, *8*, 731. [CrossRef] [PubMed]
10. Spierer, O.; Felix, E.; McClellan, A.L.; Parel, J.M.; Gonzalez, A.; Feuer, W.J.; Sarantopoulos, C.D.; Levitt, R.C.; Ehrmann, K.; Galor, A. Corneal Mechanical Thresholds Negatively Associate with Dry Eye and Ocular Pain Symptoms. *Investig. Opthalmol. Vis. Sci.* **2016**, *57*, 617–625. [CrossRef]
11. Levitt, A.E.; Galor, A.; Weiss, J.S.; Felix, E.R.; Martin, E.R.; Patin, D.J.; Sarantopoulos, K.D.; Levitt, R.C. Chronic Dry Eye Symptoms after LASIK: Parallels and Lessons to be Learned from other Persistent Post-Operative Pain Disorders. *Mol. Pain* **2015**, *11*, 21. [CrossRef]
12. Rosenthal, P.; Baran, I.; Jacobs, D.S. Corneal pain without stain: Is it real? *Ocul. Surf.* **2009**, *7*, 28–40. [CrossRef]
13. Mc Monnies, C.W. The potential role of neuropathic mechanisms in dry eye syndromes. *J. Optom.* **2017**, *10*, 5–13. [CrossRef] [PubMed]
14. Guerrero-Moreno, A.; Baudouin, C.; Parsadaniantz, S.M.; Goazigo, A.R.-L. Morphological and Functional Changes of Corneal Nerves and Their Contribution to Peripheral and Central Sensory Abnormalities. *Front. Cell. Neurosci.* **2020**, *14*, 436. [CrossRef] [PubMed]
15. Tsubota, K.; Pflugfelder, S.C.; Liu, Z.; Baudouin, C.; Kim, H.M.; Messmer, E.M.; Kruse, F.; Liang, L.; Carreno-Galeano, J.T.; Rolando, M.; et al. Defining Dry Eye from a Clinical Perspective. *Int. J. Mol. Sci.* **2020**, *21*, 9271. [CrossRef]
16. Dieckmann, G.; Borsook, D.; Moulton, E. Neuropathic corneal pain and dry eye: A continuum of nociception. *Br. J. Ophthalmol.* **2021**. [CrossRef]
17. Moshirfar, M.; Benstead, E.E.; Sorrentino, P.M.; Tripathy, K. *StatPearls*; StatPearls Publishing: Treasure Island, FL, USA, 2021.
18. Aragona, P.; Giannaccare, G.; Mencucci, R.; Rubino, P.; Cantera, E.; Rolando, M. Modern approach to the treatment of dry eye, a complex multifactorial disease: A P.I.C.A.S.S.O. board review. *Br. J. Ophthalmol.* **2020**, *105*, 446–453. [CrossRef]
19. Giannaccare, G.; Versura, P.; Buzzi, M.; Primavera, L.; Pellegrini, M.; Campos, E.C. Blood derived eye drops for the treatment of cornea and ocular surface diseases. *Transfus. Apher. Sci.* **2017**, *56*, 595–604. [CrossRef]
20. Bernabei, F.; Roda, M.; Buzzi, M.; Pellegrini, M.; Giannaccare, G.; Versura, P. Blood-Based Treatments for Severe Dry Eye Disease: The Need of a Consensus. *J. Clin. Med.* **2019**, *8*, 1478. [CrossRef] [PubMed]
21. Harnisch, J.P.; Hoffmann, F.; Dumitrescu, L. Side-effects of local anesthetics on the corneal epithelium of the rabbit eye. *Graefe's Arch. Clin. Exp. Ophthalmol.* **1975**, *197*, 71–81. [CrossRef]
22. Joubert, F.; Guerrero-Moreno, A.; Fakih, D.; Reboussin, E.; Gaveriaux-Ruff, C.; Acosta, M.C.; Gallar, J.; Sahel, J.A.; Bodineau, L.; Baudouin, C.; et al. Topical treatment with a mu opioid receptor agonist alleviates corneal allodynia and corneal nerve sensitization in mice. *Biomed. Pharmacother.* **2020**, *132*, 110794. [CrossRef]
23. Reaux-Le Goazigo, A.; Poras, H.; Ben-Dhaou, C.; Ouimet, T.; Baudouin, C.; Wurm, M.; Melik Parsadaniantz, S. Dual enkephalinase inhibitor PL265: A novel topical treatment to alleviate corneal pain and inflammation. *Pain* **2019**, *160*, 307–321. [CrossRef]
24. Yang, D.J.; Lee, K.S.; Ko, C.M.; Moh, S.H.; Song, J.; Hur, L.C.; Cheon, Y.W.; Yang, S.H.; Choi, Y.H.; Kim, K.W. Leucine-enkephalin pro-motes wound repair through the regulation of hemidesmosome dynamics and matrix metalloprotease. *Peptides* **2016**, *76*, 57–64. [CrossRef]
25. Hossain, A.; Heron, D.; Davenport, I.; Huckaba, T.; Graves, R.; Mandal, T.; Muniruzzaman, S.; Wang, S.; Bhattacharjee, P.S. Protective effects of bestatin in the retina of streptozotocin-induced diabetic mice. *Exp. Eye Res.* **2016**, *149*, 100–106. [CrossRef] [PubMed]
26. Versura, P.; Giannaccare, G.; Pellegrini, M.; Sebastiani, S.; Campos, E.C. Neurotrophic keratitis: Current challenges and future prospects. *Eye Brain* **2018**, *10*, 37–45. [CrossRef] [PubMed]

27. Bourcier, T.; Acosta, M.C.; Borderie, V.; Borras, F.; Gallar, J.; Bury, T.; Laroche, L.; Belmonte, C. Decreased corneal sensitivity in patients with dry eye. *Investig. Ophthalmol. Vis. Sci.* **2005**, *46*, 2341–2345. [CrossRef]
28. Peyman, G.A.; Rahimy, M.H.; Fernandes, M.L. Effects of morphine on corneal sensitivity and epithelial wound healing: Implications for topical ophthalmic analgesia. *Br. J. Ophthalmol.* **1994**, *78*, 138–141. [CrossRef]
29. Chen, H.-T.; Chen, K.-H.; Hsu, W.-M. Toxic keratopathy associated with abuse of low-dose anesthetic: A case report. *Cornea* **2004**, *23*, 527–529. [CrossRef] [PubMed]
30. Wisner, A.; Dufour, E.; Messaoudi, M.; Nejdi, A.; Marcel, A.; Ungeheuer, M.N.; Rougeot, C. Human Opiorphin, a natural antino-ciceptive modulator of opioid-dependent pathways. *Proc. Natl. Acad. Sci. USA* **2006**, *103*, 17979–17984. [CrossRef] [PubMed]
31. Rougeot, C.; Messaoudi, M. Identification of human opiorphin, a natural antinociceptive modulator of opioid dependent pathways. *Med. Sci.* **2007**, *23*, 33–35.
32. Power, I. An update on analgesics. *Br. J. Anaesth.* **2011**, *107*, 19–24. [CrossRef] [PubMed]
33. Salarić, I.; Sabalic, M.; Alajbeg, I. Opiorphin in burning mouth syndrome patients: A case-control study. *Clin. Oral Investig.* **2016**, *21*, 2363–2370. [CrossRef] [PubMed]
34. Ozdogan, M.S.; Gungormus, M.; Yusufoglu, S.I.; Ertem, S.Y.; Sonmez, C.; Orhan, M. Salivary opiorphin in dental pain: A potential biomarker for dental disease. *Arch. Oral Biol.* **2018**, *99*, 15–21. [CrossRef] [PubMed]
35. Ozdogan, S.; Sonmez, C.; Yolcu, D.; Gungormus, M. Tear Opiorphin Levels in Ocular Pain Caused by Corneal Foreign Body. *Cornea* **2020**, *39*, 1377–1380. [CrossRef] [PubMed]
36. Mennini, N.; Mura, P.; Nativi, C.; Richichi, B.; Mannelli, L.D.C.; Ghelardini, C. Injectable liposomal formulations of opiorphin as a new therapeutic strategy in pain management. *Futur. Sci. OA* **2015**, *1*, FSO2. [CrossRef]
37. Popik, P.; Kamysz, E.; Kreczko, J.; Wrobel, M. Human opiorphin: The lack of physiological dependence, tolerance to antinociceptive effects and abuse liability in laboratory mice. *Behav. Brain Res.* **2010**, *213*, 88–93. [CrossRef]
38. Rougeot, C.; Robert, F.; Menz, L.; Bisson, J.-F.; Messaoudi, M. Systemically active human opiorphin is a potent yet non-addictive analgesic without drug tolerance effects. *J. Physiol. Pharmacol.* **2020**, *61*, 483–490.
39. Ghelardini, C.; Giotti, A.; Gualtieri, F.; Matucci, R.; Romanelli, M.; Scapecchi, S.; Teodori, E.; Bartolini, A. Presynaptic auto- and hetero-receptors in the cholinergic regulation of pain. In *Trends in Receptor Research*; Angeli, P., Gulini, U., Quaglia, W., Eds.; Edizioni Elsevier: Amsterdam, The Netherlands, 1992; pp. 95–114.
40. Tian, X.-Z.; Chen, J.; Xiong, W.; He, T.; Chen, Q. Effects and underlying mechanisms of human opiorphin on colonic motility and nociception in mice. *Peptides* **2009**, *30*, 1348–1354. [CrossRef]
41. Mencucci, R.; Strazzabosco, G.; Cristofori, V.; Alogna, A.; Bortolotti, D.; Gafà, R.; Cennamo, M.; Favuzza, E.; Trapella, C.; Gentili, V.; et al. GlicoPro, Novel Standardized and Sterile Snail Mucus Extract for Multi-Modulative Ocular Formulations: New Perspective in Dry Eye Disease Management. *Pharmaceutics* **2021**, *13*, 2139. [CrossRef]

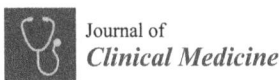

Review

The Role of the Stromal Extracellular Matrix in the Development of Pterygium Pathology: An Update

Javier Martín-López [1], Consuelo Pérez-Rico [2], Selma Benito-Martínez [1,3,4], Bárbara Pérez-Köhler [1,3,4], Julia Buján [1,4] and Gemma Pascual [1,3,4,*]

1   Departamento de Medicina y Especialidades Médicas, Facultad de Medicina y Ciencias de la Salud, Universidad de Alcalá, 28805 Alcalá de Henares, Spain; javier.martinlopez@gmail.com (J.M.-L.); selma.benito@uah.es (S.B.-M.); barbara.perez@uah.es (B.P.-K.); mjulia.bujan@uah.es (J.B.)
2   Departamento de Cirugía, Ciencias Médicas y Sociales, Facultad de Medicina y Ciencias de la Salud, Universidad de Alcalá, 28805 Alcalá de Henares, Spain; cinta.perezrico@gmail.com
3   Biomedical Networking Research Centre on Bioengineering, Biomaterials and Nanomedicine (CIBER-BBN), 28029 Madrid, Spain
4   Ramón y Cajal Health Research Institute (IRYCIS), 28034 Madrid, Spain
*   Correspondence: gemma.pascual@uah.es

Citation: Martín-López, J.; Pérez-Rico, C.; Benito-Martínez, S.; Pérez-Köhler, B.; Buján, J.; Pascual, G. The Role of the Stromal Extracellular Matrix in the Development of Pterygium Pathology: An Update. *J. Clin. Med.* **2021**, *10*, 5930. https://doi.org/10.3390/jcm10245930

Academic Editor: Vincenzo Scorcia

Received: 19 November 2021
Accepted: 15 December 2021
Published: 17 December 2021

Publisher's Note: MDPI stays neutral with regard to jurisdictional claims in published maps and institutional affiliations.

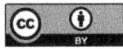

Copyright: © 2021 by the authors. Licensee MDPI, Basel, Switzerland. This article is an open access article distributed under the terms and conditions of the Creative Commons Attribution (CC BY) license (https://creativecommons.org/licenses/by/4.0/).

Abstract: Pterygium is a benign fibrovascular lesion of the bulbar conjunctiva with frequent involvement of the corneal limbus. Its pathogenesis has been mainly attributed to sun exposure to ultraviolet-B radiation. Obtained evidence has shown that it is a complex and multifactorial process which involves multiple mechanisms such as oxidative stress, dysregulation of cell cycle checkpoints, induction of inflammatory mediators and growth factors, angiogenic stimulation, extracellular matrix (ECM) disorders, and, most likely, viruses and hereditary changes. In this review, we aim to collect all authors' experiences and our own, with respect to the study of fibroelastic ECM of pterygium. Collagen and elastin are intrinsic indicators of physiological and pathological states. Here, we focus on an in-depth analysis of collagen (types I and III), as well as the main constituents of elastic fibers (tropoelastin (TE), fibrillins (FBNs), and fibulins (FBLNs)) and the enzymes (lysyl oxidases (LOXs)) that carry out their assembly or crosslinking. All the studies established that changes in the fibroelastic ECM occur in pterygium, based on the following facts: An increase in the synthesis and deposition of an immature form of collagen type III, which showed the process of tissue remodeling. An increase in protein levels in most of the constituents necessary for the development of elastic fibers, except FBLN4, whose biological roles are critical in the binding of the enzyme LOX, as well as FBN1 for the development of stable elastin. There was gene overexpression of TE, FBN1, FBLN5, and LOXL1, while the expression of LOX and FBLN2 and -4 remained stable. In conclusion, collagen and elastin, as well as several constituents involved in elastic fiber assembly are overexpressed in human pterygium, thus supporting the hypothesis that there is dysregulation in the synthesis and crosslinking of the fibroelastic component, constituting an important pathogenetic mechanism for the development of the disease.

Keywords: ocular surface disease; pterygium pathology; extracellular matrix disorders; collagen; elastin

1. Introduction

Pterygium is a benign fibrovascular lesion of the bulbar conjunctiva, which is related to chronic sun exposure, with frequent involvement of the corneal limbus that can invade the cornea. It usually shows a triangular wing shape, with the vertex opposite the base and directed toward the pupil and the base more frequently located in the nasal area toward the caruncle (Figure 1), although it can also arise from the temporal region. Pterygium can be unipolar if it affects only the nasal or temporal area of the conjunctiva or bipolar if it affects both. Similarly, it can develop in a single eye or appear bilaterally.

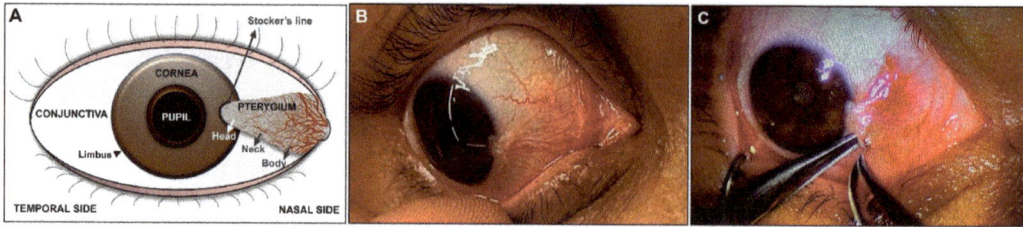

Figure 1. Surgical procedures. (**A**) Scheme of the pathology of a unipolar pterygium developing on the nasal side of the conjunctiva. Different areas in the anatomy of the eye and pterygium have been identified; (**B**) preoperative appearance in a grade II pterygium patient that exceeds the limbus and approaches the pupillary area; (**C**) beginning of the surgical process of pterygium excision in the cornea.

2. Clinical Diagnosis and Histopathological Characterization of Pterygium

Mild cases are usually asymptomatic; however, as the process progresses, it can cause symptoms in the form of redness, dry eyes, irritation, changes in ocular refraction, and vision problems. If left untreated, symptoms may increase in severity over time and may lead to significant vision loss due to infiltrative corneal growth.

Three parts of pterygium are defined: head, neck, and body (Figure 1). The head is a gray, flat, and avascular area at the apex. A pigmented line called the Stocker's line is located at its anterior border, and it is associated with long-standing cases. The neck connects the head and the body, where finely branched neovessels are located. The body is located in the bulbar conjunctiva with vessels straight and radial to the apex. Generally, the head is firmly attached to the cornea, while the body can be separated from the anterior ocular surface.

One of the clinical classifications of pterygium is based on the extent to which it covers the corneal surface. Thus, it is possible to distinguish between four grades: grade I, invades the corneal limbus; grade II, exceeds the limbus and approaches the pupillary area; grade III, reaches the pupil; and grade IV, exceeds the pupil.

Tan et al. [1] morphologically classified pterygium into three categories: atrophic, fleshy, and intermediate. In the atrophy category, episcleral vessels below the pterygium body are easily distinguished. In the fleshy category, pterygium shows a greater thickness so that the episcleral vessels below the body are not visualized. In the intermediate category, the vessels can be seen with difficulty.

In the histopathological characterization of pterygium, the epithelial tissue does not present significant differences with respect to healthy conjunctiva. It usually shows varying degrees of acanthosis or alterations in keratinization in the form of parakeratosis or hyperkeratosis. On the contrary, the stroma is classically described as a thickening of the connective tissue, and it is characterized by elastotic changes in the thickness of the subepithelial stroma and associated lymphocyte-predominant inflammation (Figure 2) with respect to healthy conjunctiva. Thus, immature or fragmented elastic fibers are observed together with collagen fibers of variable thicknesses and mature-looking lymphocytes together with some scattered macrophages in the tissue.

In the subepithelial tissue of pterygium, large areas of extracellular matrix (ECM) with fibrillar and amorphous material can be observed, which are not observed in healthy conjunctiva. These areas do not have an affinity for eosin or for Masson's trichrome light green dye, thus, discarding their collagenous nature. These areas show some basophilia or appear without evident staining, and they are identified based on elastotic alterations (Figure 2). In the subepithelial tissue, angiogenesis is very evident, and in the stromal tissue, a large number of blood vessels are observed. The lymphatic vessels are also very patent, dilated, and numerous.

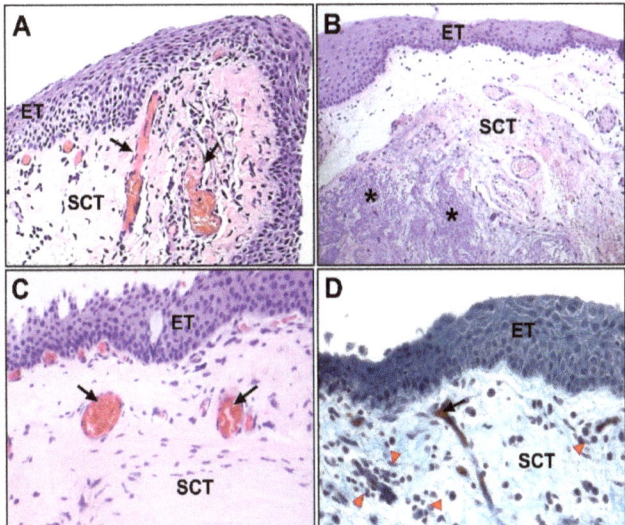

Figure 2. (**A**) Hematoxylin and eosin-stained image of healthy conjunctival tissue (×100); (**B**) amorphous and fibrillar material (*) can be observed in the subepithelial zones of pterygium (×100); (**C**) no amorphous or fibrillar material can be observed in normal conjunctival tissue (×200); (**D**) presence of lymphocytic infiltrate (▶) near the vascular vessels in the subepithelial connective tissue of pterygium (×200). (ET, epithelial tissue; SCT, subepithelial connective tissue; →, blood vessels).

3. Epidemiology and Pathogenesis of Pterygium

There is a higher prevalence of pterygium development in countries near the equator, i.e., up to 22% of the general population, whereas 2% prevalence has been estimated in populations from other latitudes [2]. A recent study with a total of 415,911 participants from 24 countries showed that the prevalence of pterygium in the total population was 12%. The lowest and highest prevalence rates were 3% in the 10- to 20-year-old group and 19.5% in those over 80 years old, respectively, and a similar prevalence was observed in men and women [3].

This pathology is more frequent in outdoor workers, and its prevalence tends to increase with age [4]. The pathogenesis of pterygium has been fundamentally attributed to damage related to sun exposure to ultraviolet-B radiation (UV-B, wavelength, 280–320 nm), although evidence has been obtained that shows it is a complex process that includes multiple mechanisms (proinflammatory or immunological modifiers of ECM, cell proliferation and survival, or proangiogenic), the release of mediators (growth factors or cytokines), and probably viruses and genetic factors [5] (Figure 3).

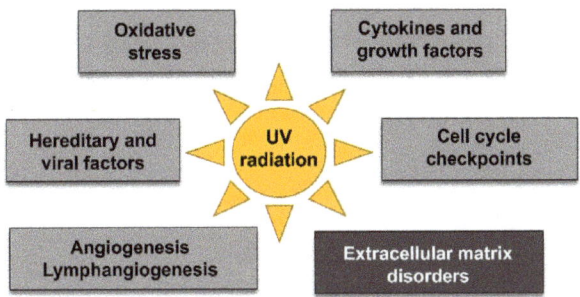

Figure 3. Summary of the multifactorial pathogenesis of pterygium.

3.1. Oxidative Stress

Chronic solar exposure causes oxidative stress, which activates growth factors related to the development of pterygium. Oxidative stress is produced by an imbalance between reactive oxygen species (ROS), which include oxygen ions, peroxides, and free radicals, and a tissue's capacity to reduce these species and repair the tissue damage that causes oxidative stress. The release of peroxides and free radicals is responsible for alterations of DNA, protein structure, and lipoperoxidation. The presence of 8-oxo-2'-deoxyguanosine, one of the classic markers of oxidative stress, has been described in pterygium samples by multiple authors [6,7].

3.2. Dysregulation of Cell Cycle Checkpoints

In the pathogenesis of pterygium, a relationship with apoptotic regulatory mechanisms that condition its formation, growth, and persistence has been described. DNA fragmentation has been demonstrated by terminal deoxynucleotidyl transferase dUTP nick end labeling (TUNEL) marking, in addition to increases in antiapoptotic proteins Bcl-2 and BAX [8], as well as survival of apoptosis inhibitor [9]. Thus, chronic sun exposure has been correlated with oxidative stress and the expression of these antiapoptotic mediators.

However, most studies on the pathogenesis of pterygium have focused on describing alterations in cell cycle control points, such as p16, p53, p27, and cyclin D1, or on the state of loss of heterozygosity that has been described more frequently than microsatellite instability type [10]. In relation to cell cycle checkpoints, various authors have identified increases in p53 [11], p16 [12], as well as p27 and cyclinD1 [13], although they do not represent the mechanism underlying the presence of a somatic mutation in the TP53 gene [14,15], for which they associate an increase in its expression with the activation of these factors via intracellular signaling pathways.

3.3. Induction of Inflammatory Mediators and Growth Factors

The vast majority of studies on the pathogenesis of pterygium have also described that the above alterations triggered a response that involved inflammatory mediators and growth factors that enhanced inflammatory and angiogenic responses. In this way, increases in the interleukins IL-1, IL-6, and IL-8 [16] and the tumor necrosis factor TNF-α [17] have been described as contributing to the recruitment of other inflammatory mediators and metalloproteases involved in pterygium pathogenesis.

However, the role of numerous growth factors in pterygium pathogenesis has also been described, such as heparin-binding epithelial growth factor (HB-EGF) [18], vascular endothelial growth factor (VEGF) [19], transforming growth factor β (TGF-β), platelet-derived growth factor (PDGF), and basic fibroblast growth factor (bFGF) [20].

3.4. Angiogenic Stimulation

Angiogenesis research has been extensively analyzed in the pathology of pterygium. Inflammation promotes angiogenesis as an additional mechanism for the repair of tissue damage from inflammatory mediators and growth factors, especially VEGF, and the reduction of thrombospondin-1 [21]. VEGF promotes endothelial migration and is related to one of the classic mechanisms that promotes angiogenesis, such as in nitric oxide-rich cellular microenvironments, through the activity of endothelial nitric oxide synthase (eNOS) and inducible nitric oxide synthase (iNOS) [22]. Our research group has shown that the formation of new blood vessels was the most relevant event, and it was correlated with increased expression of vascular endothelial CD31 and an elevated blood/lymphatic vessel ratio. The presence of high levels of VEGF-A in both vessel networks and ECM in human pterygium tissue may have a major impact on angiogenesis in this pathological tissue [23].

3.5. Viruses and Hereditary Changes

Due to the influence of human papilloma virus (HPV) serotypes in various conjunctival pathologies (squamous papilloma and a subgroup of dysplasias and squamous carcinomas), its role in the proliferation of pterygium has been hypothesized, with discrepancies in the geographic distribution and serotypes described by different authors. However, a clear pathogenic association between pterygium and HPV- or herpes simplex (HSV)-type viral infections has not been established [24,25]. Viruses encode proteins that inactivate p53, which leads to chromosomal instability and increases the likelihood of cell progression to malignancy, although its implication remains controversial.

Moreover, specific hereditary traits involved in the pathogenesis of pterygium have not been described, and little evidence of family association has been observed. However, some authors have suggested that there could be an autosomal dominant inheritance pattern with incomplete penetrance [5]. Few studies have analyzed hereditary factors, and in most cases, the influence of an environmental or occupational factor is not ruled out before considering genetic alterations [2].

3.6. Extracellular Matrix Disorders

The ECM is a group of extracellular components secreted by stromal cells that provide structural and biochemical support to the cellular environment. Aberrant expression of ECM proteins may be directly associated with proliferative growth of pterygium. Tissue damage from chronic sun exposure and the activation of inflammatory mediators increase the expression of matrix metalloproteases (MMP-1, MMP-2, MMP-3, MMP-7, MMP-8, MMP-9, MMP-14, and MMP-15), which leads to modification/remodeling of the ECM [26,27]. These alterations may be an initial change in the development of pterygium at the level of the limbus in which the components of the stromal connective tissue, elastin, and tropoelastin (TE) are altered [28]. The fibrovascular tissue that makes up pterygium is characterized by an increase in elastin and myofibroblasts, which plays a critical role in the migration and growth of pterygium [29].

Due to the scarcity of studies related to the latter mechanism implicated in the development of pterygium pathology, in this study, we focus on ECM disorders and review the most studied ECM constituents, with a special emphasis on updating and summarizing the main findings obtained by our research group, whose members have many years of experience in the study of the collagen and elastic components of different soft tissues, including pterygium.

4. Role of ECM in Tissue Repair and Pathological Processes

ECM is a coordinated network composed of multiple molecules that make up a three-dimensional structure with physical properties that play a fundamental role in cell adhesion, structure, and tissue and organ support. However, the interconnection of these molecules and their functional interactions represent microenvironmental signals that influence cell differentiation, proliferation, survival and migration.

ECM also has a dynamic role in physiological mechanisms, such as tissue repair or healing, or in pathological contexts, such as cancer, in which ECM changes are induced by multiple mediators and growth factors, which condition various effects, such as stimulation of angiogenesis and inflammatory responses and promotion of stromal invasion that can lead to an excessive accumulation of proteins or differentiation of cellular components.

There are multiple cells that collaborate in the promotion of an unstructured matrix, such as endothelial cells, pericytes, cancer-associated fibroblasts (CAFs), and immune cells. One of the mechanisms identified is an increase in the activity of the lysyl oxidase (LOX) enzymes, which promotes crosslinking of collagen and its interaction with ECM components and increases rigidity [30].

The enzymes responsible for the degradation of ECM are MMPs, hyaluronidases, disintegrins, ADAMs, ADAMTS, as well as plasminogen activators and proteases such as granzymes and intracellular cathepsins. The degradation of the ECM coexists with the production of new elements and their accumulation. Fibroblasts are the main source of matrix components, although remodeling is a process involving multiple cells. The alteration of normal remodeling is an initiating factor in pathological processes and their progression.

Fibroblasts are involved in the synthesis of ECM components, and they can acquire contractile capacity and can participate in the secretion of cytokines and matrix mediators. They play a fundamental role in tissue repair and healing processes, in which activated fibroblasts produce myofibroblasts through the expression of α-smooth muscle actin (α-SMA) filaments mediated by the activation of the SMAD2 protein.

Fibroblasts participate in the pathogenesis of pterygium via their activation to myofibroblasts, their secretion of mediators and their interactions with other ECM elements. The magnitude of tissue damage and aberrations in the activation and functionality of fibroblasts, either in their proliferation, production of collagen or elastic fibers, and migration or differentiation to myofibroblasts, are among the mechanisms involved in the alteration of tissue repair and the pathological processes of ocular fibrosis.

5. ECM and Its Pathogenic Mechanisms in the Development of Pterygium

In the pathogenesis of pterygium, epithelial cells are proposed to be responsible for an alteration in the balance between proliferation and apoptosis, which conditions a stromal overgrowth of activated fibroblasts, thereby, promoting angiogenesis, inflammation, and aberrant elastin and collagen accumulation in ECM. Furthermore, pterygium epithelial cells show characteristics involved in the epithelium-mesenchymal transition, such as the loss of E-cadherin and the nuclear accumulation of β-catenin [31]. Other models of epithelial-mesenchymal transition from epithelial cells have shown how the expression of epithelial markers is reduced and the expression of mesenchymal markers increases [32]. Phenotypic changes induce morphological changes in cell interactions and functions. Among the mechanisms described are the change from E-cadherin to N-cadherin and the expression of α-SMA or other mesenchymal markers or transcription factors, such as vimentin, FSP-1 (fibroblast specific protein 1), Snail, Slug, TWIST, and ZEB1 [33]. Thus, it has been postulated that myofibroblasts are derived from keratinocytes [34], progenitor cells of the limbus [35], orbital fibroadipose tissue [36], or cells from bone marrow [37].

Elevated levels of TGF-β expression have been reported in pterygium samples [20] and in cultures of isolated pterygium fibroblasts [38]. Antifibrotic treatments in other organs have led to studies that evaluated the efficacy of such treatments, for example, the expression of TGF-β in cultured pterygium fibroblasts has been inhibited, and a decrease in cell proliferation, migration, and collagen synthesis has been observed [39]. Treatment with human amniotic membrane grafts suppresses the expression of TGF-β2, TGF-β3, and TGFBR receptors in cultured pterygium fibroblasts, with the consequent inhibition of contractility [40]. Moreover, a reduction in α-SMA expression in cultured pterygium fibroblasts [41] has led to improved healing.

A number of studies have relatively frequently reported the role of other ECM components in pterygium not related to fibroblasts or TGF-β, such as MMPs [29], different growth factors (PDGF, bFGF, HB-EGFM, and VEGF) [18,38], or inflammatory mediators, such as IL-6 and IL-8 [42].

The activities of various enzymes, such as cyclooxygenases (COX), lipoxygenases, or cytochrome P450, have also been described in relation to increases in proinflammatory mediators [43], although the expression of LOX has not been characterized in relation to processes such as elastogenesis.

In the field of ophthalmological research, alterations in elastogenesis have been evaluated mainly in corneal diseases, such as macular degeneration with respect to fibulins (FBLNs) or fibrillins (FBNs) [44,45], in the dysfunction of LOX-like 1 (LOXL1) action in glaucoma models related to exfoliation syndrome [46,47], or in keratoconus [48].

Experimental studies of pterygium in which alterations in essential components for elastogenesis have been characterized are scarce [49] and have not described alterations in the expression and functionality of TE, LOXs, or proteins of the family of FBLNs or FBNs.

As our research group is a pioneer in the analysis of the elastic component in the pathogenesis of pterygium, all the results obtained by our group about alterations found exclusively at the level of the fibroelastic component of pterygium are shared below, with special emphasis on the constituents and the assembly and reticulation process of the elastic fiber.

6. Fibroelastic Alterations in Pterygium ECM

The ECM of pterygium includes fibrillar elements, such as collagens and elastic fibers and an amorphous component (proteoglycans, multi-adhesive glycoproteins, and glycosaminoglycans) that constitutes the ground substance.

These components interact in a complex way with each other as well as with other elements of the matrix and various cell types (such as endothelial, immune, or epithelial cells). Interactions occur through surface receptors, such as integrins, discoidin domain receptors (DDRs), cell surface proteoglycans (such as syndecans), and hyaluronan receptors (such as CD44). In addition, they interact with different growth factors and with MMP enzymes that maintain the integrity and remodel the composition of the ECM.

In this case, we focus on the in-depth analysis of the two main fibrillar elements of the ECM, collagen fibers (types I and III), as well as the main constituents of elastic fibers (TE, FBNs, and FBLNs), and the enzymes (LOXs) that carry out their assembly or crosslinking.

6.1. Collagen

Collagen is the most abundant component of the ECM, and it is also present in pericellular regions. It is synthesized from fibroblasts, which also have a role in its spatial arrangement and organization. Collagen is formed from three polypeptide chains called alpha chains, which can be organized to create homodimeric or heterodimeric triple helices. The α chains are formed from triplets of Gly-X-Y, with X and Y representing the amino acids proline and hydroxyproline, respectively. The triple helices crosslink to form crosslinked collagen fibrils in the ECM.

Fibrillar collagens are found in multiple tissues that confer tensile strength and are involved in cellular functions, such as cell migration and adhesion, angiogenesis, and tissue development and repair.

In the eye, the cornea is the anatomical structure with the greatest presence of collagen [50]. The corneal stroma accounts for 90% of the stroma and is composed of an abundant amount of collagen, especially type I, although the presence of multiple types of collagens has been identified, most at the stromal level (types II, III, V, XIII, etc.). Regarding the conjunctiva, the predominant collagen is type VII collagen at the level of the basement membrane, where it forms anchor fibrils, which have also been identified in the basement or Bowman membrane of the cornea or at the level of the limbus [51,52], and the predominant types in subepithelial connective tissue are I and III.

Our research group has carried out different studies to evaluate the expression of different types of collagens in pterygium tissue [53]. Through observations with polarized light, Sirius red staining has made it possible to jointly assess type I and III collagens and to identify the location and balance of both types in healthy conjunctiva and pterygium. This technique is based on the orientation and interaction between the sulfone groups of the dye and the amine groups of lysine and hydroxylysine and guanidine groups of arginine in the collagen fibers, and the colors differ depending on the degree of collagen maturity. Collagen type I (mature collagen) stains reddish orange whereas collagen type III (immature collagen) stains yellow–green.

The two types of collagens are located in the ECM of the subepithelial stromal tissue of both types of tissue samples. In healthy conjunctiva samples, collagens type I and III are present in similar proportions, while in pterygium samples, the most immature form of collagen (type III) is increased, thus, indicating a new process of synthesis and deposition of collagen and suggesting a process of tissue formation and remodeling (Figure 4). In deep areas, the collagen fibers infiltrate and distribute as a reticulum between the amorphous fibrillar areas of the pterygium samples. These areas with a fibrillar or amorphous component are not stained by Sirius red; thus, they appear without staining under the light microscope and with a translucent appearance under polarized light, which indicates that these structures do not have a collagenous nature, and therefore correspond to immature or fragmented elastic fibers (Figure 4).

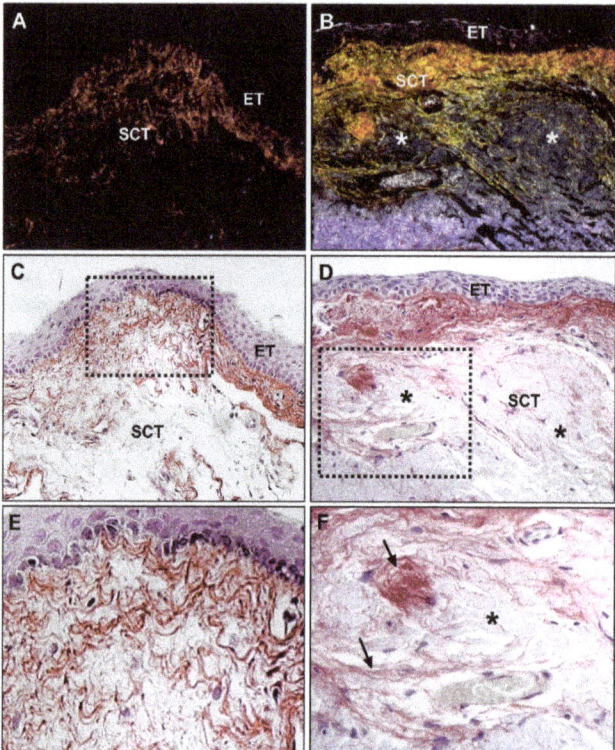

Figure 4. Photomicrographs of Sirius red staining observed under polarized light of (**A**) conjunctival and (**B**) pterygium tissue, showing expression of collagen I (mature) in red and collagen III (immature) in yellow, in the subepithelial connective tissue of both specimens (×200); (**C**) conjunctival and (**D**) pterygium tissue images of the same samples stained with Sirius red observed under normal light, where collagen expression appears in red (×200); (**E,F**) magnification of the squared area from the (**C,D**) image showing collagen fibers (→) (×400). (ET, epithelial tissue; SCT, subepithelial connective tissue; *, areas of amorphous and fibrillar material accumulation; →, collagen fibers).

6.2. Elastin and Elastogenesis

The elastic fibers of the ECM are formed by a compact network with two main components, with the majority represented by elastin together with a network of microfibrils of fibrillins [54]. Elastin is another structural protein closely related to collagen that provides elasticity to tissues and stability to ECM components. In its development and operation, TE, FBNs, FBLNs, LOXs, and other associated proteins are necessary (Figure 5).

Elastic fibers are assembled in developmental stages and represent stable structures [55]; however, tissue damage and pathological processes can cause their degradation by MMPs, which releases elastin fragments that promote monocyte chemotaxis and fibroblasts that will activate changes in the ECM together with incorrect repair and abnormal functioning of the fibers [56].

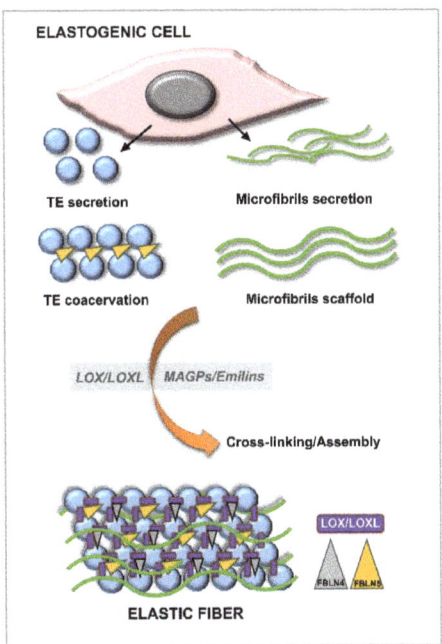

Figure 5. Process of elastogenesis and the molecular interactions among the different components of the elastic fiber. Functions of LOX/LOXL, fibulin-4 (FBLN4), and fibulin-5 (FBLN5) during coacervation, crosslinking, and assembly have been shown.

6.2.1. Tropoelastin

Elastin is an insoluble polymer composed of monomeric subunits of tropoelastin TE that are crosslinked with a framework of fibrillin microfibrils that form elastic fibers. TE contains hydrophobic residues rich in valine and glycine that are responsible for the elastic properties of fibers, and it also contains other smaller lysine domains, the latter of which are modified by LOX or LOXL. Essential for the correct formation of elastin is its extensive crosslinking by LOX enzymes that oxidize selective lysine residues to align to form desmosine and isodesmosine crosslinks that stabilize the elastin polymer and render it insoluble.

However, in addition to elastin, elastic fibers are made up of various microfibrils whose main function is to form a necessary framework for the configuration of elastic fibers, including MAGP (microfibril-associated glycoproteins), LTBP (latent TGFβ binding protein), interface molecules, and especially, FBN1 (predominantly) and FBN2 glycoproteins [57,58] (Figure 5).

An immunohistochemical analysis has been performed and revealed the presence of TE in the stroma of healthy conjunctiva, and showed how the expression of this elastic component was reduced. Large areas of low density were observed with minimal expression of TE and slight marking in some thin fibrillar elements of the ECM. Therefore, these results showed the predominance of the collagen component and nonfibrillar matrix over the elastic component in healthy conjunctiva. In contrast, the expression of TE was significantly increased in pterygium, where it was observed in the subepithelial tissue as large areas with degenerative changes or immature formations of elastic fibers. The labeling was located in the amorphous material and thickened and tortuous fibers of the subepithelial connective tissue (Figure 6).

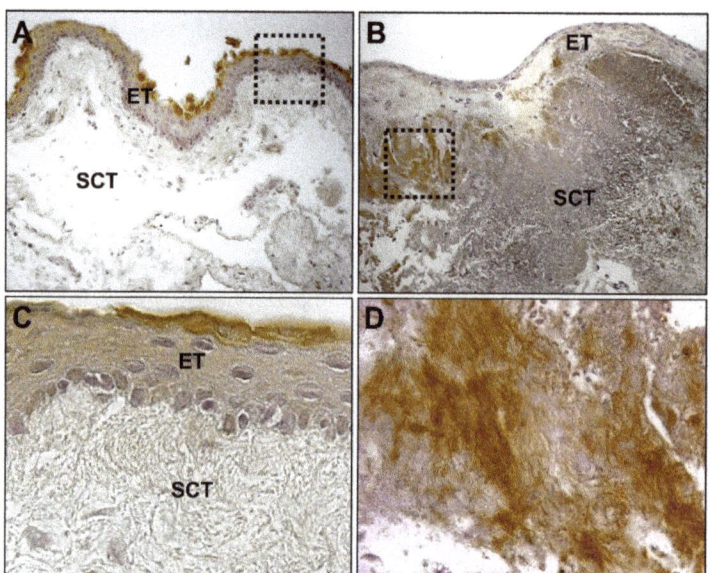

Figure 6. Images of immunohistochemical tropoelastin staining show an increased expression in pathologic tissue: (**A**) Conjunctival tissue (×100); (**B**) pterygium (×100); (**C,D**) detailed view of the squared section in (**A,B**), respectively (×630). (ET, epithelial tissue; SCT, subepithelial connective tissue).

The mRNA analysis results for TE correlated with the immunohistochemical findings and showed a significant increase ($p < 0.001$) in the pterygium group as compared with healthy conjunctiva, with gene expression increasing approximately 2.8 times in the active pterygium group (Figure 7).

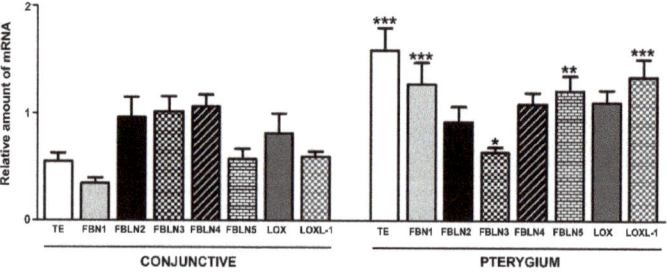

Figure 7. Relative quantification of tropoelastin (TE), fibrillin-1 (FBN1), fibulin-2 (FBLN2), fibulin-3 (FBLN3), fibulin-4 (FBLN4), fibulin-5 (FBLN5), LOX and LOXL1 messenger ribonucleic acid (mRNA) in conjunctival and pterygium tissue. Gene expression was normalized with glyceraldehyde 3-phosphate dehydrogenase (GAPDH). (* $p < 0.05$, ** $p < 0.01$, and *** $p < 0.001$).

6.2.2. Fibrillins

FBNs are extracellular glycoproteins that compose the microfibrils on which elastin is deposited, and they are located within and on the periphery of the elastic fiber. In addition to being the predominant component of the fibril framework of elastic fibers, they interact closely with TE and integrins. Three isoforms, FBN1, -2, and -3, have been described and are characterized by an amino acid region together with cysteine domains that bind TGF-β and calcium domains that bind EGF. While FBN2 and FBN3 are mainly expressed in the embryonic period, FBN1 appears in both embryonic and adult tissues.

Mutations in the fibrillin genes cause alterations in elastogenesis and connective tissue disorder conditions, such as Marfan syndrome or Weill-Marchesani syndrome if mutations occur in the FBN1 gene, or congenital contractural arachnodactyly (Beals syndrome) if the FBN2 gene is altered.

Very low levels of FBN1 have been observed in the stroma of healthy conjunctiva. However, the pathological population showed a significant increase in FBN1 immunostaining in the ECM (Figure 8). Gene expression for FBN1 has been revealed by quantitative PCR techniques and was also increased in this pathological population, where it was four times higher than that found in conjunctiva samples ($p < 0.001$) (Figure 7).

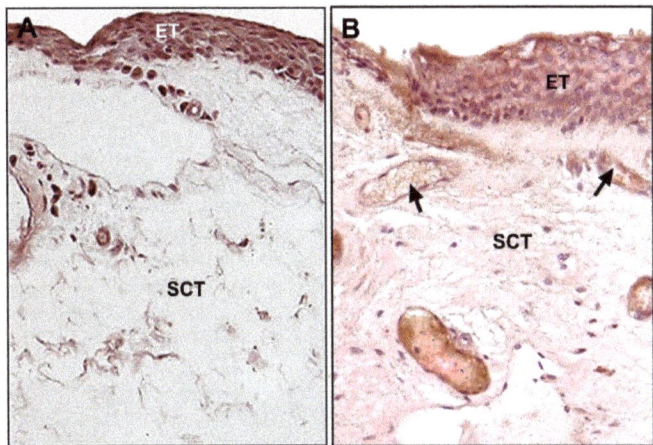

Figure 8. Photomicrographs show immunohistochemical staining for fibrillin-1: (**A**) Conjunctival tissue (×400); (**B**) pterygium (×400). Fibrillin-1 expression was increased in pathologic tissue. (ET, epithelial tissue; SCT, subepithelial connective tissue; →, blood vessels).

6.2.3. Fibulins

Since the discovery of fibulin-1 [59], seven members of the FBLNs family have been described in the last 30 years [60,61], and they have been functionally characterized both in vitro and in physiological and pathogenic states. They are divided into class I and class II based on their length and the structure of their domains. Specifically, class II FBLNs (FBLN3, FBLN4, and FBLN5) behave as short FBLNs of the elastogenic type (due to the presence of a calcium domain that binds to EGF similar to that of FBN1), thus, exerting a fundamental role in the development of elastic fibers [62]. The most important biological role in elastogenesis corresponds to FBLN4 and -5. FBLN5 has a greater capacity to bind TE than FBLN4, and it also has a greater capacity to enhance the formation of elastic fibers. However, the biological role of FBLN4 in elastin development appears to be critical, because FBLN4 knockout animal models are lethal during gestation and the neonatal period [63–65], while FBLN5 knockouts are capable of living with progressively accumulating defects of the elastic fibers [66,67].

FBLNs are necessary for the assembly and function of elastin, and they are also capable of binding integrins and establishing cell and ECM interactions. For example, FBLN1 interacts with cytoskeletal proteins and has been identified around fibroblasts in in vitro and embryonic models [68]. FBLN2 is able to bind elastin to FBN1 and to participate in its anchoring to the fibrillin microfibril network, while FBLN3 interacts by binding elastic fibers to basement membranes.

In elastogenesis, the interactions of TE with FBLN4 and FBLN5 are critical for binding LOX enzymes and FBN1 and for forming stable elastin.

We have been pioneers in the analysis of the most important FBLNs in the development of elastic fibers (FBLN2, -3, -4, and -5). Our studies have shown that a significant increase in FBLN2 expression generally occurred in the subepithelial tissue of pterygium. Immunostaining in the stromal area occurred in the ECM, and it was relatively more intense around the blood and lymphatic vessels and in the areas of fibrillar or amorphous material accumulation (Figure 9A,B). As compared with TE, FBLN2 gene expression did not increase in the pathological samples as compared with healthy conjunctiva, with both groups presenting very similar values ($p > 0.05$) (Figure 7).

Our studies have also shown that healthy conjunctiva presented similar expression patterns for FBLN3 and FBLN2, with FBLN3 colocalizing with FBLN2, although a difference was observed in the more intense labeling in areas of the subepithelial connective tissue in contact with the basal epithelium. However, we found that the expression of FBLN3 in pterygium increased significantly and spread homogeneously throughout the subepithelial connective tissue; moreover, a significant increase in FBLN3 expression was observed in areas closer to the blood and lymphatic vessels (Figure 9C,D). The expression of mRNA in healthy patients was very similar to that of FBLN2; however, in pterygium, the expression was decreased approximately 1.5 times as compared with that of healthy samples ($p < 0.05$) (Figure 7).

The results of our immunohistochemical studies have shown that, contrary to FBLN2 and FBLN3, no differences were observed in FBLN4 protein expression between the healthy and pathological groups; both groups showed similar labeling in the subepithelial connective tissue, and the expression was very low (Figure 10A,B). Similar to the immunohistochemical study, no differences were found in the expression of the gene for FBLN4 and both study groups showed similar values for the relative amount of the messenger (Figure 7).

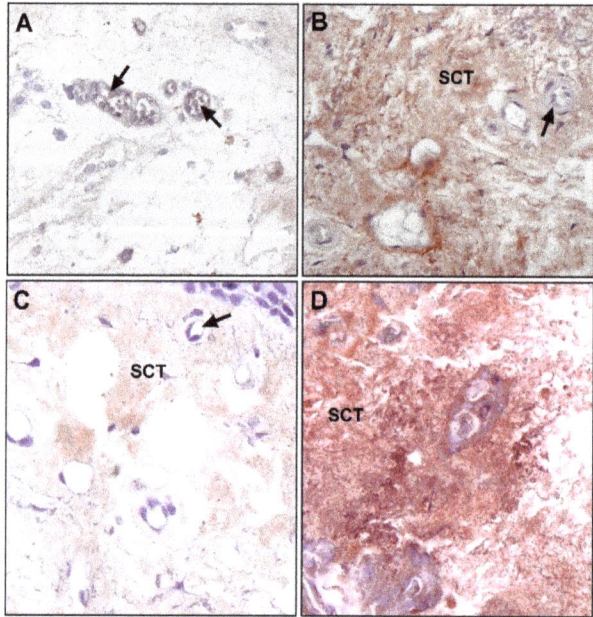

Figure 9. Expression of fibulin-2 localized in the subepithelial connective tissue in both (**A**) conjunctival and (**B**) pterygium tissue (×630); (**C**) fibulin-3 expression in conjunctival sample (×630); (**D**) positive labeling for fibulin-3 in pterygium tissue (×630). Higher expression levels of fibulin-2 and fibulin-3 were observed in pterygium with respect to the conjunctiva. (SCT, subepithelial connective tissue; →, blood vessels).

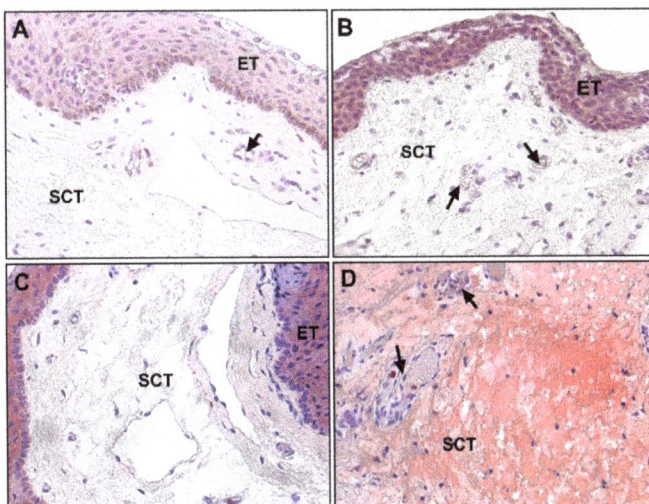

Figure 10. Fibulin-4 expression in (**A**) conjunctival and (**B**) pterygium samples (×400). Immunohistochemical staining of fibulin-5 expression in (**C**) conjunctival and (**D**) pterygium tissue (×400). Fibulin-4 expression was similar between the healthy and pathological groups. In contrast, increased expression of fibulin-5 was localized in the pterygium subepithelial connective tissue. (ET, epithelial tissue; SCT, subepithelial connective tissue; →, blood vessels).

The subepithelial connective tissue shows weak immunolabeling for FBLN5 in healthy conjunctiva, while the levels are significantly increased in pterygium, which show very marked areas of degenerative elastogenic changes or immature fiber formation (Figure 10C,D).

In general, the mRNA levels of FBLN5 coincide with significantly higher protein expression, by approximately 2.5 times in a pathological population vs. healthy conjunctiva ($p < 0.01$) (Figure 7).

6.2.4. Lysyl Oxydases

Lysyl oxidases (LOXs) are the enzymes responsible for the assembly of collagen and elastin, which form the desmosine bonds. They belong to a heterogeneous family of amino oxidases that oxidize the amino substrate to aldehyde. LOX and four isoforms of LOXL, (namely, LOXL1, LOXL2, LOXL3, and LOXL4) have been described as performing such oxidization, and they are synthesized in their inactive proenzyme form. They all share the C-terminal catalytic region in common and are differentiated by the N-terminal region. Its main substrates are collagen fibers and TE, oxidizing lysine or hydroxylysine residues into lysine or hydroxylysine for TE and collagen fibers, respectively. These aldehydes can react spontaneously to form the covalent bonds that confer resistance to collagen fibers and elasticity to elastic fibers. However, other more specific functions have been described for these enzymes, such as the possible roles they play in the control of cell adhesion and growth determined by domains such as the "cytokine-like" receptor domain [69].

Elastin crosslinking is another critical point for the synthesis of polymerized insoluble elastin. This process is mediated by the LOX family of enzymes, and in vitro models have shown that interactions occurred with proteins of the FBLN family [70]. In this way, FBLN4 mediated the binding of TE to LOX [71], while FBLN5 did so by interacting with LOXL1 [72,73]. Its role was critical in identifying lethality in LOX knockout models [74] due to rupture of the aorta and diaphragm due to incomplete elastin crosslinking.

The protein expression of LOX showed immunostaining that appeared mainly in the ECM and was significantly higher in pterygium (Figure 11A,B). This result is perfectly justifiable given the participation of both enzymes LOX and LOXL in the crosslinking of collagen and elastin, forming complex crosslinks essential for the stabilization of collagen fibrils and for the integrity and functionality of mature elastin.

In contrast, the mRNA expression did not correlate with the protein expression and was not increased in pterygium (Figure 7).

Taking into consideration that FBLN4 is capable of binding to TE and FBN1, thereby, mediating the maturation and crosslinking of elastic fibers through strong LOX binding and directing the deposition of elastin in microfibrils, in pathological samples, the difference in protein expression between FBLN4 and LOX (which is increased) is not argued. This reduced expression of FBLN4 could be one of the factors associated with the development of elastotic alterations and the immature and fragmented elastic fibers observed in pterygium pathology.

Our experience shows that immunohistochemical labeling for LOXL1 presents an expression pattern very similar to that of LOX. It appears mainly in the subepithelial matrix in both samples, although higher expression is observed in the pathological samples. Given that LOXL-1 seems to be necessary more specifically in the crosslinking of TE that participates in the formation, maintenance, and remodeling of elastic fibers, particularly during dynamic processes, the increase of this protein in the ECM of pterygium would be totally justified (Figure 11C,D).

As compared with LOX, the relative amount of LOXL1 mRNA was correlated with protein expression and showed a significant increase of approximately two-fold in pterygium as compared with healthy conjunctiva ($p < 0.001$) (Figure 7).

This same pattern of expression and the increase in protein expression observed in the pathological samples of FBLN5 corresponded to the analysis of LOXL1. Considering that FBLN5 was capable of binding TE and FBN1 and mediated their assembly through its interaction with LOXL1 as well as promoted the aggregation of TE molecules by coacervation, LOXL1/FBLN5 colocalization has been fully proven.

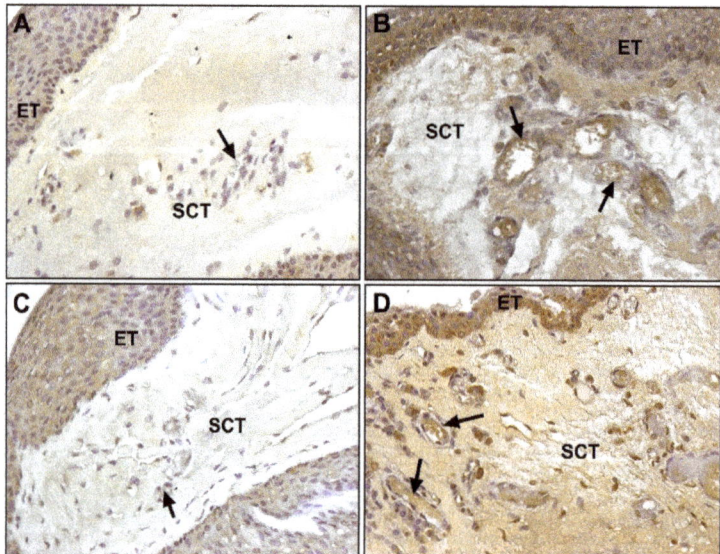

Figure 11. Immunohistochemical labeling for LOX in (**A**) conjunctival and (**B**) pterygium tissue (×400). LOXL1 expression in (**C**) conjunctival and (**D**) pterygium tissue (×400). LOX and LOXL1 can be observed in the subepithelial matrix in both samples, with a higher expression in pterygium. (ET, epithelial tissue; SCT, subepithelial connective tissue; →, blood vessels).

7. Discussion

Collagen and elastin, the main components of the ECM, are intrinsic indicators of physiological and pathological states. To understand healthy and diseased tissues in pterygium pathogenesis, an investigation of the modification of these main structural proteins is necessary, which is what we have tried to summarize in this review article.

Due to the pathogenic relationship between chronic exposure to solar radiation and the development of pterygium, studies have focused on how this chronic exposure to solar radiaiton activates the expression of inflammatory mediators and cytokines [75] in addition to matrix metalloproteases [76] that produce conformational changes in the matrix components identified in pterygium samples. However, in addition to inflammatory mediators and metalloproteases, the expression of growth factors, such as HB-EGF [77], which is involved in tissue or bFGF healing processes, has been described, as reported in recurrent pterygium [38]. This inflammatory microenvironment leads to the cooperative activation of other growth factors and other pathogenic mechanisms, such as angiogenesis, as well as the activation and functionality of stromal fibroblasts [78], which acquire a myofibroblast phenotype involved in the activation of various signaling pathways, such as mTOR [79], which modifies the composition of the ECM. Previous studies have indicated that the basal cells of the limbus and stromal fibroblasts secrete TGF-β, and thereby synthesize elastic material [80], and produce several types of MMPs similar to those reported in tumor models [81].

Gene and protein expression studies are also optimal tools to elucidate the pathogenic mechanisms involved in the development of pterygium. The data reported based on microarray analyses have included the relationship of miR-125 with fibroblast proliferation and the production of ECM components [82], the influence of miR-218-5p on EGFR expression and its activity on the PI3K/AKT/mTOR signaling pathway involved in cell proliferation and migration [83], the influence of miR-21 on the PTEN/AKT pathway [84], and the influence of miR-143-3p, miR-181-2-3p, miR-377-5p, and miR-411a-5p on pterygium fibroblasts [85].

In addition to modifications at the promoter level, studies have shown that the pathogenesis of pterygium may be related to the DNA methylation state, which would imply alterations in the genes involved in the expression of proteins, such as CD24, MMP-2, or TGM-2, which play essential roles in wound healing and development [86]. Therefore, these epigenetic changes could determine the recurrence of lesions after surgery.

Characteristically, the histopathological description of pterygium has indicated a highly vascularized subepithelial stromal tissue with the presence of morphological changes in collagen and elastic fibers consisting of hypertrophic and elastotic fibers, respectively. Fibroblastic activation induced by sun exposure was initially postulated to first affect the correct configuration of the elastic fibers and to cause abnormal maturation, which is called elastodysplasia, and then lead to secondary degenerative changes, such as elastodystrophy [49].

These fibroelastic changes are not exclusive to the pathology of the ocular surface and are frequently identified at the level of the superficial dermis in the histopathology of actinic keratosis-type skin lesions or in skin carcinomas related to sun exposure [87,88].

In the eye, elastin, together with collagen, is one of the main stromal components of the cornea, the cribriform plate, and the peripapillary sclera, and both the epithelium and the corneal endothelium have been reported to synthesize fibrillar components involved in the synthesis of elastin. A decrease in precursor components in the final stages of life is characteristic [89] and has been related to the development of glaucoma [90,91].

Few models of ophthalmological diseases have been developed in which the influence of the degradation and configuration of elastic fibers on their development has been studied. One model is the pathogenesis of involutional ectropion and entropion, in which a significant loss of elastic fibers and overexpression of MMP-2, MMP-7, and MMP-9 has been identified [92].

In addition to vascular proliferation, one of the most obvious morphological characteristics of pterygium is the presence of these changes at the level of the elastic fibers; however, few studies have directly focused on the elastic component and changes that occurred around its configuration or degradation in the primary disease, such as in recurrences.

For the proper configuration of the elastic matrix to occur, the monomeric form of elastin, TE, will develop multiple complex interactions with the entire series of associated proteins, which include FBNs, FBLNs, and matrix-associated glycoproteins (MAGPs) [93]. Therefore, TE is a common ligand for these proteins, and as observed in our studies, colocalization in their expression pattern occasionally occurs.

Our studies showed general increases in the TE, FBN1, FBLN5, and LOXL1 mRNA levels in pterygium as compared with in control conjunctiva, although this was not observed in the FBLN2, -3, -4, and LOX analyses. However, at the protein level, we identified an increase in all of their levels except for FBLN4 and the immature form of collagen.

Regarding the expression of TE, our results agree with those described by other groups [28] that have also found high levels of expression of this protein in pterygium. This may be the result of mutations in the untranslated region but not in the coding sequence of TE mRNA, which would lead to errors in DNA polymerase activity and a massive accumulation of abnormal elastic fibers. However, inconsistent with our results, the protein expression did not correlate with the mRNA, which was justified as a posttranscriptional modification of the TE. This discrepancy may be because their studies were carried out in cell populations of fibroblasts obtained from pterygium subjected to UV radiation and those of our group were conducted on fresh pathological tissue.

Therefore, in the pathology of pterygium, the protein expression of the mentioned elastic components increases but they do not assemble correctly, thus, producing dysfunctional elastic fibers at the stromal level, which macroscopically and clinically translate into inelastic tissue in its fresh state. This change leads to a loss of functionality that could contribute to the development of other ocular pathologies, such as astigmatism induced by various mechanisms, such as the accumulation of tear film on the leading edge of pterygium or the mechanical traction exerted by it at the level of the cornea [94].

Regarding the expression of FBN1, our results confirmed an increase in mRNA levels in pterygium with respect to the normal conjunctiva at the transcriptional level, although this increase was only discretely significant at the level of protein expression, possibly indicating the existence of messenger degradation or alterations at the translational level.

Other ocular diseases that affect the elastic component, and more specifically the microfibrils of FBN1, include myopia and ectopia lentis; both ophthalmological pathologies are frequently observed in Marfan syndrome, which involves defects in the microfibrils of FBN1. Glaucoma is also associated with this syndrome, although the form of this pathology has not been well characterized [95].

FBLNs are matrix proteins capable of directing the deposition of TE on microfibrils. Different studies have revealed that FBLN4 and FBLN5 were essential for the formation of elastic fibers [67,96], and mutations in both molecules could cause cutis laxa, an inherited disorder associated with degeneration of elastic fibers leading to sagging skin, vascular tortuosity, and pulmonary emphysematous changes [97]. FBLN4 is expressed during early embryogenesis and is necessary for normal vascular, pulmonary, and skin development. Experimental studies on mice lacking FBLN4 have shown that the mice did not form elastic fibers and die perinatally. However, the absence of FBLN5 causes a less severe phenotype, identifying fragmented and irregular elastic fibers in the skin, lungs, and aorta.

Although differences in the distribution of microfibrils have been identified in eye diseases, such as keratoconus [98], limited ophthalmological research has focused on the mechanisms involved in the assembly of elastin, and no studies have directly focused on pterygium. Our group pioneered the analysis of these proteins in pterygium and showed that they have very important roles in the assembly of elastic fibers and participate in various supramolecular structures with binding sites to various proteins, including TE, fibrillin, and proteoglycans.

In our studies, all the FBLNs analyzed, except FBLN4, showed an increase in their protein expression in pterygium as compared with healthy conjunctivae. However, the messenger was only increased in FBLN5, and in the case of FBLN3, the expression even decreased. These results can be explained by the degradation of the mRNA. Thus, protein overexpression may be the result of mechanisms at the posttranscriptional level. However, the results obtained in relation to FBLN4, whose biological role is critical in binding to the LOX enzyme and FBN1 for the development of stable elastin, did not show any type of alteration as compared with the controls. Staying at normal levels could imply the effect of maturation and crosslinking of the rest of the overexpressed components, which could be related to the development of the disease.

Molecular studies have associated fibulin expression with disorders that affect multiple organs, including the eye [99]. These authors demonstrated a significant association between sequence variations in a member of the FBLN gene family and age-related macular degeneration, the most common cause of irreversible vision loss diseases in the developed world [44]. Studies have shown that these proteins were key in stabilizing the structure of the cornea and were synthesized by corneal cells at the epithelium or endothelium level [100].

LOXs are considered to be the main enzymes involved in collagen and elastin crosslinking in the ECM. The most important finding related to LOXs in ophthalmological research is associated with ocular pseudoexfoliation syndrome, which conditions the development and progression of glaucoma [101]. The research results provide evidence of a primary alteration in the LOXL1 gene (polymorphisms rs1048661 and rs3825942) that constitutes a risk factor involved in the alteration of elastic fiber homeostasis. Among the genetic factors, LOXL1 polymorphism constitutes the main genetic risk identified for the development of the disease [102]. In fact, it has been reported that LOXL1 knockout mice developed ocular pseudoexfoliation syndrome traits, which related decreased enzyme activity to a predisposition to the disease [103]. In addition, exposing cultures obtained from Tenon's capsule fibroblasts with high- and low-risk haplotypes of LOXL1 to factors such as ultraviolet radiation, hypoxia, oxidative stress states, or TGF-β has been shown to produce a significant increase in the expression levels of LOXL1 proteins and other elastin constituents, such as FBN1 and FBLN4. Therefore, it has been postulated that genetic factors in combination with other factors, particularly TGF-β activity and oxidative stress, could cooperate in the development of pseudoexfoliation syndrome [104–106].

According to studies of LOX and LOXL1, other related components in elastogenesis and ocular exfoliation syndrome have recently been reported. In fact, the presence of FBLN5 polymorphisms rs7149187: G > A and rs929608: T > C has been associated with high-risk variants in the development of the disease [107]. Therefore, the study of the components involved in the synthesis of elastin is an area of great interest in ophthalmological research.

Gene expression analyses have shown clear differences between primary pterygium and healthy conjunctiva [108]. Among the positively regulated genes, some encoded proteins involved in wound healing and components of the ECM, including different types of collagens, LOXL1, and various structural proteins. This was consistent with our RT-PCR results that showed a significant increase in LOXL1 mRNA in disease that was associated with a corresponding level of protein overexpression.

In our case, overexpressed LOXL1 mRNA and protein levels were identified in pterygium, but, in the case of LOX, the messenger remained stable and only the protein levels showed a significant increase in pterygium pathology. Related to this last result, we must remember that a selective role for LOXL1 has been proposed in elastin but not in collagen metabolism based on desmosine and hydroxyproline levels, which represent elastin and collagen crosslinks, respectively. The authors of one study reported significantly lower desmosine levels in various tissues with mutated LOXL1, while hydroxyproline levels remained unchanged. This apparently showed that one of the main substrates of LOX was collagen I. However, LOXL1, but not LOX, was specifically targeted to elastogenesis sites [72], showing that LOXL1 was closely related to elastic fibers, while LOX is more widely distributed.

Recently, transcriptional profiling to identify the key genes and pathways of pterygium and transcriptome analysis of mRNAs have been performed, indicating that differentially expressed RNAs were associated with ECM organization, blood vessel morphogenesis, and focal adhesion and that the upregulated genes were mainly associated with the ECM, cell adhesion, or migration [109,110].

In summary, taking into consideration all the studies carried out by our research group on the pathogenesis of pterygium throughout our scientific career, we can establish that the changes in the fibroelastic component of the ECM that occur in pterygium are based on the following:

- Increased synthesis and deposition of collagen fibers favor the immature form of collagen type III, and thus show a process of tissue remodeling;
- Increased protein levels in most of the constituents necessary for the development of elastic fibers, except FBLN4, whose biological roles are critical in the binding of the enzyme LOX and FBN1 for the development of stable elastin;
- Gene overexpression of TE, FBN1, FBLN5, and LOXL1, while the expression levels of LOX, as well as FBLN2 and -4, are comparable to those of controls.

Future research in this regard is strongly recommended, since, in our opinion, the FBLN4 and the LOX protein family should be considered to be important targets for the development of future therapies for treating diseases involving remodeling of extracellular matrix.

8. Conclusions

In conclusion, we can affirm that the two most important fibrillar proteins of the ECM of the conjunctival stroma, collagen, and elastin, as well as several constituents involved in elastic fiber assembly are overexpressed in human pterygium; thus, supporting the hypothesis that there is dysregulation in the synthesis and crosslinking of the fibroelastic component, constituting an important pathogenetic mechanism for the development of the disease.

Author Contributions: Conceptualization, J.M.-L. and G.P.; investigation, J.M.-L., C.P.-R., B.P.-K. and J.B.; writing—original draft preparation, G.P.; writing and review, S.B.-M., B.P.-K. and G.P.; editing, S.B.-M. and G.P.; supervision, C.P.-R., J.B. and G.P.; funding acquisition, G.P. All authors have read and agreed to the published version of the manuscript.

Funding: Financial support from the CIBER-BBN is acknowledged.

Institutional Review Board Statement: Not applicable.

Informed Consent Statement: Not applicable.

Data Availability Statement: Not applicable.

Conflicts of Interest: The authors declare no conflict of interest.

References

1. Tan, D.T.; Chee, S.P.; Dear, K.B.; Lim, A.S. Effect of pterygium morphology on pterygium recurrence in a controlled trial comparing conjunctival autografting with bare sclera excision. *Arch. Ophthalmol.* **1997**, *115*, 1235–1240, Erratum in *Arch. Ophthalmol.* **1998**, *116*, 552. [CrossRef]
2. Saw, S.M.; Tan, D. Pterygium: Prevalence, demography and risk factors. *Ophthalmic Epidemiol.* **1999**, *6*, 219–228. [CrossRef]
3. Rezvan, F.; Khabazkhoob, M.; Hooshmand, E.; Yekta, A.; Saatchi, M.; Hashemi, H. Prevalence and risk factors of pterygium: A systematic review and meta-analysis. *Surv. Ophthalmol.* **2018**, *63*, 719–735. [CrossRef]
4. Luthra, R.; Nemesure, B.B.; Wu, S.Y.; Xie, S.H.; Leske, M.C.; Barbados Eye Studies Group. Frequency and risk factors for pterygium in the Barbados Eye Study. *Arch. Ophthalmol.* **2001**, *119*, 1827–1832. [CrossRef]
5. Chui, J.; Di Girolamo, N.; Wakefield, D.; Coroneo, M.T. The pathogenesis of pterygium: Current concepts and their therapeutic implications. *Ocul. Surf.* **2008**, *6*, 24–43. [CrossRef]

6. Kau, H.C.; Tsai, C.C.; Lee, C.F.; Kao, S.C.; Hsu, W.M.; Liu, J.H.; Wei, Y.H. Increased oxidative DNA damage, 8-hydroxydeoxyguanosine, in human pterygium. *Eye* **2006**, *20*, 826–831. [CrossRef] [PubMed]
7. Perra, M.T.; Maxia, C.; Corbu, A.; Minerba, L.; Demurtas, P.; Colombari, R.; Murtas, D.; Bravo, S.; Piras, F.; Sirigu, P. Oxidative stress in pterygium: Relationship between p53 and 8- hydroxydeoxyguanosine. *Mol. Vis.* **2006**, *12*, 1136–1142.
8. Tan, D.T.; Tang, W.Y.; Liu, Y.P.; Goh, H.S.; Smith, D.R. Apoptosis and apoptosis related gene expression in normal conjunctiva and pterygium. *Br. J. Ophthalmol.* **2000**, *84*, 212–216. [CrossRef] [PubMed]
9. Maxia, C.; Perra, M.T.; Demurtas, P.; Minerba, L.; Murtas, D.; Piras, F.; Corbu, A.; Gotuzzo, D.C.; Cabrera, R.G.; Ribatti, D.; et al. Expression of survivin protein in pterygium and relationship with oxidative DNA damage. *J. Cell Mol. Med.* **2008**, *12*, 2372–2380, Erratum in *J. Cell Mol. Med.* **2009**, *13*, 207–209. [CrossRef] [PubMed]
10. Detorakis, E.T.; Sourvinos, G.; Tsamparlakis, J.; Spandidos, D.A. Evaluation of loss of heterozygosity and microsatellite instability in human pterygium: Clinical correlations. *Br. J. Ophthalmol.* **1998**, *82*, 1324–1328. [CrossRef]
11. Tan, D.T.; Lim, A.S.; Goh, H.S.; Smith, D.R. Abnormal expression of the p53 tumor suppressor gene in the conjunctiva of patients with pterygium. *Am. J. Ophthalmol.* **1997**, *123*, 404–405. [CrossRef]
12. Chen, P.L.; Cheng, Y.W.; Chiang, C.C.; Tseng, S.H.; Chau, P.S.; Tsai, Y.Y. Hypermethylation of the p16 gene promoter in pterygia and its association with the expression of DNA methyltransferase 3b. *Mol. Vis.* **2006**, *12*, 1411–1416.
13. Tong, L. Expression of p27(KIP1) and cyclin D1, and cell proliferation in human pterygium. *Br. J. Ophthalmol.* **2008**, *92*, 157. [CrossRef] [PubMed]
14. Tsai, Y.Y.; Cheng, Y.W.; Lee, H.; Tsai, F.J.; Tseng, S.H.; Chang, K.C. P53 gene mutation spectrum and the relationship between gene mutation and protein levels in pterygium. *Mol. Vis.* **2005**, *11*, 50–55. [PubMed]
15. Schneider, B.G.; John-Aryankalayil, M.; Rowsey, J.J.; Dushku, N.; Reid, T.W. Accumulation of p53 protein in pterygia is not accompanied by TP53 gene mutation. *Exp. Eye Res.* **2006**, *82*, 91–98. [CrossRef]
16. Di Girolamo, N.; Kumar, R.K.; Coroneo, M.T.; Wakefield, D. UVB-mediated induction of interleukin-6 and -8 in pterygia and cultured human pterygium epithelial cells. *Investig. Ophthalmol. Vis. Sci.* **2002**, *43*, 3430–3437.
17. Hong, S.; Choi, J.Y.; Lee, H.K.; Seong, G.J.; Seo, K.Y.; Kim, E.K.; Byeon, S.H. Expression of neurotrophic factors in human primary pterygeal tissue and selective TNF-alpha induced stimulation of ciliary neurotrophic factor in pterygeal fibroblasts. *Exp. Toxicol. Pathol.* **2008**, *60*, 513–520. [CrossRef] [PubMed]
18. Nolan, T.M.; Di Girolamo, N.; Coroneo, M.T.; Wakefield, D. Proliferative effects of heparin binding epidermal growth factor-like growth factor on pterygium epithelial cells and fibroblasts. *Investig. Ophthalmol. Vis. Sci.* **2004**, *45*, 110–113. [CrossRef] [PubMed]
19. Jin, J.; Guan, M.; Sima, J.; Gao, G.; Zhang, M.; Liu, Z.; Fant, J.; Ma, J.X. Decreased pigment epithelium-derived factor and increased vascular endothelial growth factor levels in pterygia. *Cornea* **2003**, *22*, 473–477. [CrossRef]
20. Kria, L.; Ohira, A.; Amemiya, T. Immunohistochemical localization of basic fibroblast growth factor, platelet derived growth factor, transforming growth factor-beta and tumor necrosis factor-alpha in the pterygium. *Acta Histochem.* **1996**, *98*, 195–201. [CrossRef]
21. Aspiotis, M.; Tsanou, E.; Gorezis, S.; Ioachim, E.; Skyrlas, A.; Stefaniotou, M.; Malamou-Mitsi, V. Angiogenesis in pterygium: Study of microvessel density, vascular endothelial growth factor, and thrombospondin-1. *Eye* **2007**, *21*, 1095–1101. [CrossRef] [PubMed]
22. Lee, D.H.; Cho, H.J.; Kim, J.T.; Choi, J.S.; Joo, C.K. Expression of vascular endothelial growth factor and inducible nitric oxide synthase in pterygia. *Cornea* **2001**, *20*, 738–742. [CrossRef]
23. Martín-López, J.; Pérez-Rico, C.; García-Honduvilla, N.; Buján, J.; Pascual, G. Elevated blood/lymphatic vessel ratio in pterygium and its relationship with vascular endothelial growth factor (VEGF) distribution. *Histol. Histopathol.* **2019**, *34*, 917–929. [CrossRef]
24. Reid, T.W.; Dushku, N. Does human papillomavirus cause pterygium? *Br. J. Ophthalmol.* **2003**, *87*, 806–808. [CrossRef]
25. Detorakis, E.T.; Sourvinos, G.; Spandidos, D.A. Detection of herpes simplex virus and human papilloma virus in ophthalmic pterygium. *Cornea* **2001**, *20*, 164–167. [CrossRef] [PubMed]
26. Dake, Y.; Mukae, R.; Soda, Y.; Kaneko, M.; Amemiya, T. Immunohistochemical localization of collagen types I, II, III, and IV in pterygium tissues. *Acta Histochem.* **1989**, *87*, 71–74. [CrossRef]
27. Naib-Majani, W.; Eltohami, I.; Wernert, N.; Watts, W.; Tschesche, H.; Pleyer, U.; Breipohl, W. Distribution of extracellular matrix proteins in pterygia: An immunohistochemical study. *Graefes Arch. Clin. Exp. Ophthalmol.* **2004**, *242*, 332–338. [CrossRef]
28. Wang, I.J.; Hu, F.R.; Chen, P.J.; Lin, C.T. Mechanism of abnormal elastin gene expression in the pinguecular part of pterygia. *Am. J. Pathol.* **2000**, *157*, 1269–1276. [CrossRef]
29. Di Girolamo, N.; McCluskey, P.; Lloyd, A.; Coroneo, M.T.; Wakefield, D. Expression of MMPs and TIMPs in human pterygia and cultured pterygium epithelial cells. *Investig. Ophthalmol. Vis. Sci.* **2000**, *41*, 671–679.
30. Bonnans, C.; Chou, J.; Werb, Z. Remodelling the extracellular matrix in development and disease. *Nat. Rev. Mol. Cell Biol.* **2014**, *15*, 786–801. [CrossRef]
31. Kato, N.; Shimmura, S.; Kawakita, T.; Miyashita, H.; Ogawa, Y.; Yoshida, S.; Higa, K.; Okano, H.; Tsubota, K. Beta-catenin activation and epithelial-mesenchymal transition in the pathogenesis of pterygium. *Investig. Ophthalmol. Vis. Sci.* **2007**, *48*, 1511–1517. [CrossRef] [PubMed]
32. Taylor, M.A.; Parvani, J.G.; Schiemann, W.P. The pathophysiology of epithelialmesenchymal transition induced by transforming growth factor-beta in normal and malignant mammary epithelial cells. *J. Mammary Gland Biol. Neoplasia* **2010**, *15*, 169–190. [CrossRef] [PubMed]

33. Zeisberg, M.; Neilson, E.G. Biomarkers for epithelial-mesenchymal transitions. *J. Clin. Investig.* **2009**, *119*, 429–1437. [CrossRef] [PubMed]
34. Torricelli, A.A.; Santhanam, A.; Wu, J.; Singh, V.; Wilson, S.E. The corneal fibrosis response to epithelial-stromal injury. *Exp. Eye Res.* **2016**, *142*, 110–118. [CrossRef]
35. Chui, J.; Coroneo, M.T.; Tat, L.T.; Crouch, R.; Wakefield, D.; Di Girolamo, N. Ophthalmic pterygium: A stem cell disorder with premalignant features. *Am. J. Pathol.* **2011**, *178*, 817–827. [CrossRef]
36. Chen, S.Y.; Mahabole, M.; Horesh, E.; Wester, S.; Goldberg, J.L.; Tseng, S.C. Isolation and characterization of mesenchymal progenitor cells from human orbital adipose tissue. *Investig. Ophthalmol. Vis. Sci.* **2014**, *55*, 4842–4852. [CrossRef]
37. Galligan, C.L.; Fish, E.N. The role of circulating fibrocytes in inflammation and autoimmunity. *J. Leukoc. Biol.* **2013**, *93*, 45–50. [CrossRef]
38. Kria, L.; Ohira, A.; Amemiya, T. Growth factors in cultured pterygium fibroblasts: Immunohistochemical and ELISA analysis. *Graefes Arch. Clin. Exp. Ophthalmol.* **1998**, *236*, 702–708. [CrossRef]
39. Lee, K.; Young Lee, S.; Park, S.Y.; Yang, H. Antifibrotic effect of pirfenidone on human pterygium fibroblasts. *Curr. Eye Res.* **2014**, *39*, 680–685. [CrossRef]
40. Lee, S.B.; Li, D.Q.; Tan, D.T.; Meller, D.C.; Tseng, S.C. Suppression of TGF-beta signaling in both normal conjunctival fibroblasts and pterygial body fibroblasts by amniotic membrane. *Curr. Eye Res.* **2000**, *20*, 325–334. [CrossRef]
41. Sha, X.; Wen, Y.; Liu, Z.; Song, L.; Peng, J.; Xie, L. Inhibition of α-smooth muscle actin expression and migration of pterygium fibroblasts by coculture with amniotic mesenchymal stem cells. *Curr. Eye Res.* **2014**, *39*, 1081–1089. [CrossRef]
42. Di Girolamo, N.; Chui, J.; Coroneo, M.T.; Wakefield, D. Pathogenesis of pterygia: Role of cytokines, growth factors, and matrix metalloproteinases. *Prog. Retin Eye Res.* **2004**, *23*, 195–228. [CrossRef] [PubMed]
43. Fox, T.; Gotlinger, K.H.; Dunn, M.W.; Lee, O.L.; Milman, T.; Zaidman, G.; Schwartzman, M.L.; Bellner, L. Dysregulated heme oxygenase-ferritin system in pterygium pathogenesis. *Cornea* **2013**, *32*, 1276–1282. [CrossRef]
44. Stone, E.M.; Braun, T.A.; Russell, S.R.; Kuehn, M.H.; Lotery, A.J.; Moore, P.A.; Eastman, C.G.; Casavant, T.L.; Sheffield, V.C. Missense variations in the fibulin 5 gene and age-related macular degeneration. *N. Engl. J. Med.* **2004**, *35*, 346–353. [CrossRef]
45. Li, F.; Xu, H.; Zeng, Y.; Yin, Z.Q. Overexpression of fibulin-5 in retinal pigment epithelial cells inhibits cell proliferation and migration and downregulates VEGF, CXCR4, and TGFB1 expression in cocultured choroidal endothelial cells. *Curr. Eye Res.* **2012**, *37*, 540–548. [CrossRef]
46. Ritch, R. Exfoliation syndrome-the most common identifiable cause of open-angle glaucoma. *J. Glaucoma* **1994**, *3*, 176–177. [CrossRef]
47. Thorleifsson, G.; Magnusson, K.P.; Sulem, P.; Walters, G.B.; Gudbjartsson, D.F.; Stefansson, H.; Jonsson, T.; Jonasdottir, A.; Jonasdottir, A.; Stefansdottir, G.; et al. Common sequence variants in the LOXL1 gene confer susceptibility to exfoliation glaucoma. *Science* **2007**, *317*, 1397–1400. [CrossRef] [PubMed]
48. Dudakova, L.; Liskova, P.; Trojek, T.; Palos, M.; Kalasova, S.; Jirsova, K. Changes in lysyl oxidase (LOX) distribution and its decreased activity in keratoconus corneas. *Exp. Eye Res.* **2012**, *104*, 74–81. [CrossRef]
49. Austin, P.; Jakobiec, F.A.; Iwamoto, T. Elastodysplasia and elastodystrophy as the pathologic bases of ocular pterygia and pinguecula. *Ophthalmology* **1983**, *90*, 96–109. [CrossRef]
50. Ihanamäki, T.; Pelliniemi, L.J.; Vuorio, E. Collagens and collagen-related matrix components in the human and mouse eye. *Prog. Retin. Eye Res.* **2004**, *23*, 403–434. [CrossRef] [PubMed]
51. Tuori, A.; Uusitalo, H.; Burgeson, R.E.; Terttunen, J.; Virtanen, I. The immunohistochemical composition of the human corneal basement membrane. *Cornea* **1996**, *15*, 286–294. [CrossRef]
52. Fukuda, K.; Chikama, T.; Nakamura, M.; Nishida, T. Differential distribution of subchains of the basement membrane components type IV collagen and laminin among the amniotic membrane, cornea, and conjunctiva. *Cornea* **1999**, *18*, 73–79. [CrossRef]
53. Pérez-Rico, C.; Pascual, G.; Sotomayor, S.; Montes-Mollón, M.Á.; Trejo, C.; Sasaki, T.; Mecham, R.; Bellón, J.M.; Buján, J. Tropoelastin and fibulin overexpression in the subepithelial connective tissue of human pterygium. *Am. J. Ophthalmol.* **2011**, *151*, 44–52. [CrossRef]
54. Mecham, R.P. Elastin synthesis and fiber assembly. *Ann. N. Y. Acad. Sci.* **1991**, *624*, 137–146. [CrossRef]
55. Wagenseil, J.E.; Mecham, R.P. New insights into elastic fiber assembly. *Birth Defects Res. C Embryo Today* **2007**, *81*, 229–240. [CrossRef]
56. Watanabe, M.; Sawai, T. Alteration of cross-linking amino acids of elastin in human aorta in association with dissecting aneurysm: Analysis using high performance liquid chromatography. *Tohoku J. Exp. Med.* **1999**, *187*, 291–303. [CrossRef] [PubMed]
57. Trask, T.M.; Trask, B.C.; Ritty, T.M.; Abrams, W.R.; Rosenbloom, J.; Mecham, R.P. Interaction of tropoelastin with the amino-terminal domains of fibrillin-1 and fibrillin-2 suggests a role for the fibrillins in elastic fiber assembly. *J. Biol. Chem.* **2000**, *275*, 24400–24406. [CrossRef] [PubMed]
58. Tiedemann, K.; Bätge, B.; Müller, P.K.; Reinhardt, D.P. Interactions of fibrillin-1 with heparin/heparan sulfate, implications for microfibrillar assembly. *J. Biol. Chem.* **2001**, *276*, 36035–36042. [CrossRef] [PubMed]
59. Argraves, W.S.; Dickerson, K.; Burgess, W.H.; Ruoslahti, E. Fibulin, a novel protein that interacts with the fibronectin receptor beta subunit cytoplasmic domain. *Cell* **1989**, *58*, 623–629. [CrossRef]
60. Argraves, W.S.; Greene, L.M.; Cooley, M.A.; Gallagher, W.M. Fibulins: Physiological and disease perspectives. *EMBO Rep.* **2003**, *4*, 1127–1131. [CrossRef] [PubMed]

61. Yanagisawa, H.; Davis, E.C. Unraveling the mechanism of elastic fiber assembly: The roles of short fibulins. *Int. J. Biochem. Cell Biol.* **2010**, *42*, 1084–1093. [CrossRef] [PubMed]
62. Visconti, R.P.; Barth, J.L.; Keeley, F.W.; Little, C.D. Codistribution analysis of elastin and related fibrillar proteins in early vertebrate development. *Matrix Biol.* **2003**, *22*, 109–121. [CrossRef]
63. McLaughlin, P.J.; Chen, Q.; Horiguchi, M.; Starcher, B.C.; Stanton, J.B.; Broekelmann, T.J.; Marmorstein, A.D.; McKay, B.; Mecham, R.; Nakamura, T.; et al. Targeted disruption of fibulin-4 abolishes elastogenesis and causes perinatal lethality in mice. *Mol. Cell Biol.* **2006**, *26*, 1700–1709. [CrossRef] [PubMed]
64. Horiguchi, M.; Inoue, T.; Ohbayashi, T.; Hirai, M.; Noda, K.; Marmorstein, L.Y.; Yabe, D.; Takagi, K.; Akama, T.O.; Kita, T.; et al. Fibulin-4 conducts proper elastogenesis via interaction with cross-linking enzyme lysyl oxidase. *Proc. Natl. Acad. Sci. USA* **2009**, *106*, 19029–19034. [CrossRef]
65. Huang, J.; Davis, E.C.; Chapman, S.L.; Budatha, M.; Marmorstein, L.Y.; Word, R.A.; Yanagisawa, H. Fibulin-4 deficiency results in ascending aortic aneurysms: A potential link between abnormal smooth muscle cell phenotype and aneurysm progression. *Circ. Res.* **2010**, *106*, 583–592. [CrossRef]
66. Nakamura, T.; Lozano, P.R.; Ikeda, Y.; Iwanaga, Y.; Hinek, A.; Minamisawa, S.; Cheng, C.F.; Kobuke, K.; Dalton, N.; Takada, Y.; et al. Fibulin5/DANCE is essential for elastogenesis in vivo. *Nature* **2002**, *415*, 171–175. [CrossRef]
67. Yanagisawa, H.; Davis, E.C.; Starcher, B.C.; Ouchi, T.; Yanagisawa, M.; Richardson, J.A.; Olson, E.N. Fibulin-5 is an elastin-binding protein essential for elastic fibre development in vivo. *Nature* **2002**, *415*, 168–171. [CrossRef]
68. Zhang, H.Y.; Timpl, R.; Sasaki, T.; Chu, M.L.; Ekblom, P. Fibulin-1 and fibulin-2 expression during organogenesis in the developing mouse embryo. *Dev. Dyn.* **1996**, *205*, 348–364. [CrossRef]
69. Csiszar, K. Lysyl oxidases: A novel multifunctional amine oxidase family. *Prog. Nucleic Acid Res. Mol. Biol.* **2001**, *70*, 1–32. [CrossRef]
70. Thomassin, L.; Werneck, C.C.; Broekelmann, T.J.; Gleyzal, C.; Hornstra, I.K.; Mecham, R.P.; Sommer, P. The Pro-regions of lysyl oxidase and lysyl oxidase-like 1 are required for deposition onto elastic fibers. *J. Biol. Chem.* **2005**, *280*, 42848–42855. [CrossRef]
71. Hirai, M.; Horiguchi, M.; Ohbayashi, T.; Kita, T.; Chien, K.R.; Nakamura, T. Latent TGF-betabinding protein 2 binds to DANCE/fibulin-5 and regulates elastic fiber assembly. *EMBO J.* **2007**, *26*, 3283–3295. [CrossRef] [PubMed]
72. Liu, X.; Zhao, Y.; Gao, J.; Pawlyk, B.; Starcher, B.; Spencer, J.A.; Yanagisawa, H.; Zuo, J.; Li, T. Elastic fiber homeostasis requires lysyl oxidase-like 1 protein. *Nat. Genet.* **2004**, *36*, 178–182. [CrossRef] [PubMed]
73. Papke, C.L.; Yanagisawa, H. Fibulin-4 and fibulin-5 in elastogenesis and beyond: Insights from mouse and human studies. *Matrix Biol.* **2014**, *37*, 142–149. [CrossRef] [PubMed]
74. Hornstra, I.K.; Birge, S.; Starcher, B.; Bailey, A.J.; Mecham, R.P.; Shapiro, S.D. Lysyl oxidase is required for vascular and diaphragmatic development in mice. *J. Biol. Chem.* **2003**, *278*, 14387–14393. [CrossRef] [PubMed]
75. Kennedy, M.; Kim, K.H.; Harten, B.; Brown, J.; Planck, S.; Meshul, C.; Edelhauser, H.; Rosenbaum, J.T.; Armstrong, C.A.; Ansel, J.C. Ultraviolet irradiation induces the production of multiple cytokines by human corneal cells. *Investig. Ophthalmol. Vis. Sci.* **1997**, *38*, 2483–2491.
76. Di Girolamo, N.; Coroneo, M.T.; Wakefield, D. UVB-elicited induction of MMP-1 expression in human ocular surface epithelial cells is mediated through the ERK1/2 MAPKdependent pathway. *Investig. Ophthalmol. Vis. Sci.* **2003**, *44*, 4705–4714. [CrossRef]
77. Nolan, T.M.; DiGirolamo, N.; Sachdev, N.H.; Hampartzoumian, T.; Coroneo, M.T.; Wakefield, D. The role of ultraviolet irradiation and heparin-binding epidermal growth factor-like growth factor in the pathogenesis of pterygium. *Am. J. Pathol.* **2003**, *162*, 567–574. [CrossRef]
78. Chen, J.K.; Tsai, R.J.; Lin, S.S. Fibroblasts isolated from human pterygia exhibit transformed cell characteristics. *In Vitro Cell Dev. Biol. Anim.* **1994**, *30*, 243–248. [CrossRef]
79. Kim, S.W.; Kim, H.I.; Thapa, B.; Nuwormegbe, S.; Lee, K. Critical Role of mTORC2-Akt signaling in TGF-β1-induced myofibroblast differentiation of human pterygium fibroblasts. *Investig. Ophthalmol. Vis. Sci.* **2019**, *60*, 82–92. [CrossRef]
80. Zhong, L.; Li, M. Transforming growth factor-beta1 induced cultured human trabecular cells to produce elastin. *Zhonghua Yan Ke Za Zhi* **1999**, *35*, 383–385. [PubMed]
81. Dushku, N.; John, M.K.; Schultz, G.S.; Reid, T.W. Pterygia pathogenesis: Corneal invasion by matrix metalloproteinase expressing altered limbal epithelial basal cells. *Arch. Ophthalmol.* **2001**, *119*, 695–706. [CrossRef] [PubMed]
82. Lan, W.; Chen, S.; Tong, L. MicroRNA-215 Regulates Fibroblast Function: Insights from a Human Fibrotic Disease. *Cell Cycle* **2015**, *14*, 1973–1984. [CrossRef]
83. Han, S.; Chen, Y.; Gao, Y.; Sun, B.; Kong, Y. MicroRNA-218-5p inhibit the migration and proliferation of pterygium epithelial cells by targeting EGFR via PI3K/Akt/mTOR signaling pathway. *Exp. Eye Res.* **2019**, *178*, 37–45. [CrossRef]
84. Li, X.; Dai, Y.; Xu, J. MiR-21 promotes pterygium cell proliferation through the PTEN/AKT pathway. *Mol. Vis.* **2018**, *24*, 485–494.
85. Lee, J.H.; Jung, S.A.; Kwon, Y.A.; Chung, J.L.; Kim, U.S. Expression of microRNAs in fibroblast of pterygium. *Int. J. Ophthalmol.* **2016**, *9*, 967–972. [CrossRef]
86. Riau, A.K.; Wong, T.T.; Lan, W.; Finger, S.N.; Chaurasia, S.S.; Hou, A.H.; Chen, S.; Yu, S.J.; Tong, L. Aberrant DNA methylation of matrix remodeling and cell adhesion related genes in pterygium. *PLoS ONE* **2011**, *6*, e14687, Erratum in *PLoS ONE* **2011**, *6*, doi:10.1371/annotation/814c14d4-eee6-44e2-bea8-cac11a0bae8f. [CrossRef]
87. Bernstein, E.F.; Chen, Y.Q.; Tamai, K.; Shepley, K.J.; Resnik, K.S.; Zhang, H.; Tuan, R.; Mauviel, A.; Uitto, J. Enhanced elastin and fibrillin gene expression in chronically photodamaged skin. *J. Investig. Dermatol.* **1994**, *103*, 182–186. [CrossRef] [PubMed]

88. Schwartz, E.; Feinberg, E.; Lebwohl, M.; Mariani, T.J.; Boyd, C.D. Ultraviolet radiation increases tropoelastin accumulation by a post-transcriptional mechanism in dermal fibroblasts. *J. Investig. Dermatol.* **1995**, *105*, 65–69. [CrossRef] [PubMed]
89. Alexander, R.A.; Garner, A. Elastic and precursor fibres in the normal human eye. *Exp. Eye Res.* **1983**, *36*, 305–315. [CrossRef]
90. Umihira, J.; Nagata, S.; Nohara, M.; Hanai, T.; Usuda, N.; Segawa, K. Localization of elastin in the normal and glaucomatous human trabecular meshwork. *Investig. Ophthalmol. Vis. Sci.* **1994**, *35*, 486–494.
91. Wei, X.; Cai, S.P.; Zhang, X.; Li, X.; Chen, X.; Liu, X. Is low dose of estrogen beneficial for prevention of glaucoma? *Med. Hypotheses* **2012**, *79*, 377–380. [CrossRef]
92. Damasceno, R.W.; Heindl, L.M.; Hofmann-Rummelt, C.; Belfort, R.; Schlötzer-Schrehardt, U.; Kruse, F.E.; Holbach, L.M. Pathogenesis of involutional ectropion and entropion: The involvement of matrix metalloproteinases in elastic fiber degradation. *Orbit* **2011**, *30*, 132–139. [CrossRef]
93. Cirulis, J.T.; Bellingham, C.M.; Davis, E.C.; Hubmacher, D.; Reinhardt, D.P.; Mecham, R.P.; Keeley, F.W. Fibrillins, fibulins, and matrix-associated glycoprotein modulate the kinetics and morphology of in vitro self-assembly of a recombinant elastin-like polypeptide. *Biochemistry* **2008**, *47*, 12601–12613. [CrossRef]
94. Mohammad-Salih, P.A.; Sharif, A.F. Analysis of pterygium size and induced corneal astigmatism. *Cornea* **2008**, *27*, 434–438. [CrossRef]
95. Kuchtey, J.; Chang, T.C.; Panagis, L.; Kuchtey, R.W. Marfan syndrome caused by a novel FBN1 mutation with associated pigmentary glaucoma. *Am. J. Med. Genet. A* **2013**, *161*, 880–883. [CrossRef]
96. Kobayashi, N.; Kostka, G.; Garbe, J.H.; Keene, D.R.; Bächinger, H.P.; Hanisch, F.G.; Markova, D.; Tsuda, T.; Timpl, R.; Chu, M.L.; et al. A comparative analysis of the fibulin protein family. Biochemical characterization, binding interactions, and tissue localization. *J. Biol. Chem.* **2007**, *282*, 11805–11816. [CrossRef]
97. Hu, Q.; Loeys, B.L.; Coucke, P.J.; De Paepe, A.; Mecham, R.P.; Choi, J.; Davis, E.C.; Urban, Z. Fibulin-5 mutations: Mechanisms of impaired elastic fiber formation in recessive cutis laxa. *Hum. Mol. Genet.* **2006**, *15*, 3379–3386. [CrossRef] [PubMed]
98. White, T.L.; Lewis, P.N.; Young, R.D.; Kitazawa, K.; Inatomi, T.; Kinoshita, S.; Meek, K.M. Elastic microfibril distribution in the cornea: Differences between normal and keratoconic stroma. *Exp. Eye Res.* **2017**, *159*, 40–48. [CrossRef] [PubMed]
99. Stone, E.M.; Lotery, A.J.; Munier, F.L.; Héon, E.; Piguet, B.; Guymer, R.H.; Vandenburgh, K.; Cousin, P.; Nishimura, D.; Swiderski, R.E.; et al. A single EFEMP1 mutation associated with both Malattia Leventinese and Doyne honeycomb retinal dystrophy. *Nat. Genet.* **1999**, *22*, 199–202. [CrossRef]
100. Ducros, E.; Berthaut, A.; Mirshahi, P.; Lemarchand, S.; Soria, J.; Legeais, J.M.; Mirshahi, M. Expression of extracellular matrix proteins fibulin-1 and fibulin-2 by human corneal fibroblasts. *Curr. Eye Res.* **2007**, *32*, 481–490. [CrossRef] [PubMed]
101. Schlötzer-Schrehardt, U.; Pasutto, F.; Sommer, P.; Hornstra, I.; Kruse, F.E.; Naumann, G.O.; Reis, A.; Zenkel, M. Genotype-correlated expression of lysyl oxidase-like 1 in ocular tissues of patients with pseudoexfoliation syndrome/glaucoma and normal patients. *Am. J. Pathol.* **2008**, *173*, 1724–1735. [CrossRef] [PubMed]
102. Chen, L.; Jia, L.; Wang, N.; Tang, G.; Zhang, C.; Fan, S.; Liu, W.; Meng, H.; Zeng, W.; Liu, N.; et al. Evaluation of LOXL1 polymorphisms in exfoliation syndrome in a Chinese population. *Mol. Vis.* **2009**, *15*, 2349–2357.
103. Wiggs, J.L.; Pasquale, L.R. Expression and regulation of LOXL1 and elastin-related genes in eyes with exfoliation syndrome. *J. Glaucoma* **2014**, *23*, S62–S63. [CrossRef]
104. Zenkel, M.; Krysta, A.; Pasutto, F.; Juenemann, A.; Kruse, F.E.; Schlötzer-Schrehardt, U. Regulation of lysyl oxidase-like 1 (LOXL1) and elastin-related genes by pathogenic factors associated with pseudoexfoliation syndrome. *Investig. Ophthalmol. Vis. Sci.* **2011**, *52*, 8488–8495. [CrossRef]
105. Zenkel, M.; Schlötzer-Schrehardt, U. Expression and regulation of LOXL1 and elastinrelated genes in eyes with exfoliation syndrome. *J. Glaucoma* **2014**, *23*, S48–S50. [CrossRef]
106. Gayathri, R.; Coral, K.; Sharmila, F.; Sripriya, S.; Sripriya, K.; Manish, P.; Shantha, B.; Ronnie, G.; Vijaya, L.; Narayanasamy, A. Correlation of Aqueous Humor Lysyl Oxidase Activity with TGF-ß Levels and LOXL1 Genotype in Pseudoexfoliation. *Curr. Eye Res.* **2016**, *41*, 1331–1338. [CrossRef]
107. Padhy, B.; Kapuganti, R.S.; Hayat, B.; Mohanty, P.P.; Alone, D.P. De novo variants in an extracellular matrix protein coding gene, fibulin-5 (FBLN5) are associated with pseudoexfoliation. *Eur. J. Hum. Genet.* **2019**, *27*, 1858–1866. [CrossRef] [PubMed]
108. Tong, L.; Chew, J.; Yang, H.; Ang, L.P.; Tan, D.T.; Beuerman, R.W. Distinct gene subsets in pterygia formation and recurrence: Dissecting complex biological phenomenon using genome wide expression data. *BMC Med. Genom.* **2009**, *2*, 14. [CrossRef]
109. Liu, X.; Zhang, J.; Nie, D.; Zeng, K.; Hu, H.; Tie, J.; Sun, L.; Peng, L.; Liu, X.; Wang, J. Comparative Transcriptomic Analysis to Identify the Important Coding and Non-coding RNAs Involved in the Pathogenesis of Pterygium. *Front. Genet.* **2021**, *15*, 646550. [CrossRef] [PubMed]
110. Chen, Y.; Wang, H.; Jiang, Y.; Zhang, X.; Wang, Q. Transcriptional profiling to identify the key genes and pathways of pterygium. *PeerJ* **2020**, *4*, 8. [CrossRef] [PubMed]

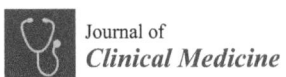

Article

Membrane of Plasma Rich in Growth Factors in Primary Pterygium Surgery Compared to Amniotic Membrane Transplantation and Conjunctival Autograft

Miriam Idoipe [1], Borja de la Sen-Corcuera [2,3], Ronald M. Sánchez-Ávila [2,*], Carmen Sánchez-Pérez [1], María Satué [1], Antonio Sánchez-Pérez [1], Gorka Orive [2,3], Francisco Muruzabal [2,3], Eduardo Anitua [2,3] and Luis Pablo [1]

[1] Ophthalmology Department, Miguel Servet University Hospital, 50009 Zaragoza, Spain; midoipe@gmail.com (M.I.); mamensp02@gmail.com (C.S.-P.); mariasatue@gmail.com (M.S.); asanch@telefonica.net (A.S.-P.); lpablo@unizar.es (L.P.)

[2] Regenerative Medicine Laboratory, Biotechnology Institute (BTI), 01007 Vitoria, Spain; bdelasen@bti-health.com (B.d.l.S.-C.); gorka.orive@bti-implant.es (G.O.); francisco.muruzabal@bti-implant.es (F.M.); eduardoan-itua@eduardoanitua.com (E.A.)

[3] Regenerative Medicine Laboratory, University Institute for Regenerative Medicine and Oral Implantology (UIRMI), 01007 Vitoria, Spain

* Correspondence: rsanchez@bti-health.com; Tel./Fax: +34-945-160-652

Abstract: This prospective and comparative study aimed to compare the use of a conjunctival autograft (CAG), plasma rich in growth factors fibrin membrane (mPRGF) or amniotic membrane transplantation (AMT) in primary pterygium surgery. Patients were assigned for surgery with CAG (group A), mPRGF (group B), or AMT (group C). Pterygium recurrence, Best Corrected Visual Acuity (BCVA), graft size (measured with anterior segment optical coherence tomography (AS-OCT)), and ocular surface symptoms (visual analogue scale (VAS) and ocular surface disease index (OSDI)) were evaluated. Thirteen eyes in group A, 26 in group B, and 10 in group C were evaluated. No changes in BCVA ($p > 0.05$) were found. Recurrence cases for groups A, B, and C were none, two, and two, respectively, and three cases of pyogenic granulomas in group A. The horizontal/vertical graft size was lower in group B vs group A ($p < 0.05$) from months 1 to 12. The improvement in VAS frequency for groups A, B, and C was: 35.5%, 86.2%, and 39.1%, respectively. The OSDI scale reduction for groups A, B, and C was: 12.7%, 39.0%, and 84.1%. The use of the three surgical techniques as a graft for primary pterygium surgery was safe and effective, showing similar results. The mPRGF graft represents an autologous novel approach for pterygium surgery.

Keywords: PRGF; pterygium surgery; amniotic membrane transplantation; conjunctival autograft; PRP; plasma rich in growth factors

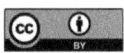

1. Introduction

Pterygium is defined as a fibrovascular formation of triangular morphology that extends from the conjunctiva to the cornea [1]. This neoformation is more frequent in the nasal sector [1], and it is characterized by inflammation and fibrosis, leading to tissue remodeling [2]. Histopathologically, it affects the conjunctival collagen, leading to elastotic degeneration; Bowman´s membrane and corneal surface destruction are observed along with stem cell alterations [2]. A higher prevalence has been found in regions located thirty-seven degrees above and below the equator, with a higher ultraviolet (UV) intensity [1]. Di Girolamo et al. [3] showed that UV radiation stimulated the expression of matrix metalloproteinase (MMP)-1 in human ocular epithelial cells. Moreover, Nolan et al. [4] found overexpression of heparin-binding epidermal growth factor (HB-EGF) in pterygial tissue caused by UV radiation, which is considered as a driving force in the development of pterygium as it is a potent mitogen. Tsai et al. [5] highlighted in their study the importance of UV-mediated oxidative DNA damage in the formation of pterygium.

The prevalence of pterygium in the worldwide population is 12%, while in Spain, it is 5.9% (95% CI: 4.3–7.9) [6,7]. The most frequent symptoms are nonspecific due to tear film alteration (irritation, burning, photophobia, tearing, and foreign body sensation). Other less frequent and more specific symptoms are pain due to ulceration or decreased visual acuity because of corneal invasion [8]. Excision surgery is the only effective procedure in the treatment of pterygium. The usual procedures, according to complexity, are simple excision [8], excision with conjunctival autograft (CAG) [8–10], excision with an amniotic membrane (AM) graft [11], excision with mitomycin C [9,12–14], excision with limbal autograft [8], and lamellar sclerokeratoplasty [8]. Pterygium surgery with CAG remains the gold standard procedure, and involves placing the donor tissue using either suture or with a biological adhesive [15]. Autograft suturing requires surgical experience and technical skills. Suzuki et al. [16] reported that the use of silk or nylon sutures causes conjunctival inflammation and the migration of Langerhans cells in the cornea. Other drawbacks are increased surgical time, patient discomfort, Dellen, symblepharon, or graft rupture [17,18].

AM grafting is a widely used technique in ocular surface surgery [19]. Preserved human AM can be used as a substrate to replace damaged mucosal surfaces and successfully reconstruct the cornea [20] or conjunctival tissues after ocular surface neoplasia excision [21], as well as to repair scleral and corneal melting and perforations [22,23] and has been successfully included in pterygium surgery [24]. AM transplantation (AMT) improves ocular surface epithelialization, reducing inflammation, vascularization, and scarring [2,19]. However, some complications, including granulomas, superior anterior scars, symblepharon, and recurrences, have been found after using these surgical techniques [25,26]. Recently, numerous investigations have shown the relevance of platelets in regeneration processes by releasing biological mediators such as growth factors [27,28]. Plasma Rich in Growth Factors (PRGF) is a standardized type of platelet-rich plasma (PRP) with specific characteristics that differentiate it from other blood-derived products [29,30]. PRGF has been used in different medical fields [31–33]. Several properties of PRGF, in addition to its autologous origin and the absence of preservatives and stabilizers offers broad applicability in the ophthalmic field by using several formulations (eye drops, injectables, fibrin membranes or fibrin clots) [34–36].

Several studies have evaluated the features of PRGF in its eye drop formulation (ePRGF); it has been well-tolerated, demonstrating proliferative, cell migration, anti-inflammatory, antibacterial and antifibrotic capabilities [34,36–38]. Several studies have been carried out to evaluate the stability and safety of ePRGF during its storage. These studies showed that ePRGF maintains its biological activity after 12 months of storage under frozen conditions, for 7 days of daily, and use even stored at room temperature. No contamination was observed in any of the different storage conditions and temperatures analyzed [39]. On the other hand, the tolerance and usefulness of autologous PRGF fibrin membrane (mPRGF) in ophthalmology have been evaluated as an adjuvant to nonpenetrating deep sclerectomy [40] or ocular surface disorders [41] with positive results. This study aims to provide information about the safety and efficacy of mPRGF as a graft for pterygium surgery, compared with CAG and AM grafts.

2. Materials and Methods

This prospective, comparative, and observational clinical study evaluates the clinical results in pterygium surgeries carried out between February 2017 and April 2019 at Miguel Servet University Hospital, Zaragoza (Spain). This study was carried out following the principles of the Declaration of Helsinki, the regional clinical research ethics committee (Aragon, Spain) approved the conduct of this study (Authorization C.P.-C.I. EC16/0031). Informed consent forms were signed by all patients included in this study.

2.1. Patients

Patients included in this study had to be over 18 years of age and have a primary pterygium diagnosis requiring excision surgery (grade 2 or greater) [1]. Patients must have visual acuity greater than 0.5 Snellen (decimal). The exclusion criteria were: eyelid or conjunctival abnormalities (trichiasis, entropion, symblepharon), blepharitis, dry eye disease, persistent epithelial defects, glaucoma, and retinal or autoimmune diseases. Patients were consecutively assigned to one of these three groups: group A (surgery performed with CAG), group B (surgery performed with fibrin membrane obtained by PRGF technique), group C (surgery performed with an AM graft, with the basement membrane facing up). In the particular case of the patients in group B, coagulation issues and thrombocytopenia were included as exclusion criteria. The type of treatment received was known only by the surgeon performing the excision and was only revealed after the follow-up time had concluded. The clinical follow-up times were the same for the three groups: days 1, 7, 15, and months 1, 3, 6, and 12; this was carried out by a surgeon who did not know the group to which the patient belongs (single blind). Data from previous studies comparing the use of conjunctival autografts and amniotic membranes were analyzed [42,43], and the calculated sample size required to detect significant differences, assuming an alpha error of 5% and a beta error of 10%, was 50 patients, including 15 patients in group A, 25 patients in group B, and 10 patients in group C, with missing cases estimated to be 10%.

2.2. Outcome Measures

The primary outcomes were pterygium recurrence, Best Corrected Visual Acuity (BCVA), and graft size. The BCVA measured with Snellen optotype (decimal) was transformed to LogMAR (Logarithm of the Minimum Angle of Resolution), and the intraocular pressure (IOP) (mmHg) was measured with a Goldmann applanation tonometer. The pterygium grade was evaluated with a slit lamp [1]: grade 1 (atrophic), grade 2 (intermediate), and grade 3 (fleshy). The pterygium recurrence was evaluated using the Solomon scale [19]. Anterior segment optical coherence tomography (AS-OCT) (DRI OCT Triton®, Topcon Europe Medical B.V, Capelle aan den Ijssel, The Netherlands) was used for the baseline measurements of the pterygium size (μm): 1. thickness of the limbus, 2. horizontal size, 3. total horizontal size, and 4. vertical size. During the postoperative follow-up, the conjunctival restoration zone was also measured with AS-OCT (μm): 1. graft central thickness, 2. graft thickness in the limbus, 3. graft horizontal size (measured between the sclerocorneal limbus to the nasal area of the excised conjunctiva), and 4. graft vertical size. Symptoms related to alterations in the ocular surface were also evaluated, including the Visual Analogue Scale (VAS) for frequency and severity, and the OSDI scale (Ocular Surface Disease Index) [44]. The presence of a conjunctival defect or other complications were also evaluated.

2.3. PRGF Preparation

For the preparation of the autologous mPRGF and ePRGF, an Endoret®-PRGF® ophthalmology kit (BTI Biotechnology Institute, S.L., Miñano, Alava, Spain) was used for each patient. Briefly, 50 mL of blood was extracted and processed following the protocol described by Anitua et al. [45]. Then, 12 mL of plasma was activated and incubated at 37 °C for one hour to obtain ePRGF. For the mPRGF preparation, fraction 2 (F2) (defined as 2 mL above the leukocyte layer) was used to obtain the mPRGF, while F1 (defined as the remaining plasma above F2) was discarded. For each membrane, 5 mL of F2 was activated and incubated at 37 °C for 20 minutes, and the obtained fibrin clot was conformed in a membrane shaper, obtaining mPRGF about 500 microns thick [41].

2.4. Surgical Procedures

The surgeries were carried out by the same surgeon (MIC). After pterygium excision, different grafts were applied to each patient. (a) Conjunctiva autograft: the superior conjunctiva was used as a donor site for the graft. The graft was placed with the epithelial side up, and the limbal edge was positioned toward the limbus. Finally, fibrin glue (Tissucol®, Baxter AG, Vienna, Austria) was applied to fix the graft. (b) PRGF membrane: the membrane was placed over the bare scleral bed. Tissucol® was applied at the scleral-PRGF membrane interface and held until complete gluing (see Figure 1). The patient received additional treatment with instilled ePRGF four times a day during the first month after the surgery. (c) Amniotic membrane graft: the AM was obtained from nonpreserved, lyophilized and cryopreserved samples on a cellulose nitrate filter. The epithelial/basement membrane side was positioned on the up side. Tissucol® was applied at the scleral-AM interface, and the AM was held until complete gluing was achieved. The postoperative treatment in all groups was the same: Chloramphenicol and Dexamethasone eye ointment for 24-hour with eye bandage and then Dexamethasone/Tobramycin eye drops with a decreasing dosage for twelve weeks.

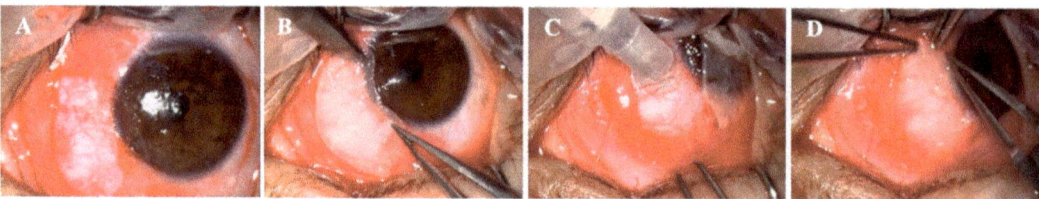

Figure 1. Use of mPRGF in pterygium surgery. (**A**) Bare sclera after pterigium surgery, (**B**) mPRGF was placed over the bare sclera and it was cut according to the size of the resected tissue, (**C**) one or two drops of fibrin glue was added to the bare sclera, and (**D**) mPRGF was placed over the fibrin glue, approximating the edges between the conjunctiva and the mPRGF to allow the gluing between them.

2.5. Statistical Analysis

The Kolmogorov–Smirnov test was performed to analyze the normal distribution. The continuous data were presented as mean, range, and standard deviation. A paired t-Student test or the Wilcoxon test was used to analyze the results obtained for all variables in each treatment group along the follow-up period. The ANOVA test, the Friedman test, or Cochran's Q (in case of proportions) was used for repeated measurements. For independent data, ANOVA test (normal distribution) and a subsequent Bonferroni post hoc analysis for multiple comparisons between groups, a Kruskal–Wallis test in the case of nonnormal distribution, and chi-square tests were applied. The statistical program SPSS version 20.0 (SPSS Inc., Chicago, IL, USA) was used for the statistical analyses. A level of $p < 0.05$ was considered significant for all statistical analysis.

3. Results

Forty-nine eyes (49 patients) with primary pterygium were included, all of them were classified as grade 2 [1] and were divided into three groups: group A (13 eyes, 26.5%), group B (26 eyes, 53.1%), and group C (10 eyes, 20.4%). The country where patients had lived the longest is presented in Table 1. Demographic data are presented in Table 2.

Table 1. The country where patients have lived the longest.

Country	Group A n (%)	Group B n (%)	Group C n (%)	Total n (%)
Ecuador	3 (6.1)	7 (14.3)	5 (10.2)	15 (30.6)
Spain *	1 (2.0)	7 (14.3)	2 (4.1)	10 (20.4)
Nicaragua	3 (6.1)	3 (6.1)	-	6 (12.2)
Colombia	2 (4.1)	2 (4.1)	-	4 (8.2)
Peru	1 (2.0)	1 (2.0)	1 (2.0)	3 (6.1)
Argelia	-	2 (4.1)	-	2 (4.1)
Brazil	1 (2.0)	-	-	1 (2.0)
Honduras	-	1 (2.0)	-	1 (2.0)
Romania	-	1 (2.0)	-	1 (2.0)

Table 1. Cont.

Country	Group A n (%)	Group B n (%)	Group C n (%)	Total n (%)
Senegal	1 (2.0)	-	-	1 (2.0)
Uruguay	-	1 (2.0)	-	1 (2.0)
Venezuela	-	-	1 (2.0)	1 (2.0)
Bolivia	-	-	1 (2.0)	1 (2.0)
France	1 (2.0)	-	-	1 (2.0)
Dominican Republic	-	1 (2.0)	-	1 (2.0)
Overall	13 (26.5)	26 (53.1)	10 (20.4)	49 (100)

* All from Zaragoza. Group A: conjunctival autograft. Group B: mPRGF. Group C: amniotic membrane.

Table 2. Demographics and sun protection.

	Group A	Group B	Group C	p-Value
Pacients, n (%)	13 (26.5)	26 (53.1)	10 (20.4)	-
Age, mean ± SD (range)	44.4 ± 12.9 (33.0–78.0)	47.5 ± 14.0 (31.0–77.0)	47.2 ± 14.0 (31.0–82.0)	0.791
Gender, M (%)	8 (61.5)	14 (53.8)	4 (40.0)	0.593
Race *				
Amerindian, n (%)	8 (61.5)	12 (46.2)	8 (80.0)	
African, n (%)	1 (7.7)	3 (11.5)	0 (0.0)	0.235
European, n (%)	4 (30.8)	11 (42.3)	2 (20.0)	
Evolution time of the pterygium, mean ± SD (range)	8.2 ± 4.6 (1.0–16.0)	6.1 ± 5.9 (1.0–30.0)	7.5 ± 5.5 (2.0–20.0)	0.503
Residence time in Zaragoza, mean ± SD (range)	16.2 ± 12.9 (1.0—50.0)	20.2 ± 22.1 (0.0–75.0)	23.8 ± 23.4 (6.0–82.0)	0.668
Hours of sun exposure per day, mean ± SD (range)	2.52 ± 3.62 (0.0–10.0)	3.92 ± 3.39 (0.0–10.0)	2.29 ± 2.57 (0.0–8.0)	0.306
Sun protection *				
None, n (%)	5 (38.5)	14 (53.8)	3 (30.0)	
Hat, n (%)	1 (7.7)	4 (15.4)	1 (10.0)	
UV filter glasses + Hat, n (%)	1 (7.7)	2 (7.7)	2 (20.0)	0.429
UV filter glasses (occasional), n (%)	1 (7.7)	0 (0.0)	0 (0.0)	
UV filter glasses (usually), n (%)	5 (38.5)	4 (15.4)	4 (40.0)	

Group A: conjunctival autograft, Group B: mPRGF, Group C: amniotic membrane, M: male, SD: standard deviation, * Percentage calculated within each group, UV: ultraviolet.

3.1. Visual Acuity and Intraocular Pressure

No changes in BCVA and IOP were observed between the baseline measurement and the end of each group's follow-up ($p > 0.05$). Furthermore, there were no significant differences among the treatment groups for BVCA and IOP at any follow-up time (see Figure 2). The IOP was maintained between 13 and 18 mmHg during follow-up in the three groups.

3.2. Pterygium Measurement (AS-OCT)

On average, the mPRGF was reabsorbed at 13 days, while the AM was reabsorbed on average at 16 days. No statistical differences were obtained between the groups ($p > 0.05$) in the postsurgical baseline measurements for any of the variables analyzed (see Table 3). However, significant differences were found among the treatment groups in each variable analyzed with AS-OCT during the follow-up time (see Table 3).

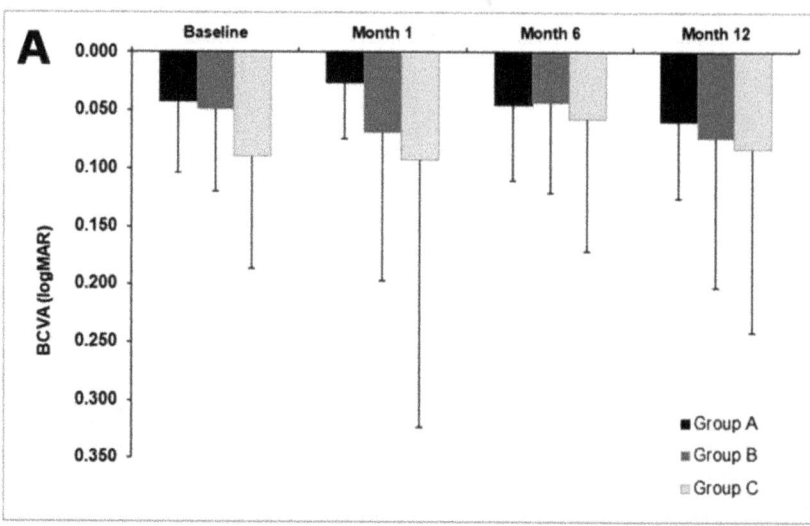
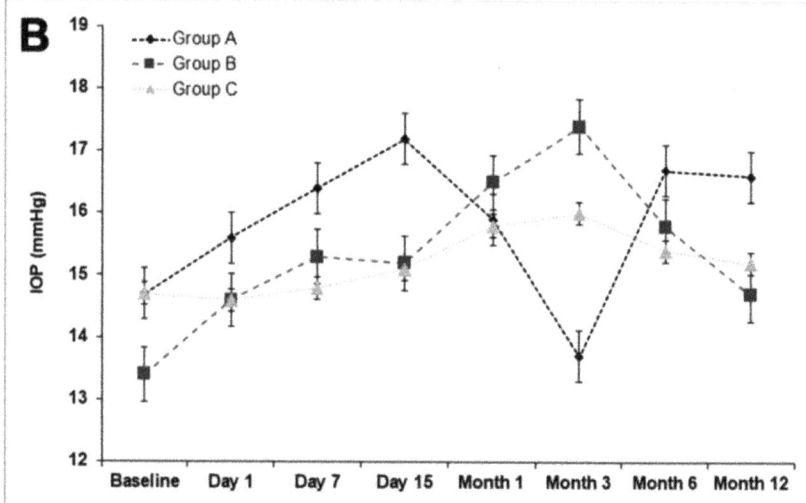

Figure 2. Visual acuity and intraocular pressure in the three treatment groups. (**A**) BCVA: best corrected visual acuity; Group A: conjunctival autograft; Group B: membrane - plasma rich in growth factors; Group C: amniotic membrane. No significant differences were found in visual acuity between the three groups ($p > 0.05$) during the follow-up time. (**B**). IOP: intraocular pressure; Group A: conjunctival autograft; Group B: membrane - plasma rich in growth factors; Group C: amniotic membrane. No significant differences were observed in IOP among the three groups ($p > 0.05$) during the entire follow-up time.

Table 3. Graft sizes in each treatment group along the follow-up period measured by AS-OCT.

		Group A Mean ± SD (μm)	Group B Mean ± SD (μm)	Group C Mean ± SD (μm)	p-Value
Thickness next to limbus	Baseline	471 ± 143	478 ± 163	424 ± 110	0.767
Horizontal size from limbus		2862 ± 964	3469 ± 1594	2387 ± 988	0.106
Total horizontal size		7755 ± 2152	7482 ± 2817	7971 ± 1878	0.876
Vertical size in limbus		6206 ± 1236	6010 ± 1666	5343 ± 2038	0.461
Graft central thickness	Day 1	611 ± 216	455 ± 240	412 ± 207	0.103
	Day 7	620 ± 257 **	359 ± 271	452 ± 155	0.020
	Day 15	356 ± 141	316 ± 286	337 ± 119	0.362
	Month 1	324 ± 131	207 ± 163	271 ± 114	0.089
	Month 3	252 ± 147 **	84 ± 148	231 ± 147 #	0.002
	Month 6	229 ± 90 **	102 ± 124	183 ± 45	0.011
	Month 12	151 ± 65	192 ± 109	190 ± 183	0.503
Graft thickness next to limbus	Day 1	459 ± 184	499 ± 417	412 ± 139	0.929
	Day 7	460 ± 232 *	248 ± 171	430 ± 183	0.005
	Day 15	365 ± 159	250 ± 193	274 ± 79	0.163
	Month 1	314 ± 114	259 ± 178	273 ± 109	0.770
	Month 3	250 ± 109 **	79 ± 118	230 ± 185 #	0.002
	Month 6	207 ± 60 *	96 ± 115	188 ± 98	0.036
	Month 12	200 ± 91	197 ± 115	116 ± 37	0.226
Graft horizontal size	Day 1	6499 ± 2192	5949 ± 2336	5645 ± 2047	0.673
	Day 7	5813 ± 1894 *	3639 ± 2554	4784 ± 945	0.044
	Day 15	5287 ± 2411	3314 ± 2523	5983 ± 1028	0.059
	Month 1	4079 ± 1309 **	1048 ± 1829	3903 ± 903 #	0.001
	Month 3	4598 ± 1492 **‡	1433 ± 2077	2626 ± 2346	0.003
	Month 6	3809 ± 1396 **	1433 ± 1908	2176 ± 1928	0.009
	Month 12	4815 ± 1426 *	1394 ± 1456	2299 ± 1970	0.003
Graft vertical size	Day 1	7356 ± 2322	7054 ± 2713	7882 ± 1153	0.651
	Day 7	7140 ± 2266	5230 ± 3640	6476 ± 1446	0.355
	Day 15	6298 ± 1619	5106 ± 3559	5983 ± 1097	0.442
	Month 1	6881 ± 959 **	4018 ± 3071	5320 ± 1906	0.007
	Month 3	6951 ± 1699 **‡‡	1649 ± 2450	3728 ± 2259	0.000
	Month 6	5926 ± 1274 **	1921 ± 2138	4762 ± 2507 #	0.000
	Month 12	5653 ± 824 *‡	2374 ± 2457	2951 ± 1702	0.019

Group A: conjunctival autograft, Group B: mPRGF, Group C: amniotic membrane, SD: standard deviation. * Significant differences between group A and B, ** very significant differences between group A and B, ‡ significant differences between group A and C, ‡‡ very significant differences between group A and C. # Significant differences between group B and C.

Figure 3 shows representative images of a clinical case of a patient treated with a PRGF membrane graft, evaluating the follow-up by OCT, the mPRGF graft was reabsorbed by the second week. Subsequently, the evaluations of the graft size were related to the regeneration of the conjunctival epithelium (see Figure 3).

Figure 4 shows several images obtained from a patient treated with mPRGF as a graft showing a complete restoration of the conjunctiva during the follow-up period (see Figure 4).

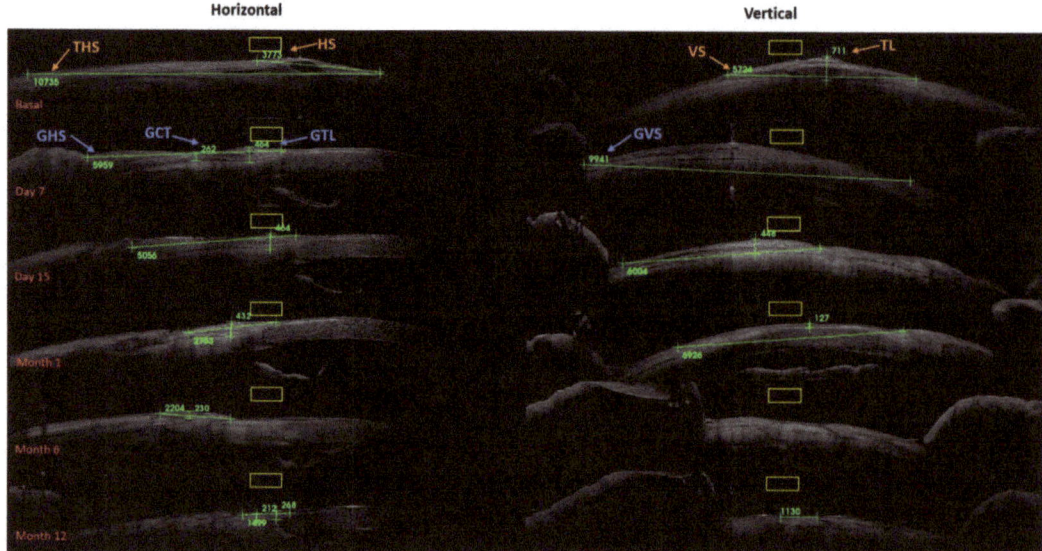

Figure 3. OCT graft measurements (μm) for mPRGF. Basal: TL: thickness of the limbus, HS: horizontal size, THS: total horizontal size, and VS: vertical size. During the postoperative follow-up, the conjunctival restoration zone was measured: GCT: graft central thickness, GTL: graft thickness in the limbus, GHS: graft horizontal size (measured between the sclerocorneal limbus to the nasal area of the excised conjunctiva), and GVS: graft vertical size.

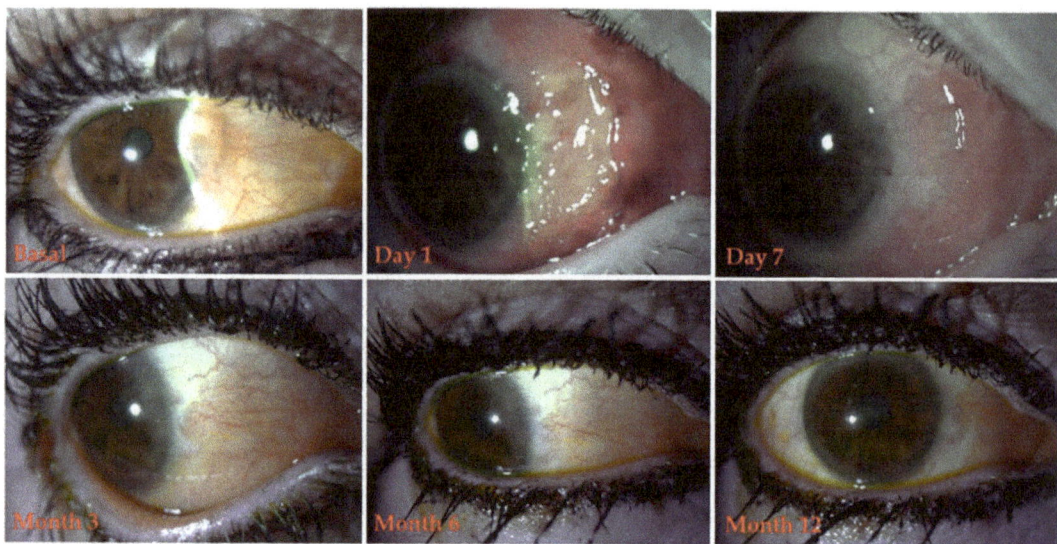

Figure 4. Clinical follow-up of a patient treated with mPRGF in pterygium surgery.

3.3. Pterygium Recurrence: Solomon Scale

Group A showed lower pterygium recurrence throughout the follow-up, in contrast to groups B and C. Group A showed differences ($p < 0.05$) compared to group B at month 1 and 3, and showed differences compared to group C in month 6. No intraoperative complications were found in the three treatment groups. A descriptive analysis for recurrence

(Solomon scale: grade 4), indicated two cases (7.7%) of the patients in the Group B (n = 26), and two cases (20.0%) of the patients in the Group C (n = 10). Moreover, during the first month of follow-up in group A, 3 cases with pyogenic granulomas were observed (see Table 4).

Table 4. Solomon scale in the different treatment groups.

	Month 1 Mean ± SD	Month 3 Mean ± SD	Month 6 Mean ± SD	Month 12 Mean ± SD
Group A	1.00 ± 0.00 *	1.08 ± 0.29 *	1.10 ± 0.32 ‡	1.00 ± 0.00
Group B	1.55 ± 0.76	2.06 ± 0.87	1.88 ± 0.96	1.91 ± 1.04
Group C	1.11 ± 0.33	2.00 ± 1.22	2.43 ± 1.13	2.17 ± 0.98

Solomon scale: grade 1 (normal appearance of the surgery area), grade 2 (presence of some fine episcleral vessels without extending beyond the limbus, without any fibrous tissue in the excised area), grade 3 (presence of additional fibrous tissue in the excised area without invading the cornea, grade 4 (represents a true recurrence with fibrovascular tissue invading the cornea). Group A: conjunctival autograft, Group B: mPRGF, Group C: amniotic membrane. SD: standard deviation. * Significant differences between group A and B ($p < 0.05$), ‡ significant differences between group A and C ($p < 0.05$).

3.4. Ocular Surface Symptom Assessment (VAS and OSDI)

The VAS frequency and severity outcomes showed no significant differences ($p > 0.05$) among the groups at any time of the follow-up time (see Figure 5). The improvement percentage in VAS frequency was 35.5% for group A, 86.2% for group B, and 39.1% for group C. The percentage improvement in VAS severity was 51.8% for group A, 79.5% for group B, and 37.1% for group C. The analysis of the OSDI questionnaire showed no significant differences among the different groups at any time of the study, except for group A and C, among which significant differences ($p < 0.05$) were observed at months 6 and 12 between both groups (see Table 5).

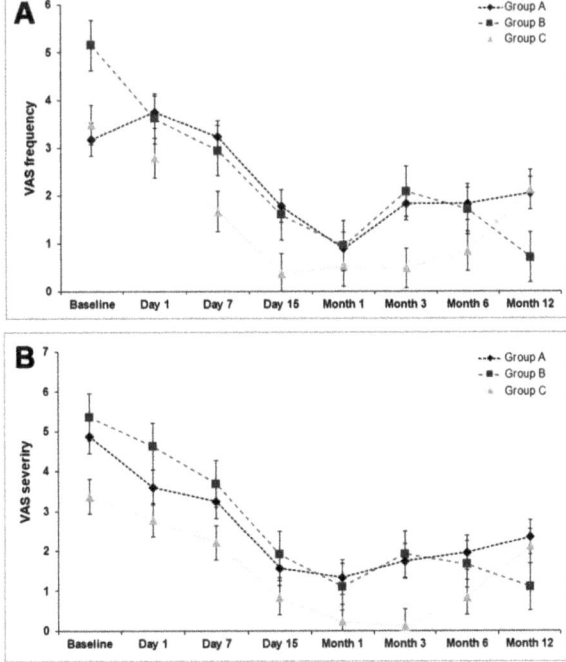

Figure 5. Visual analog scale. (**A**) Frequency. Group A: conjunctival autograft, Group B: membrane-plasma rich in growth factors, Group C: amniotic membrane. (**B**) Severity. Group A: conjunctival autograft, Group B: membrane-plasma rich in growth factors, Group C: amniotic membrane.

Table 5. Ocular surface disease index (OSDI) outcomes obtained in each treatment group at each time point of the follow-up.

	Baseline Mean ± SD	Day 7 Mean ± SD	Day 15 Mean ± SD	Month 1 Mean ± SD	Month 3 Mean ± SD	Month 6 Mean ± SD	Month 12 Mean ± SD
Group A	36.82 ± 26.00	36.45 ± 23.24	23.87 ± 18.61	19.60 ± 21.95	22.85 ± 22.85	31.31 ± 24.70	41.48 ± 27.34
Group B	33.92 ± 26.18	42.39 ± 25.60	26.62 ± 25.23	22.41 ± 21.76	20.04 ± 23.11	19.93 ± 23.46	20.68 ± 24.65
Group C	37.12 ± 26.18	38.85 ± 30.99	12.62 ± 14.79	5.72 ± 6.68	8.59 ± 14.51	7.87 ‡ ± 13.97	5.90 ‡ ± 9.72

Group A: Conjunctival autograft, Group B: mPRGF, Group C: amniotic membrane, SD: standard deviation. ‡ Significant differences between group A and C ($p < 0.05$).

The reduction percentage in total OSDI score was 12.7% for group A, 39.0% for group B, and 84.1% for group C, and this change was significant ($p < 0.05$) in group B and group C, but not in group A ($p > 0.05$) (see Table 6). Group B showed significant differences ($p < 0.05$) in 6 symptoms (sensitivity to light, sensation of grit, eye pain, use of computer or screen, watching TV, and wind) with improvement in the OSDI score. However, group C showed only significant differences ($p < 0.05$) in two symptoms (blurred vision and low vision) and group A showed no differences ($p > 0.05$) in any symptoms.

Table 6. Results of the OSDI questionnaire: by symptom groups.

		Baseline Mean (Range)	Month 12 Mean (Range)	*p*-Value
Group A	Light sensitivity	2.08 (0–4)	2.00 (0–4)	0.41
	Grit feeling	2.15 (0–4)	1.50 (0–4)	0.34
	Eye pain	1.00 (0–4)	1.17 (0–4)	1.00
	Blurry vision	0.77 (0–3)	1.00 (0–2)	0.49
	Bad vision	0.69 (0–3)	1.00 (0–4)	0.59
	Read	1.08 (0–4)	2.50 (0–4)	0.24
	Night driving	0.88 (0–4)	0.40 (0–2)	0.32
	Use of computer or screen	0.92 (0–4)	1.33 (0–4)	0.85
	Watch TV	1.08 (0–4)	1.50 (0–4)	0.56
	Wind	2.38 (0–4)	2.83 (0–4)	0.79
	Very dry environments	2.46 (0–4)	2.50 (0–4)	1.00
	Air conditioning	1.92 (0–4)	1.83 (0–4)	0.79
	Total OSDI score	36.82 (0–93)	41.48 (6–61)	0.35
Group B	Light sensitivity	1.57 (0–4)	0.92 (0–3)	≤0.01 *
	Grit feeling	1.78 (0–4)	0.83 (0–3)	0.02 *
	Eye pain	0.91 (0–4)	0.67 (0–3)	≤0.01 *
	Blurry vision	0.83 (0–3)	1.80 (0–4)	0.19
	Bad vision	0.48 (0–3)	0.73 (0–4)	0.16
	Read	1.30 (0–4)	0.92 (0–4)	0.06
	Night driving	0.50 (0–4)	0.40 (0–3)	1.00
	Use of computer or screen	1.48 (0–4)	0.50 (0–3)	0.04 *
	Watch TV	1.22 (0–4)	0.83 (0–4)	0.03 *
	Wind	2.65 (0–4)	1.50 (0–4)	≤0.01 *
	Very dry environments	1.78 (0–4)	0.75 (0–3)	0.06
	Air conditioning	1.25 (0–4)	0.58 (0–3)	0.42
	Total OSDI score	33.9 (0–77)	20.7 (0–66)	≤0.01 *
Group C	Light sensitivity	1.50 (0–4)	0.33 (0–1)	0.11
	Grit feeling	2.30 (0–4)	0.67 (0–3)	0.06
	Eye pain	0.70 (0–3)	0.0 (0–0)	0.32
	Blurry vision	1.60 (0–4)	0.17 (0–1)	0.03 *
	Bad vision	1.60 (0–4)	0.17 (0–1)	0.03 *
	Read	1.00 (0–4)	0.17 (0–1)	1.00
	Night driving	1.00 (0–4)	0.00 (0–0)	1.00
	Use of computer or screen	0.78 (0–4)	0.20 (0–1)	0.32
	Watch TV	0.40 (0–4)	0.17 (0–1)	0.32
	Wind	2.40 (0–4)	0.50 (0–2)	0.07
	Very dry environments	2.40 (0–4)	0.17 (0–1)	0.10
	Air conditioning	1.50 (0–4)	0.17 (0–1)	0.10
	Total OSDI score	37.1 (6–75)	5.9 (0.25)	0.03 *

OSDI: ocular surface disease index; Group A: conjunctival autograft; Group B: mPRGF (membrane of plasma rich in growth factors); Group C: amniotic membrane; * *p* value < 0.05.

4. Discussion

Surgical techniques for pterygium treatment have been improved over the years; nowadays, it is necessary to achieve the closure of the tissue defect, avoid recurrence, improve symptoms of the ocular surface, and increase life quality of patients [8,13,14]. To treat ocular defects and reduce the risk of ocular perforation, many techniques have been used in the past, including AMT, tissue adhesives (collagen, fibrin), animal-based tissue patches, limbal stem cell transplants, conjunctival autograft transplants or keratoplasty surgery [46,47]. The recurrence rate is the main result obtained in most clinical studies; meanwhile, the efficacy and safety results are evaluated using different surgical techniques. In our study, the primary outcome was pterygium recurrence, a fact that is consistent with the interests of current research [15].

In recent years, the field of ocular surface tissue regeneration has experienced significant progress. Some examples include the use of tissue replacements and auto-, allo- and xeno-grafts for limbal cell therapy, or pterygium surgery, either alone or in combination with a temporary graft such as an AM [48–50]. These grafts are not always useful, mainly due to the imbalance between demand and tissue availability and the immunological response between the donor tissue and the host [49,50]. Moreover, the use of allogeneic fibrin glues may potentially present certain biosafety risks, in the case of the AM, these risks will be enhanced due to its also allogeneic origin as one of its main disadvantages, along with the requirement of a tissue bank. Accordingly, using a safe and effective autologous tissue as a graft would be highly desirable, avoiding the risk of viral or prion transmission. In this sense, mPRGF provides a fibrin scaffold used as a regenerative and physical support membrane in many ocular defects. PRGF technology has a standardized protocol that guarantees the reproducibility of the treatment, the availability of direct costs related to its preparation and use, and immediate availability in the surgery room. Furthermore, it is also important to highlight that ePRGF is obtained during the same mPRGF preparation process and can be used as a postsurgical treatment, thus increasing the periodical availability of growth factors [34].

The main PRGF feature responsible for most of its biological effects is the sustained release of growth factors. However, the absence of leukocytes and antibacterial, anti-inflammatory, and anti-fibrotic activity are also essential characteristics of PRGF [35,51]. The growth factor release from the platelet's alpha granules is mediated by calcium chloride, which activates fibrinogen and is converted to fibrin, and then begins to develop a three-dimensional acellular matrix with high stability [35,51]. Moreover, being mPRGF a leukocyte-free formulation potentially avoids faster fibrin degradation kinetics and a more significant proinflammatory response. It has been demonstrated that this mPRGF fibrin matrix retains trapped in the fibrin clot, almost 30% of the amount of growth factors remained trapped after eight days of incubation, for sustained release [35,51].

Nonetheless, this sustained release has shown an increment of the proliferation and migration activity of corneal keratocytes and conjunctival fibroblasts and the reduction of the TGF β1–induced myofibroblast differentiation reducing the number of α-SMA positive cells. This inhibition limits the fibrosis pathways, which is especially relevant in the pathogenesis of pterygium and its tissue remodeling [35,38,51,52]. Several studies have evaluated the potential benefits of mPRGF alone or in combination with other membranes like AM [34,41], showing a stable closure of the corneal defect in all patients treated with PRGF with no evidence of infection, inflammation, or pain [34,41].

In this study, no differences in BCVA and IOP were observed in the intergroup and intragroup analysis. In the anatomical evaluation, a progressive and sustained decrease in the size (horizontal and vertical) and thickness of the conjunctiva was observed in group B. In a study carried out by Zhang et al. [53] in 771 healthy subjects, a full conjunctiva thickness of 240.1 ± 29.8 μm was shown. In another study, the progression of the graft thickness in 40 pterygium surgery patients showed a graft thickness of 430 ± 127 μm in the primary pterygium group and 461 ± 178 μm in the recurrent group at one week after surgery and a graft thickness of 109 ± 15 μm and 107 ± 18 μm at month three, postoperatively [54]. The results obtained in the present study showed similar initial postsurgical thicknesses among the three groups for the graft placement area, most likely due to similar iatrogenic reasons in all procedures. All groups underwent a gradual size and thickness decrease, group B was the first to show graft thickness outcomes similar to those reported in healthy subjects at month 1 [53]. Moreover, there were significant differences between group B and the other two groups in month 3, with the mPRGF group achieving the lowest graft thickness outcomes. These findings might have been caused by a combined effect of autologous fibrin degradation and conjunctival tissue remodeling. When a fibrin graft is applied for wound healing purposes, it is invaded by surrounding cells, which will produce a new extracellular matrix to replace the fibrin meshwork, and the new tissue formation will be regulated by the gradual degradation of the fibrin clot (fibrinolytic process) [55]. The use of AS-OCT as a diagnostic and follow-up aid in ocular surface diseases such as pterygium or conjunctival tumors is increasingly common [56,57].

During the healing process in the mPRGF and AM groups, it is suggested that the degradation of the fibrin meshwork occurs, leading to a graft tissue replacement. A study carried out by Oscar Gris et al. [58] established that AM degradation may take a mean of 12.5 days (3 to 34 days). These results are similar to the use of mPRGF for the surgery of ocular surface disorders, in which complete mPRGF reabsorption occurred after a mean of 12.67 days [41]. Moreover, part of the fibroblast cells will be transformed into myofibroblasts during the wound healing process, favoring epithelial and endothelial cell migration through the graft and promoting wound contraction [59]. However, the persistence of myofibroblastic cells after wound healing could lead to the development of scarring tissue. Interestingly, it has been demonstrated that PRGF formulations reduce the number of myofibroblasts and modulate their action during wound healing, improving tissue regeneration and avoiding fibrosis formation [60–62]. Further studies are needed to determine the optimal graft size and degradation kinetics to avoid the risk of fast degradation that could compromise the pterygium surgery results.

The gold standard for pterygium surgery is excision with conjunctiva autograft, observing a recurrence between 1.9–8%. On the other hand, in a meta-analysis it was found that the graft with an amniotic membrane has greater recurrence (3.7–40.9%) than surgery with a conjunctival autograft (2.6–17.7%) [63]. In our study, for the Solomon scale, the overall results showed no statistical differences among the three groups at 12 months of follow-up ($p > 0.05$), showing that the three surgical techniques are similar in pterygium recurrence rates.

A clinical study with 108 patients comparing the use of platelet-rich fibrin (PRF) grafts and limbal conjunctival autografts (LCA) in pterygium surgery has recently been published, and it was observed that the surgery time was shorter in the PRF group (25.0 ± 4.2 min) than in the LCA group (36.5 ± 6.3 min) ($p < 0.001$) [64]. The use of mPRGF could decrease the surgical time compared to the conjunctival autograft group, since conjunctival dissection is not necessary; we believe that the surgical time would be similar to that of the amniotic membrane group.

In terms of ocular surface symptoms, the mPRGF group showed a higher percentage of improvement in VAS frequency (86.2%) and VAS severity (79.5%) compared to the other treatment groups. Similar results were observed in other studies treating several ocular surface diseases with PRGF, in which improvement of the VAS was demonstrated [34,36–38,41]. For the OSDI questionnaire, significant improvement was observed in the AM group than in the CAG group. However, no significant differences were showed between AM and mPRGF groups. Regarding the categories of symptoms, the mPRGF group obtained significant improvement ($p < 0.05$) in 6 of the twelve categories. However, the AM group only improved in 2 categories ($p < 0.05$), and the CAG group did not improve in any. One of the categories that improved with mPRGF treatment was eye pain. Several studies in different medical areas reported pain improvement after using PRGF [34,36]. The absence of leukocytes and endocannabinoid-mediated analgesic effects may be two of the main reasons for the pain reduction scores after PRGF treatment [35,65].

This study has some limitations, such as the fact that it was carried out at a single center, with a small cohort, and lacks inflammation biomarker measurements. Further studies are needed to determine the optimal surgical approach of mPRGF in graft placement and thickness. The results show that mPRGF is a safe and effective treatment for primary pterygium surgery, which produces an autologous graft in an agile way and contributes to preserve the patient´s healthy conjunctiva.

5. Conclusions

This is the first clinical study evaluating these three surgical techniques (CAG, AM, and mPRGF) to the best of our knowledge. The results obtained in this study suggest that the three evaluated techniques are effective in achieving tissue coverage. Therefore, mPRGF is a safe and effective treatment for primary pterygium surgery, allowing the production of an autologous graft quickly, without the need of a tissue bank and while avoiding iatrogenesis in healthy conjunctiva. This new surgical approach may be relevant for those cases of pterygium that require large excisions or with insufficient healthy conjunctiva.

Author Contributions: Conceptualization, M.I., B.d.l.S.-C. and L.P.; methodology, M.I., B.d.l.S.-C. and L.P.; software, M.I., B.d.l.S.-C. and R.M.S.-Á.; validation, M.I., B.d.l.S.-C. and L.P.; formal analysis, M.I., R.M.S.-Á. and F.M.; investigation, M.I., C.S.-P., M.S., A.S.-P. and L.P.; resources, M.I.; B.d.l.S.-C. and L.P.; data curation, M.I.; B.d.l.S.-C.; R.M.S.-Á. and F.M.; writing—original draft preparation, M.I.; B.d.l.S.-C.; R.M.S.-Á. and F.M., writing—review and editing, M.I.; B.d.l.S.-C.; R.M.S.-Á. and F.M., visualization, M.I.; B.d.l.S.-C.; R.M.S.-Á. and F.M., supervision, G.O., E.A. and L.P.; project administration, M.I.; B.d.l.S.-C. and L.P., funding acquisition, B.d.l.S.-C., E.A. and L.P. All authors have read and agreed to the published version of the manuscript.

Funding: This clinical research received funding from the Institute of Biotechnology (BTI), Vitoria, Spain, to carry it out.

Institutional Review Board Statement: The study was conducted according to the guidelines of the Declaration of Helsinki. The approval of the regional clinical research ethics committee (Aragon, Spain) was obtained (authorization C.P.-C.I. EC16/0031).

Informed Consent Statement: Informed consent was obtained from all subjects involved in this study.

Data Availability Statement: The data used to support this study's findings are available by contacting the corresponding author upon request.

Conflicts of Interest: The authors declare the following competing financial interest(s): E.A. is the Scientific Director of Biotechnology Institute; B.d.l.S.-C., R.M.S.-Á., G.O., and F.M. are scientists at BTI Biotechnology Institute. The other authors declare no conflicts of interest in developing this study.

References

1. Tan, D.T.; Chee, S.P.; Dear, K.B.; Lim, A.S. Effect of pterygium morphology on pterygium recurrence in a controlled trial comparing conjunctival autografting with bare sclera excision. *Arch. Ophthalmol.* **1997**, *115*, 1235–1240. [CrossRef]
2. Solomon, A.S. Pterygium. *Br. J. Ophthalmol.* **2006**, *90*, 665–666. [CrossRef] [PubMed]
3. Di Girolamo, N.; Coroneo, M.T.; Wakefield, D. UVB-elicited induction of MMP-1 expression in human ocular surface epithelial cells is mediated through the ERK1/2 MAPK-dependent pathway. *Invest. Ophthalmol. Vis. Sci.* **2003**, *44*, 4705–4714. [CrossRef]
4. Nolan, T.M.; Di Girolamo, N.; Sachdev, N.H.; Hampartzoumian, T.; Coroneo, M.T.; Wakefield, D. The role of ultraviolet irradiation and heparin-binding epidermal growth factor-like growth factor in the pathogenesis of pterygium. *Am. J. Pathol.* **2003**, *162*, 567–574. [CrossRef]
5. Tsai, Y.-Y.; Cheng, Y.-W.; Lee, H.; Tsai, F.-J.; Tseng, S.-H.; Lin, C.-L.; Chang, K.-C. Oxidative DNA damage in pterygium. *Mol. Vis.* **2005**, *11*, 71–75. [PubMed]
6. Rezvan, F.; Khabazkhoob, M.; Hooshmand, E.; Yekta, A.; Saatchi, M.; Hashemi, H. Prevalence and risk factors of pterygium: A systematic review and meta-analysis. *Surv. Ophthalmol.* **2018**, *63*, 719–735. [CrossRef]
7. Viso, E.; Gude, F.; Rodriguez-Ares, M.T. Prevalence of pinguecula and pterygium in a general population in Spain. *Eye* **2011**, *25*, 350–357. [CrossRef]
8. Iradier, M.T. Cirugía del Pterigión. In *Monografía de la Sociedad Española de Oftalmología*; Macline: Madrid, Spain, 2006.
9. Akinci, A.; Zilelioglu, O. Comparison of limbal-conjunctival autograft and intraoperative 0.02% mitomycin-C for treatment of primary pterygium. *Int. Ophthalmol.* **2007**, *27*, 281–285. [CrossRef] [PubMed]

10. Ozdamar, Y.; Mutevelli, S.; Han, U.; Ileri, D.; Onal, B.; Ilhan, O.; Karakaya, J.; Zilelioglu, O. A comparative study of tissue glue and vicryl suture for closing limbal-conjunctival autografts and histologic evaluation after pterygium excision. *Cornea* **2008**, *27*, 552–558. [CrossRef] [PubMed]
11. Ozer, A.; Yildirim, N.; Erol, N.; Yurdakul, S. Long-term results of bare sclera, limbal-conjunctival autograft and amniotic membrane graft techniques in primary pterygium excisions. *Int. J. Ophthalmol. Z. Augenheilkd.* **2009**, *223*, 269–273. [CrossRef]
12. Benitez-Herreros, J.; Perez-Rico, C.; Montes-Mollon, M.A.; Gomez-San-Gil, Y.; Teus-Guezala, M.A. Endothelial cells analysis after intraoperative mitomycin-C adjuvant pterygium simple excision surgery: A pilot study. *Arch. Soc. Esp. Oftalmol.* **2010**, *85*, 11–15. [CrossRef]
13. Koranyi, G.; Artzen, D.; Seregard, S.; Kopp, E.D. Intraoperative mitomycin C versus autologous conjunctival autograft in surgery of primary pterygium with four-year follow-up. *Acta Ophthalmol.* **2012**, *90*, 266–270. [CrossRef] [PubMed]
14. Mastropasqua, L.; Carpineto, P.; Ciancaglini, M.; Enrico Gallenga, P. Long term results of intraoperative mitomycin C in the treatment of recurrent pterygium. *Br. J. Ophthalmol.* **1996**, *80*, 288–291. [CrossRef] [PubMed]
15. Clearfield, E.; Muthappan, V.; Wang, X.; Kuo, I.C. Conjunctival autograft for pterygium. *Cochrane Database Syst. Rev.* **2016**, *2*, CD011349. [CrossRef] [PubMed]
16. Suzuki, T.; Sano, Y.; Kinoshita, S. Conjunctival inflammation induces Langerhans cell migration into the cornea. *Curr. Eye Res.* **2000**, *21*, 550–553. [CrossRef]
17. Elwan, S.A.M. Comparison between sutureless and glue free versus sutured limbal conjunctival autograft in primary pterygium surgery. *Saudi J. Ophthalmol. Off. J. Saudi Ophthalmol. Soc.* **2014**, *28*, 292–298. [CrossRef]
18. Kim, H.H.; Mun, H.J.; Park, Y.J.; Lee, K.W.; Shin, J.P. Conjunctivolimbal autograft using a fibrin adhesive in pterygium surgery. *Korean J. Ophthalmol.* **2008**, *22*, 147–154. [CrossRef] [PubMed]
19. Solomon, A.; Pires, R.T.; Tseng, S.C. Amniotic membrane transplantation after extensive removal of primary and recurrent pterygia. *Ophthalmology* **2001**, *108*, 449–460. [CrossRef]
20. Tseng, S.C.; Prabhasawat, P.; Barton, K.; Gray, T.; Meller, D. Amniotic membrane transplantation with or without limbal allografts for corneal surface reconstruction in patients with limbal stem cell deficiency. *Arch. Ophthalmol.* **1998**, *116*, 431–441. [CrossRef]
21. Hanada, K.; Nishikawa, N.; Miyokawa, N.; Yoshida, A. Long-term outcome of amniotic membrane transplantation combined with mitomycin C for conjunctival reconstruction after ocular surface squamous neoplasia excision. *Int. Ophthalmol.* **2017**, *37*, 71–78. [CrossRef]
22. Krysik, K.; Dobrowolski, D.; Wylęgała, E.A.; Lyssek-Boroń, A. Amniotic Membrane as a Main Component in Treatment Supporting Healing and Patch Grafts in Corneal Melting and Perforations. *J. Ophthalmol.* **2020**, *2020*, 4238919. [CrossRef]
23. Ma, D.H.-K.; Wang, S.-F.; Su, W.-Y.; Tsai, R.J.-F. Amniotic membrane graft for the management of scleral melting and corneal perforation in recalcitrant infectious scleral and corneoscleral ulcers. *Cornea* **2002**, *21*, 275–283. [CrossRef] [PubMed]
24. Trinh, T.; Mimouni, M.; Mednick, Z.; Einan-Lifshitz, A.; Cohen, E.; Santaella, G.; Sorkin, N.; Slomovic, A. Outcomes of Ipsilateral Simple Limbal Epithelial Transplantation, Tenonectomy, Mitomycin and Amniotic Membrane Transplantation for Treatment of Recurrent Pterygium. *Cornea* **2020**, *43–47*. [CrossRef] [PubMed]
25. Koranyi, G.; Seregard, S.; Kopp, E.D. Cut and paste: A no suture, small incision approach to pterygium surgery. *Br. J. Ophthalmol.* **2004**, *88*, 911–914. [CrossRef] [PubMed]
26. Bhandari, V.; Rao, C.L.; Ganesh, S.; Brar, S. Visual outcome and efficacy of conjunctival autograft, harvested from the body of pterygium in pterygium excision. *Clin. Ophthalmol.* **2015**, *9*, 2285–2290. [CrossRef]
27. Pietrzak, W.S.; Eppley, B.L. Platelet rich plasma: Biology and new technology. *J. Craniofac. Surg.* **2005**, *16*, 1043–1054. [CrossRef]
28. Anitua, E.; Andia, I.; Ardanza, B.; Nurden, P.; Nurden, A.T. Autologous platelets as a source of proteins for healing and tissue regeneration. *Thromb. Haemost.* **2004**, *91*, 4–15. [CrossRef]
29. Freire, V.; Andollo, N.; Etxebarria, J.; Duran, J.A.; Morales, M.-C. In vitro effects of three blood derivatives on human corneal epithelial cells. *Invest. Ophthalmol. Vis. Sci.* **2012**, *53*, 5571–5578. [CrossRef] [PubMed]
30. Weibrich, G.; Kleis, W.K.G.; Hitzler, W.E.; Hafner, G. Comparison of the platelet concentrate collection system with the plasma-rich-in-growth-factors kit to produce platelet-rich plasma: A technical report. *Int. J. Oral Maxillofac. Implants* **2005**, *20*, 118–123.
31. Anitua, E. The use of plasma-rich growth factors (PRGF) in oral surgery. *Pract. Proced. Aesthet. Dent.* **2001**, *13*, 487–493.
32. Cobos, R.; Aizpuru, F.; Parraza, N.; Anitua, E.; Orive, G. Effectiveness and efficiency of platelet rich plasma in the treatment of diabetic ulcers. *Curr. Pharm. Biotechnol.* **2015**, *16*, 630–634. [CrossRef]
33. Sanchez, M.; Anitua, E.; Azofra, J.; Aguirre, J.J.; Andia, I. Intra-articular injection of an autologous preparation rich in growth factors for the treatment of knee OA: A retrospective cohort study. *Clin. Exp. Rheumatol.* **2008**, *26*, 910–913. [PubMed]
34. Anitua, E.; Muruzabal, F.; Tayebba, A.; Riestra, A.; Perez, V.L.; Merayo-Lloves, J.; Orive, G. Autologous serum and plasma rich in growth factors in ophthalmology: Preclinical and clinical studies. *Acta Ophthalmol.* **2015**, *93*, e605-14. [CrossRef] [PubMed]
35. Anitua, E.; Nurden, P.; Prado, R.; Nurden, A.T.; Padilla, S. Autologous fibrin scaffolds: When platelet- and plasma-derived biomolecules meet fibrin. *Biomaterials* **2019**, *192*, 440–460. [CrossRef] [PubMed]
36. Anitua, E.; Muruzabal, F.; de la Fuente, M.; Merayo, J.; Duran, J.; Orive, G. Plasma Rich in Growth Factors for the Treatment of Ocular Surface Diseases. *Curr. Eye Res.* **2016**, *41*, 875–882. [CrossRef]
37. Merayo-Lloves, J.; Sanchez, R.M.; Riestra, A.C.; Anitua, E.; Begona, L.; Orive, G.; Fernandez-Vega, L. Autologous Plasma Rich in Growth Factors Eyedrops in Refractory Cases of Ocular Surface Disorders. *Ophthalmic Res.* **2015**, *55*, 53–61. [CrossRef]

38. Anitua, E.; de la Fuente, M.; Muruzabal, F.; Riestra, A.; Merayo-Lloves, J.; Orive, G. Plasma rich in growth factors (PRGF) eye drops stimulates scarless regeneration compared to autologous serum in the ocular surface stromal fibroblasts. *Exp. Eye Res.* **2015**, *135*, 118–126. [CrossRef]
39. Anitua, E.; de la Fuente, M.; Muruzábal, F.; Merayo-Lloves, J. Short- and Long-Term Stability of Plasma Rich in Growth Factors Eye Drops. *Cornea* **2021**, *40*, 107–112. [CrossRef]
40. Rodriguez-Agirretxe, I.; Freire, V.; Muruzabal, F.; Orive, G.; Anitua, E.; Diez-Feijoo, E.; Acera, A. Subconjunctival PRGF Fibrin Membrane as an Adjuvant to Nonpenetrating Deep Sclerectomy: A 2-Year Pilot Study. *Ophthalmic Res.* **2018**, *59*, 45–52. [CrossRef]
41. Sanchez-Avila, R.M.; Merayo-Lloves, J.; Riestra, A.C.; Berisa, S.; Lisa, C.; Sanchez, J.A.; Muruzabal, F.; Orive, G.; Anitua, E. Plasma rich in growth factors membrane as coadjuvant treatment in the surgery of ocular surface disorders. *Medicine* **2018**, *97*, e0242. [CrossRef]
42. Prabhasawat, P.; Barton, K.; Burkett, G.; Tseng, S.C. Comparison of conjunctival autografts, amniotic membrane grafts, and primary closure for pterygium excision. *Ophthalmology* **1997**, *104*, 974–985. [CrossRef]
43. Ghanavati, S.Z.; Shousha, M.A.; Betancurt, C.; Perez, V.L. Combined conjunctival autograft and overlay amniotic membrane transplantation; A novel surgical treatment for pterygium. *J. Ophthalmic Vis. Res.* **2014**, *9*, 399–403. [CrossRef]
44. Schiffman, R.M.; Christianson, M.D.; Jacobsen, G.; Hirsch, J.D.; Reis, B.L. Reliability and validity of the Ocular Surface Disease Index. *Arch. Ophthalmol.* **2000**, *118*, 615–621. [CrossRef]
45. Anitua, E.; Muruzabal, F.; De la Fuente, M.; Merayo-Lloves, J.; Orive, G. Effects of heat-treatment on plasma rich in growth factors-derived autologous eye drop. *Exp. Eye Res.* **2014**, *119*, 27–34. [CrossRef] [PubMed]
46. Yuan, S.; Fan, G. Stem cell-based therapy of corneal epithelial and endothelial diseases. *Regen. Med.* **2015**, *10*, 495–504. [CrossRef]
47. Samoila, O.; Gocan, D. Clinical Outcomes From Cultivated Allogenic Stem Cells vs. Oral Mucosa Epithelial Transplants in Total Bilateral Stem Cells Deficiency. *Front. Med.* **2020**, *7*, 43. [CrossRef] [PubMed]
48. Bernardo, M.E.; Avanzini, M.A.; Perotti, C.; Cometa, A.M.; Moretta, A.; Lenta, E.; Del Fante, C.; Novara, F.; de Silvestri, A.; Amendola, G.; et al. Optimization of in vitro expansion of human multipotent mesenchymal stromal cells for cell-therapy approaches: Further insights in the search for a fetal calf serum substitute. *J. Cell. Physiol.* **2007**, *211*, 121–130. [CrossRef]
49. Fernandez-Buenaga, R.; Aiello, F.; Zaher, S.S.; Grixti, A.; Ahmad, S. Twenty years of limbal epithelial therapy: An update on managing limbal stem cell deficiency. *BMJ Open Ophthalmol.* **2018**, *3*, e000164. [CrossRef]
50. Coquelin, L.; Fialaire-Legendre, A.; Roux, S.; Poignard, A.; Bierling, P.; Hernigou, P.; Chevallier, N.; Rouard, H. In vivo and in vitro comparison of three different allografts vitalized with human mesenchymal stromal cells. *Tissue Eng. Part A* **2012**, *18*, 1921–1931. [CrossRef]
51. Anitua, E.; Zalduendo, M.M.; Alkhraisat, M.H.; Orive, G. Release kinetics of platelet-derived and plasma-derived growth factors from autologous plasma rich in growth factors. *Ann. Anat.* **2013**, *195*, 461–466. [CrossRef]
52. Anitua, E.; Sanchez, M.; Merayo-Lloves, J.; De la Fuente, M.; Muruzabal, F.; Orive, G. Plasma rich in growth factors (PRGF-Endoret) stimulates proliferation and migration of primary keratocytes and conjunctival fibroblasts and inhibits and reverts TGF-beta1-Induced myodifferentiation. *Invest. Ophthalmol. Vis. Sci.* **2011**, *52*, 6066–6073. [CrossRef]
53. Zhang, X.; Li, Q.; Xiang, M.; Zou, H.; Liu, B.; Zhou, H.; Han, Z.; Fu, Z.; Zhang, Z.; Wang, H. Bulbar conjunctival thickness measurements with optical coherence tomography in healthy chinese subjects. *Invest. Ophthalmol. Vis. Sci.* **2013**, *54*, 4705–4709. [CrossRef] [PubMed]
54. Ozgurhan, E.B.; Kara, N.; Bozkurt, E.; Gencer, B.; Yuksel, K.; Demirok, A. Comparison of conjunctival graft thickness after primary and recurrent pterygium surgery: Anterior segment optical coherence tomography study. *Indian J. Ophthalmol.* **2014**, *62*, 675–679. [CrossRef] [PubMed]
55. Heher, P.; Mühleder, S.; Mittermayr, R.; Redl, H.; Slezak, P. Fibrin-based delivery strategies for acute and chronic wound healing. *Adv. Drug Deliv. Rev.* **2018**, *129*, 134–147. [CrossRef]
56. Nampei, K.; Oie, Y.; Kiritoshi, S.; Morota, M.; Satoh, S.; Kawasaki, S.; Nishida, K. Comparison of ocular surface squamous neoplasia and pterygium using anterior segment optical coherence tomography angiography. *Am. J. Ophthalmol. Case Rep.* **2020**, *20*, 100902. [CrossRef] [PubMed]
57. Lozano García, I.; Romero Caballero, M.D.; Sellés Navarro, I. High resolution anterior segment optical coherence tomography for differential diagnosis between corneo-conjunctival intraepithelial neoplasia and pterygium. *Arch. Soc. Esp. Oftalmol.* **2020**, *95*, 108–113. [CrossRef] [PubMed]
58. Gris, O.; del Campo, Z.; Wolley-Dod, C.; Güell, J.L.; Bruix, A.; Calatayud, M.; Adán, A. Amniotic membrane implantation as a therapeutic contact lens for the treatment of epithelial disorders. *Cornea* **2002**, *21*, 22–27. [CrossRef] [PubMed]
59. Duffield, J.S.; Lupher, M.; Thannickal, V.J.; Wynn, T.A. Host responses in tissue repair and fibrosis. *Annu. Rev. Pathol.* **2013**, *8*, 241–276. [CrossRef]
60. Maltseva, O.; Folger, P.; Zekaria, D.; Petridou, S.; Masur, S.K. Fibroblast growth factor reversal of the corneal myofibroblast phenotype. *Invest. Ophthalmol. Vis. Sci.* **2001**, *42*, 2490–2495. [PubMed]
61. Netto, M.V.; Mohan, R.R.; Sinha, S.; Sharma, A.; Dupps, W.; Wilson, S.E. Stromal haze, myofibroblasts, and surface irregularity after PRK. *Exp. Eye Res.* **2006**, *82*, 788–797. [CrossRef] [PubMed]
62. Anitua, E.; Muruzabal, F.; Alcalde, I.; Merayo-Lloves, J.; Orive, G. Plasma rich in growth factors (PRGF-Endoret) stimulates corneal wound healing and reduces haze formation after PRK surgery. *Exp. Eye Res.* **2013**, *115*, 153–161. [CrossRef]
63. Chu, W.K.; Choi, H.L.; Bhat, A.K.; Jhanji, V. Pterygium: New insights. *Eye* **2020**, *34*, 1047–1050. [CrossRef] [PubMed]

64. Yang, N.; Xing, Y.; Zhao, Q.; Zeng, S.; Yang, J.; Du, L. Application of Platelet-rich Fibrin Grafts Following Pterygium Excision. *Int. J. Clin. Pract.* **2021**, e14560. [CrossRef] [PubMed]
65. Anitua, E.; Zalduendo, M.M.; Prado, R.; Alkhraisat, M.H.; Orive, G. Morphogen and proinflammatory cytokine release kinetics from PRGF-Endoret fibrin scaffolds: Evaluation of the effect of leukocyte inclusion. *J. Biomed. Mater. Res. Part A* **2015**, *103*, 1011–1020. [CrossRef] [PubMed]

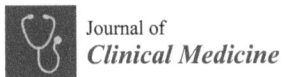

Article

Comparative Analysis of Corneal Parameters in Swept-Source Imaging between DMEK and UT-DSAEK Eyes

Anna Machalińska [1,*,†], Agnieszka Kuligowska [1,†], Bogna Kowalska [1] and Krzysztof Safranow [2]

1 First Department of Ophthalmology, Pomeranian Medical University, 70-111 Szczecin, Poland; agnieszka.kaleta91@gmail.com (A.K.); bogna.kowalska96@gmail.com (B.K.)
2 Department of Biochemistry and Medical Chemistry, Pomeranian Medical University, 70-111 Szczecin, Poland; chrissaf@mp.pl
* Correspondence: annam@pum.edu.pl; Tel.: +48-91-483-8600
† Anna Machalińska and Agnieszka Kuligowska contributed equally to this work.

Abstract: Background: The need to provide a comparative analysis of corneal parameter changes compared to their preoperative values between Descemet membrane endothelial keratoplasty (DMEK) and ultrathin Descemet stripping automated endothelial keratoplasty (UT-DSAEK) patients. Methods: The study included 24 eyes after UT-DSAEK and 24 eyes after DMEK. Visual acuity, endothelial cell count (ECC), central corneal thickness (CCT), mean keratometry (MK), mean astigmatism (MA), astigmatism asymmetry (AA) and higher-order aberrations (HOAs) were assessed at baseline and 1, 3, 6 and 12 months after the surgery. Results: From the 3rd month post operation, ECC was higher in the DMEK eyes than in the UT-DSAEK eyes ($p = 0.01$). In a bivariate analysis that was adjusted for age, DMEK was associated with a smaller decrease in posterior MK at the 1-month ($\beta = -0.49$, $p = 0.002$), 3-month ($\beta = -0.50$, $p < 0.001$), 6-month ($\beta = -0.58$, $p < 0.001$) and 12-month ($\beta = -0.49$, $p < 0.001$) follow-up visits. There were no significant differences in changes in anterior or combined surface MK throughout the observation period. Accordingly, no significant differences in changes in MA, AA or HOAs compared to the baseline values were identified between the eyes after DMEK and UT-DSAEK at any follow-up time point. Conclusions: UT-DSAEK seemed to be an easier and safer technique than DMEK while maintaining similar outcomes regarding irregular astigmatism and total keratometry values.

Keywords: UT-DSAEK; DMEK; keratometry; astigmatism; HOA

1. Introduction

The introduction of endothelial keratoplasty (EK) has revolutionized corneal transplantation over almost the past two decades. Descemet stripping automated endothelial keratoplasty (DSAEK), which is a procedure that involves the selective removal of the dysfunctional endothelium, followed by the transplantation of donor corneal endothelium, Descemet membrane (DM) and a portion of donor corneal stroma, replaced penetrating keratoplasty (PK). Accordingly, Descemet membrane endothelial keratoplasty (DMEK), comprising the selective transplantation of a donor button that is composed of endothelium and DM without the posterior stroma, replaced DSAEK as the most common type of corneal transplantation [1,2].

In 2013, Busin et al. pointed out that ultrathin Descemet stripping automated endothelial keratoplasty (UT-DSAEK) might be a procedure that shares the improved visual outcome and lower immunologic rejection rate of DMEK over DSAEK while minimizing all types of postoperative complications. It was also highlighted that, similar to DSAEK and unlike DMEK, UT-DSAEK can be performed for all types of eyes, even those with complicated anatomy or poor anterior chamber visualization [3].

There are only a few studies that compared DMEK and UT-DSAEK, and they mainly focused on visual acuity outcomes, contrast sensitivity, endothelial cell loss or complication

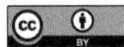

rates [4–10]. Some studies also compared the patient-recorded outcome measures between both techniques [6,10–12]. Chamberlain et al. documented that DMEK had superior visual acuity results with similar complication rates compared with UT-DSAEK at 3, 6 and 12 months post surgery in patients with isolated endothelial dysfunction [9]. In contrast, reports from other groups provided evidence that DMEK and UT-DSAEK did not differ significantly in terms of visual acuity [4,6,8]. Mencucci et al. emphasized that DMEK and UT-DSAEK show no difference in postoperative best-corrected visual acuity (BCVA), although DMEK has a better performance in terms of contrast sensitivity and overall patient satisfaction [7].

Only a few studies have compared higher-order aberrations, astigmatism, corneal pachymetry and keratometry using either Schleimpfung cameras or tomographs with corneal topographers between eyes that have undergone either DMEK or UT-DSAEK. The concomitantly growing popularity of anterior segment optical coherent tomography (AS-OCT) has caused the use of this device in clinical practice to become increasingly frequent. To the best of our knowledge, to date, there have been no studies that compared corneal topographic parameters between eyes that underwent DMEK and UT-DSAEK in swept-source AS-OCT. Bearing in mind the above, our aim was to create a study to provide an analysis of corneal parameter changes in patients who underwent DMEK and UT-DSAEK using an AS-OCT device.

2. Materials and Methods

This study included 24 consecutive eyes that had undergone UT-DSAEK and 24 consecutive eyes that had undergone DMEK due to various causes of endothelial decompensation (Fuchs endothelial corneal dystrophy or pseudophakic bullous keratopathy). The subjects that were enrolled in the study were patients that were operated on at the First Ophthalmology Clinic in Szczecin in 2018–2020 and then followed up at 1, 3, 6 and 12 months after the surgery. All participants underwent a complete ophthalmologic examination, including the following: best-corrected distance visual acuity with Snellen charts (Remote-Controlled Chart Monitor, CC-100, Topcon, Tokyo, Japan), slit lamp biomicroscopy, IOP measurements and a detailed fundus examination after pupil mydriasis. Corneal quality parameters were measured with swept-source AS-OCT at each following visit.

2.1. Donor Characteristics

Donor corneas were obtained with the multiorgan procurement method and in the dissecting room during autopsies. Corneoscleral buttons were hypothermically stored in Eusol-C medium (Alchimia, Ponte San Nicolò, Italy) at 2–6 °C at the West Pomeranian Eye Tissue Bank in Szczecin. The prestorage evaluation of the endothelium was performed using specular microscopy (Konan CellCheck EB-10; Konan Medical USA Inc., Irvine, CA, USA). All corneas had an endothelial cell count of at least 2800 cells/mm^2.

2.2. Surgical Techniques

Each surgery was performed by the same surgeon. All subjects underwent prophylactic basal laser iridectomy (Optimis Fusion, Quantel Medical, Cournon-d'Auvergne, France) before endothelial keratoplasty to minimize the risk of postoperative pupillary block. Subjects with retinal diseases that significantly affected visual acuity were excluded from the study. All procedures were performed with peribulbar block.

UT-DSAEK grafts were prepared with the single-pass technique using a MORIA One Use microkeratome. The donor tissue was mounted on an artificial anterior chamber (AAC), which maintained a continuous intracameral pressure of 200 mmHg (Moria S.A., Antony, France). After ensuring adequate pressure in the AAC system, central corneal thickness measurements were taken using an ultrasound iPac Pachymeter (Reichert, Inc., Depew, NY, USA). An appropriate microkeratome head was chosen, and the cut was performed at a deliberately slow speed. The anterior cap was removed, and the residual stromal bed was again measured. The AAC was carefully disassembled, avoiding any trauma to the endothelium.

The donor's rolled endothelial graft was inserted using a Busin glide through a 3.2 mm clear corneal incision (Moria S.A., Antony, France). After centering the graft, the anterior chamber was filled with air to allow for a perfect adherence of the donor flap to the receiving tissue.

The preparation of the DMEK graft and surgery was performed following the 'no-touch' technique, as described previously [13].

All patients were instructed to keep a supine position after the surgery till the control of the flap position was done on the first postoperative day. In the case of a pupillary block or ocular hypertension, topical mydriatics were administered, and if this was insufficient, a small quantity of air was released from the AC in the operating theatre. The postoperative treatment for both groups was a topical antibiotic given 4 times a day for 1 week and topical preservative-free dexamethasone sodium phosphate 8 times a day for the first month. The topical steroid was tapered down to one drop every other day and then discontinued over 1 year. The graft thickness in all UT-DSAEK eyes was below 100 μm (mean graft thickness at the 12-month follow-up visit was 66.09 ± 18.61 μm).

2.3. AS-OCT Measurements

Both the corneal thickness and keratometry values were determined using a swept-source anterior segment OCT CASIA2 (Tomey, Nagoya, Japan). During the entire observation period, the CASIA2 was placed in the same room under the same lighting conditions. All measurements were taken by trained operators, who also held the subjects' eyelids gently to avoid pressure on the globe. The scan was performed using the autoalignment function. The CASIA2 measurements were obtained with the corneal map mode of the anterior segment module from the OCT images using the built-in software and measurement tools provided by the manufacturers. The CASIA software automatically defined the intraocular structures and generated measurement values. The images were analyzed using built-in 2D analysis software that automatically calculated the measurements, along with the structural outlines and reference lines. The outline tracer was edited where needed.

Central corneal thickness (μm), mean keratometry values (D), astigmatism power (D) and axis (°), astigmatism asymmetry (D) and higher-order aberration power (D) were recorded and analyzed at different time points after surgery using the Fourier Analysis 3D/2D function. Measurements were read from both the anterior and posterior surfaces of the cornea, and the total values were taken into account. All parameters were assessed in 3 and 6 mm diameter optical zones (OZs). The image quality was assessed during the acquisition by the operator. Only measurements that were well-centered and with high-quality indexes were included in the study.

2.4. Statistical Analysis

Statistical analysis was conducted using Statistica software. Since most of the analyzed variables showed distributions that were significantly different from normal distributions (Shapiro–Wilk test, $p < 0.05$), non-parametric tests were used. The Wilcoxon signed-rank test was used to compare the preoperative and postoperative values. The Mann–Whitney U test was applied to analyze the differences between the groups. The correlations between the baseline variables and the corneal parameters were analyzed with Spearman's rank correlation coefficient (Rs). Bivariate analysis, including surgical technique and patient's age as independent variables, and change of a parameter relative to its baseline value as the dependent variable, was performed using a general linear model (GLM). Standardized beta values (β) were presented to show the strength of association between the surgical technique and the follow-up parameter changes. A p-value of less than 0.05 was considered to be statistically significant. The statistical power of the study at the 0.05 significance level with 24 subjects in each study group was sufficient to detect with 80% probability the real effect size corresponding to the difference between the groups equal to ± 0.83 SD and associations between variables within groups with a real effect size corresponding to the correlation coefficient of ±0.54 [14].

3. Results

3.1. Characteristics of the Study Groups

Forty-eight eyes of 43 patients were assigned to DMEK (n = 24) or UT-DSAEK (n = 24). Table 1 provides the preoperative characteristics of the study groups. The study groups were matched for sex (p = 0.55) and the DMEK group was younger than the UT-DSAEK group (p = 0.01). At the baseline, there were no significant differences between the groups in the values of corneal topographic parameters, i.e., the mean keratometry (MK) values, astigmatism power and asymmetry (AA) and the values of higher-order aberrations (HOAs). Accordingly, the groups did not differ in preoperative central corneal thickness measurements.

Table 1. Preoperative characteristics of the study groups (mean values ± SD). Statistically significant p-values are shown in bold.

			UT-DSAEK	DMEK	p
Recipient age (y)			74.96 ± 10.43	66.25 ± 11.23	**0.01**
Recipient sex (m/f)			9/13	5/16	0.55
Indications for the surgery (FECD/PBK)			14/10	21/3	n/a
Baseline BCVA			0.11 ± 0.12	0.22 ± 0.15	**0.01**
Donor graft ECC (cells/mm^2)			3129.96 ± 242.48	3057.83 ± 317.73	0.26
Baseline CCT (μm)			730.04 ± 92.67	698.92 ± 89.61	0.20
Baseline mean keratometry (D)	Anterior	3 mm OZ	49.55 ± 1.58	49.36 ± 2.72	1.00
		6 mm OZ	48.96 ± 1.39	48.89 ± 1.97	0.78
	Posterior	3 mm OZ	−6.05 ± 0.51	−6.02 ± 0.69	0.90
		6 mm OZ	−5.99 ± 0.43	−6.00 ± 0.59	0.97
	Total	3 mm OZ	43.66 ± 1.71	43.48 ± 2.94	1.00
		6 mm OZ	43.12 ± 1.44	43.04 ± 2.06	0.89
Baseline mean astigmatism (D)	Anterior	3 mm OZ	1.35 ± 0.95	1.52 ± 0.81	0.34
		6 mm OZ	1.19 ± 0.78	1.28 ± 0.52	0.29
	Posterior	3 mm OZ	0.27 ± 0.18	0.36 ± 0.19	0.10
		6 mm OZ	0.24 ± 0.13	0.30 ± 0.16	0.14
	Total	3 mm OZ	1.43 ± 0.96	1.63 ± 0.94	0.47
		6 mm OZ	1.22 ± 0.77	1.35 ± 0.59	0.28
Baseline astigmatism asymmetry (D)	Anterior	3 mm OZ	1.48 ± 1.10	1.88 ± 1.97	0.65
		6 mm OZ	1.71 ± 1.10	2.06 ± 1.80	0.73
	Posterior	3 mm OZ	0.51 ± 0.25	0.56 ± 0.55	0.60
		6 mm OZ	0.59 ± 0.28	0.66 ± 0.60	0.62
	Total	3 mm OZ	1.72 ± 1.10	2.10 ± 1.97	0.97
		6 mm OZ	1.95 ± 1.06	2.38 ± 1.80	0.66
Baseline higher-order aberrations (D)	Anterior	3 mm OZ	0.82 ± 0.61	0.74 ± 0.65	0.40
		6 mm OZ	0.88 ± 0.73	0.70 ± 0.52	0.32
	Posterior	3 mm OZ	0.22 ± 0.15	0.19 ± 0.15	0.40
		6 mm OZ	0.21 ± 0.13	0.19 ± 0.15	0.46
	Total	3 mm OZ	0.89 ± 0.57	0.77 ± 0.68	0.11
		6 mm OZ	0.94 ± 0.72	0.75 ± 0.57	0.17

UT-DSAEK—ultrathin Descemet membrane automated endothelial keratoplasty, DMEK—Descemet membrane endothelial keratoplasty, FECD—Fuchs endothelial corneal dystrophy, PBK—pseudophakic bullous keratopathy, BCVA—best-corrected visual acuity, ECC—endothelial cell count, CCT—central corneal thickness, n/a—not applicable.

Three patients in the UT-DSAEK group were lost at the 12-month follow-up point. No graft failures or rejections were observed in this study. In four eyes after UT-DSAEK and three eyes after DMEK surgery, a postoperative graft detachment was observed. All of them were recorded in the first 24 h after surgery, with one exception: one DMEK graft detachment took place one week after surgery. In this case, the patient admitted to not following the postoperative recommendations. All detached grafts were successfully attached due to intracameral SF_6 or air injection. In four eyes after DMEK, there was a need to partially remove SF_6 from the anterior chamber in the first 24 h after surgery due to the elevated intraocular pressure (IOP). No further complications in those eyes were observed.

3.2. Postoperative Changes in BCVA and ECC in DMEK and UT-DSAEK Eyes

The mean baseline BCVA was 0.22 in the DMEK arm and 0.11 in the UT-DSAEK arm ($p = 0.01$). Up to 6 months post operation, the BCVA improved in both treatment groups to a similar extent from baseline. After adjusting for age, the change in BCVA did not differ significantly between DMEK and UT-DSAEK patients at the 1-month follow-up visit ($\beta = -0.25$, $p = 0.12$), 3-month follow-up visit ($\beta = -0.04$, $p = 0.76$) or 6-month follow-up visit ($\beta = -0.22$, $p = 0.06$). In contrast, at the 12-month follow-up visit, the postoperative increase in the BCVA was higher in the DMEK group (median = 1.00) than in the UT-DSAEK group (median = 0.6, $p < 0.001$). This difference remained significant in the multivariate analysis that was performed using a GLM after an adjustment for age ($\beta = -0.37$, $p = 0.006$).

Regarding the ECC, we observed no differences in the donor endothelial cell count (median = 3045.50 cells/mm^2 in the DMEK group and median = 3140 cells/mm^2 in the UT-DSAEK group, $p = 0.26$). From 3 months post operation, the endothelial cell density was higher in the DMEK eyes than in the UT-DSAEK eyes (median = 1470.50 cells/mm^2 and median = 1156 cells/mm^2, $p = 0.009$, respectively, at the 3-month follow-up visit; median = 1384 cells/mm^2 and median = 1146 cells/mm^2, $p = 0.005$, respectively, at the 6-month follow-up visit; median = 1304.5 cells/mm^2 and median = 1113 cells/mm^2, $p = 0.07$, respectively, at the 12-month follow-up visit).

3.3. Postoperative Analysis of AS-OCT Corneal Parameters in DMEK and UT-DSAEK Eyes Compared to Baseline

First, we analyzed the changes in corneal surface parameters compared to baseline recordings for the DMEK and UT-DSAEK groups separately. Tables 2 and 3 provide the corneal topography values of the postoperative pachymetry, keratometry, astigmatism and aberration parameters that were obtained for the DMEK and UT-DSAEK groups of eyes, respectively. A significant decrease in CCT compared to baseline recordings was observed at all follow-up time points in both the DMEK and UT-DSAEK groups.

At 1, 3, 6 and 12 months after DMEK surgery, there were no significant differences in anterior surface mean keratometry values compared to the baseline in the 3.0 and 6.0 mm diameter optical zones (6.0 mm diameter—data not shown). For the posterior surface, MK values were lower at all follow-up time points than preoperative values. Interestingly, for the combined corneal surface, there were no differences in MK values between those recorded at 6 and 12 months post operation and the baseline. Contrary to the DMEK group, in the UT-DSEAK group, we observed a significant decrease in MK recordings for both the anterior and posterior corneal surfaces, as well as for total corneas in both the 3.0 and 6.0 mm diameter OZs as early as 1 month post operation (6.0 mm diameter—data not shown). Finally, the combined surface MK values were significantly lower at 12 months post operation than the preoperative values (mean difference = -1.42 ± 1.87 D for the 3 mm OZ).

Regarding the astigmatism power, in the DMEK group, we observed a significant decrease for the posterior and total corneas from 3 months post operation and the anterior corneal surface from 6 months post operation. In contrast, in the UT-DSAEK eyes, the astigmatism power remained unchanged until 6 months post operation and decreased for the anterior and total corneas only at 12 months post operation. The magnitude of the posterior astigmatism in the UT-DSAEK eyes remained unchanged throughout the observation period. Interestingly, we found no significant changes in the astigmatism axis at 1, 3, 6 and 12 months after surgery compared to the baseline in either the DMEK or UT-DSAEK group.

Table 2. Changes in the central corneal thickness (CCT), mean keratometry, astigmatism magnitude, astigmatism asymmetry and higher-order aberration power compared to the baseline in the 3 mm corneal optical zone after Descemet membrane endothelial keratoplasty (DMEK). Statistically significant values are shown in bold.

		Baseline	1 Month		3 Months		6 Months		12 Months	
		Median (IQR)	Median (IQR)	p	Median (IQR)	p	Median (IQR)	p	Median (IQR)	p
Corneal thickness (μm)	Apex	680.5 (129)	503 (69)	**<0.001**	498 (56)	**<0.001**	507 (51)	**<0.001**	517.5 (42.5)	**<0.001**
	Thinnest	618.5 (70)	490 (69)	**<0.001**	486.5 (44)	**<0.001**	493 (42)	**<0.001**	508 (43)	**<0.001**
Mean keratometry (D)	Anterior	49.96 (4.96)	48.34 (2.85)	0.50	48.11 (2.90)	0.36	49.02 (2.68)	0.54	49.26 (2.68)	0.36
	Posterior	−6.06 (0.89)	−6.47 (0.40)	**<0.001**	−6.37 (0.35)	**0.02**	−6.32 (0.41)	0.06	−6.34 (0.31)	**0.03**
	Total	43.88 (4.46)	42.07 (2.18)	0.24	41.92 (2.29)	0.19	42.76 (2.21)	0.31	42.92 (2.31)	0.17
Mean astigmatism (D)	Anterior	1.47 (1.01)	1.58 (1.28)	0.9	0.93 (0.83)	0.06	0.92 (0.68)	**0.02**	0.88 (0.90)	**0.03**
	Posterior	0.30 (0.30)	0.28 (0.20)	0.44	0.22 (0.13)	**0.03**	0.19 (0.13)	**0.001**	0.18 (0.14)	**0.001**
	Total	1.31 (1.57)	1.63 (1.15)	0.79	0.89 (0.825)	**0.03**	0.93 (0.6)	**0.02**	0.835 (0.51)	**0.02**
Astigmatism asymmetry (D)	Anterior	1.11 (1.79)	1.00 (0.59)	**0.01**	0.57 (0.44)	**0.004**	0.50 (0.29)	**<0.001**	0.49 (0.30)	**<0.001**
	Posterior	0.43 (0.54)	0.24 (0.23)	**0.01**	0.18 (0.09)	**0.002**	0.15 (0.1)	**<0.001**	0.13 (0.09)	**<0.001**
	Total	1.41 (1.69)	0.78 (0.66)	**0.001**	0.62 (0.42)	**0.002**	0.51 (0.32)	**<0.001**	0.55 (0.39)	**<0.001**
Higher-order aberrations (D)	Anterior	0.48 (0.98)	0.34 (0.37)	0.08	0.28 (0.19)	**0.007**	0.28 (0.15)	**0.006**	0.22 (0.10)	**<0.001**
	Posterior	0.18 (0.16)	0.09 (0.05)	**0.002**	0.08 (0.06)	**0.003**	0.08 (0.06)	**0.003**	0.07 (0.05)	**0.004**
	Total	0.46 (0.85)	0.37 (0.33)	**0.046**	0.27 (0.15)	**0.001**	0.27 (0.1)	**<0.001**	0.21 (0.08)	**<0.001**

When analyzing the irregular corneal astigmatism with the asymmetry of astigmatic components and HOAs, we observed similar patterns of decrease in both the UT-DSAEK and DMEK subgroups. At 1, 3, 6 and 12 months after surgery in both investigated groups, the values of the astigmatism asymmetry and HOAs decreased significantly compared to the preoperative values.

3.4. Comparative Analysis of Postoperative Corneal Surface Parameters between DMEK and UT-DSAEK Eyes

Figure 1 shows the postoperative corneal parameters, as evaluated using swept-source AS-OCT, including pachymetry, keratometry, astigmatism magnitude and asymmetry, as well as HOAs in the different corneal zones after UT-DSAEK and DMEK.

Table 3. Changes in the central corneal thickness (CCT), mean keratometry, astigmatism magnitude, astigmatism asymmetry and higher-order aberration power compared to the baseline in the 3 mm corneal optical zone after ultrathin Descemet stripping automated endothelial keratoplasty (UT-DSAEK). Statistically significant values are shown in bold.

		Baseline	1 Month		3 Months		6 Months		12 Months	
		Median (IQR)	Median (IQR)	p	Median (IQR)	p	Median (IQR)	p	Median (IQR)	p
Corneal thickness (μm)	Apex	696 (100)	600.5 (50)	**<0.001**	567 (63)	**<0.001**	577 (71)	**<0.001**	590 (62)	**<0.001**
	Thinnest	656 (84)	572 (49)	**<0.001**	544 (58)	**<0.001**	553 (69)	**<0.001**	558 (53)	**<0.001**
Mean keratometry (D)	Anterior	49.31 (2.32)	48.38 (2.14)	**0.008**	49.09 (2.15)	0.06	48.85 (1.38)	**0.02**	48.86 (1.64)	0.13
	Posterior	−6.02 (0.97)	−7.12 (0.86)	**<0.001**	−6.94 (0.27)	**<0.001**	−6.89 (0.27)	**<0.001**	−6.85 (0.24)	**<0.001**
	Total	43.53 (2.16)	41.37 (2.21)	**<0.001**	42.22 (2.16)	**0.002**	42.01 (1.43)	**<0.001**	42.14 (1.29)	**0.004**
Mean astigmatism (D)	Anterior	1.28 (1.46)	1 (1.23)	0.57	0.83 (0.65)	0.11	0.82 (0.66)	0.12	0.61 (0.65)	**0.017**
	Posterior	0.23 (0.24)	0.23 (0.23)	0.98	0.21 (0.2)	0.4	0.17 (0.21)	0.24	0.18 (0.11)	0.24
	Total	1.32 (1.41)	0.79 (1.32)	0.42	0.9 (0.84)	0.11	0.87 (0.73)	0.13	0.78 (0.4)	**0.02**
Astigmatism asymmetry (D)	Anterior	1.02 (1.03)	0.63 (0.59)	**0.01**	0.69 (0.93)	**0.002**	0.52 (0.67)	**<0.001**	0.49 (0.41)	**<0.001**
	Posterior	0.5 (0.22)	0.36 (0.25)	0.54	0.3 (0.32)	**0.001**	0.29 (0.17)	**<0.001**	0.25 (0.21)	**<0.001**
	Total	1.38 (1.4)	0.87 (0.69)	**0.02**	0.74 (0.66)	**0.001**	0.62 (0.52)	**<0.001**	0.41 (0.23)	**<0.001**
Higher-order aberrations (D)	Anterior	0.63 (0.71)	0.41 (0.25)	**0.007**	0.27 (0.09)	**<0.001**	0.22 (0.13)	**<0.001**	0.23 (0.06)	**<0.001**
	Posterior	0.19 (0.18)	0.14 (0.13)	0.43	0.1 (0.08)	**0.002**	0.09 (0.05)	**<0.001**	0.09 (0.04)	**0.002**
	Total	0.73 (0.69)	0.45 (0.16)	**0.001**	0.31 (0.18)	**<0.001**	0.26 (0.11)	**<0.001**	0.24 (0.1)	**<0.001**

Throughout the observation period, we found no differences in the values of any parameters for the anterior and total corneas between the DMEK and UT-DSAEK eyes. Importantly, the values of the posterior mean keratometry and the magnitudes of the back astigmatism asymmetry and HOAs were significantly lower in the DMEK group than in the UT-DSAEK group at all follow-up time points. No differences in astigmatism power for either the anterior or posterior region or the total cornea were observed at any time point between the analyzed groups of eyes.

Subsequently, we compared the changes in corneal surface parameters at postoperative follow-up time points relative to the preoperative values between the DMEK and UT-DSAEK groups. Regarding the pachymetry, we found no differences in the CCT changes at the 1-, 3- and 6-month follow-up visits between the study groups. Exclusively, at the 12-month follow-up visit, the decrease in the CCT was larger in the DMEK eyes ($\beta = +0.32$, $p = 0.04$) in the multivariate analysis performed using a GLM after an adjustment for age. A multivariate analysis of keratometry changes in the DMEK and UT-DSAEK eyes, after an adjustment for age, revealed that DMEK was an independent variable that was associated with a smaller decrease in posterior mean keratometry at the 1-month ($\beta = -0.49$, $p = 0.002$),

3-month ($\beta = -0.50$, $p < 0.001$), 6-month ($\beta = -0.58$, $p < 0.001$) and 12-month ($\beta = -0.49$, $p < 0.001$) follow-up visits in both the 3 and 6 mm optical zones. There were no significant differences in changes in anterior surface or combined surface MK between the UT-DSAEK and DMEK groups throughout the observation period. Regarding the astigmatism power, there were no significant differences in the anterior, posterior surface or combined surface astigmatism changes between the UT-DSAEK and DMEK groups, with one exception: posterior astigmatism decreases at the 6- and 12-month follow-up visits were larger in the DMEK group ($\beta = +0.40$, $p = 0.01$) in the multivariate analysis that was performed using a GLM after an adjustment for age. Accordingly, no significant differences in changes in astigmatism asymmetry and HOAs compared to baseline values were identified between the eyes from the DMEK and UT-DSAEK groups at any follow-up time point.

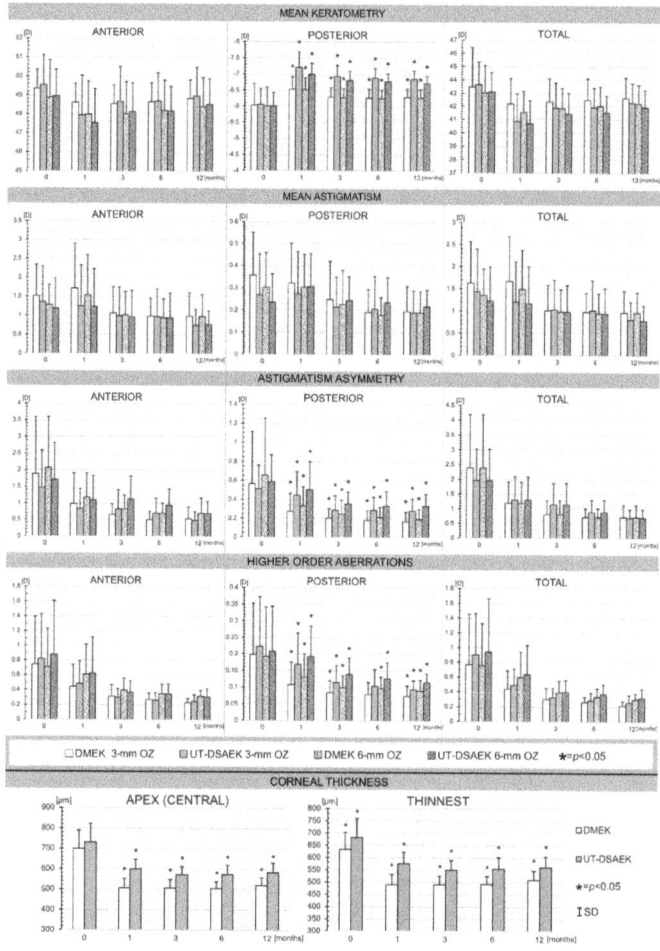

Figure 1. Bar graphs showing the pre- and postoperative mean values of the corneal parameters, which were evaluated using swept-source AS-OCT: mean keratometry, mean astigmatism, astigmatism asymmetry, higher-order aberrations and corneal thickness at the baseline and 1, 3, 6 and 12 months after Descemet membrane endothelial keratoplasty (DMEK) versus ultrathin Descemet stripping automated endothelial keratoplasty (UT-DSAEK) measured in 3 and 6 mm optical zones (OZs). * $p < 0.05$.

3.5. Correlations between BCVA and Corneal Parameters at Subsequent Follow-Up Points

Next, we investigated the potential relationships between the corneal parameters and BCVA. We found that the baseline BCVA determined the postoperative corneal thickness at the 12-month follow-up in both the UT-DSAEK and DMEK groups. Accordingly, we observed a positive correlation between the preoperative BCVA and changes in the CCT at the 1-month (Rs = +0.59, p = 0.003), 3-month (Rs = +0.54, p = 0.006), 6-month (Rs = +0.57, p = 0.004) and 12-month (Rs = +0.52, p = 0.01) follow-up visits in the DMEK eyes. Analogous correlations were observed in the UT-DSAEK eyes at 1 month (Rs = +0.59, p = 0.01), 3 months (Rs = +0.58, p = 0.006), 6 months (Rs = +0.46, p = 0.04) and 12 months (Rs = +0.33, p = 0.17) post operation.

To identify the corneal surface aberrations that most affected the BCVA at subsequent postoperative visits, we investigated the associations between the BCVA and topographic characteristics of the cornea in both the DMEK and UT-DSAEK groups (Table 4). In the UT-DSAEK eyes, we observed a negative correlation between the BCVA and astigmatism power at 3, 6 and 12 months post operation. Accordingly, the BCVA was negatively correlated with the astigmatism asymmetry throughout the observation period. No such correlations were found in the DMEK group.

Table 4. The correlations between the best-corrected visual acuity (BCVA) and the magnitudes of the keratometry, astigmatism, astigmatism asymmetry and higher-order aberrations that were obtained in the 3 mm optical zones in the eyes after Descemet membrane endothelial keratoplasty (DMEK) and ultrathin Descemet stripping automated endothelial keratoplasty (UT-DSAEK) procedures. Correlations were calculated for the baseline state and then for 4 consecutive time points, i.e., 1, 3, 6 and 12 months, after the surgery. Statistically significant values are shown in bold.

Correlation		Baseline		1 Month		3 Months		6 Months		12 Months	
		UT-DSAEK	DMEK	UT-DSAEK	DMEK	UT-DSAEK	DMEK	UT-DSAEK	DMEK	UT-DSAEK	DMEK
Mean keratometry	Anterior	+0.13	+0.17	−0.10	+0.03	+0.11	−0.29	−0.08	+0.01	**+0.41**	+0.22
	Posterior	+0.32	+0.24	+0.36	+0.19	+0.34	**+0.52**	+0.31	+0.26	**+0.54**	+0.04
	Total	+0.09	+0.18	−0.01	+0.02	+0.15	−0.22	−0.03	+0.09	**+0.45**	+0.32
Mean astigmatism	Anterior	**−0.45**	+0.11	**−0.45**	−0.08	**−0.43**	−0.22	**−0.53**	−0.29	−0.39	−0.03
	Posterior	−0.17	−0.22	−0.17	−0.09	+0.02	+0.08	+0.16	−0.03	−0.27	−0.04
	Total	**−0.41**	+0.05	**−0.41**	−0.12	−0.39	−0.27	**−0.50**	−0.29	**−0.54**	−0.20
Astigmatism asymmetry	Anterior	**−0.52**	−0.19	−0.26	+0.18	**−0.54**	−0.29	−0.40	−0.39	**−0.58**	−0.36
	Posterior	**+0.44**	−0.10	**−0.58**	−0.33	−0.35	−0.21	−0.34	−0.34	−0.03	−0.34
	Total	−0.31	−0.19	−0.39	+0.18	**−0.43**	−0.17	−0.14	−0.15	+0.06	+0.03
Higher-order aberrations	Anterior	**−0.46**	−0.03	+0.01	+0.06	−0.33	−0.32	−0.32	−0.10	−0.14	−0.04
	Posterior	−0.28	−0.26	−0.26	−0.02	−0.09	−0.05	−0.15	**−0.49**	−0.16	−0.14
	Total	**−0.41**	−0.08	−0.11	−0.05	−0.31	−0.30	**−0.42**	−0.01	−0.29	−0.04

3.6. Correlations between CCT Change and Changes in Corneal Parameters Compared to Baseline Values

We also analyzed the potential associations between the changes in selected corneal parameters at selected time points post operation. We found that decreases in the magnitudes of the astigmatism, HOA and AA values for the total and posterior cornea throughout the observation period, as well as the anterior corneal surface at 6 and 12 months post operation (Table 5), were positively associated with a decrease in the CCT in the DMEK eyes. Interestingly, in the UT-DSAEK eyes, an analogous relationship was observed only between changes in the CCT and HOAs.

Table 5. The correlations between the central corneal thickness (CCT) change and changes in the magnitudes of the keratometry, astigmatism, astigmatism asymmetry and higher-order aberrations that were obtained in 3 mm optical zones (OZs) in the eyes after Descemet membrane endothelial keratoplasty (DMEK) and ultrathin Descemet stripping automated endothelial keratoplasty (UT-DSAEK) procedures. Correlations were calculated for 4 consecutive time points, i.e., 1, 3, 6 and 12 months after the surgery. Statistically significant values are shown in bold.

Correlation		1 Month		3 Months		6 Months		12 Months	
		UT-DSAEK	DMEK	UT-DSAEK	DMEK	UT-DSAEK	DMEK	UT-DSAEK	DMEK
Mean keratometry change	Anterior	+0.43	−0.002	+0.01	−0.05	+0.06	−0.03	+0.05	+0.17
	Posterior	−0.15	−0.01	−0.11	−0.08	−0.02	−0.09	+0.14	−0.003
	Total	+0.38	+0.04	+0.02	−0.05	+0.04	−0.04	+0.07	+0.16
Mean astigmatism change	Anterior	−0.12	+0.28	−0.15	**+0.45**	−0.03	**+0.47**	+0.15	**+0.65**
	Posterior	−0.01	**+0.64**	−0.05	**+0.54**	−0.0005	**+0.48**	+0.06	**+0.64**
	Total	−0.08	+0.39	−0.07	**+0.46**	−0.03	**+0.52**	+0.22	**+0.72**
Astigmatism asymmetry change	Anterior	+0.36	+0.15	+0.33	+0.07	+0.11	−0.22	+0.22	−0.05
	Posterior	+0.01	+0.28	+0.13	**+0.47**	+0.11	+0.38	+0.11	**+0.50**
	Total	+0.20	**+0.67**	+0.18	**+0.60**	+0.31	**+0.57**	+0.22	**+0.65**
Higher-order aberrations change	Anterior	−0.05	**+0.44**	+0.26	**+0.47**	+0.27	**+0.50**	+0.18	**+0.58**
	Posterior	**+0.52**	**+0.75**	**+0.74**	**+0.75**	**+0.76**	**+0.61**	**+0.77**	**+0.72**
	Total	+0.20	**+0.45**	+0.38	**+0.54**	**+0.44**	**+0.64**	+0.18	**+0.66**

4. Discussion

In recent years, endothelial corneal transplantation has evolved to become the method of choice for the treatment of endothelial damage. Although DMEK seems to offer better and faster visual and refractive results, controversy still exists regarding whether it is a better technique than UT-DSAEK and NT-DSAEK, which are easier techniques and have similar outcomes to DMEK.

The results of this study provided a comparison of a wide range of topographic outcomes between DMEK and UT-DSAEK during a 1-year follow-up period. Compared with the UT-DSAEK results, lower mean posterior keratometry, lower posterior astigmatism, lower posterior astigmatism asymmetry and fewer posterior corneal HOAs were found after DMEK. Nevertheless, total corneal parameters were comparable after both procedures.

The results of this study indicated significant differences in posterior surface MK values between the keratoplasty techniques, which occurred after surgery. Compared to DMEK, we noted the steeper posterior corneal curvature in the UT-DSAEK group. This finding is consistent with the results of previous studies. Both Torras-Sanvicens et al. and Goldich et al. analyzed the mean anterior and posterior keratometry values and, similarly to us, found significant differences in the posterior keratometry in favor of DMEK [6,15]. Importantly, the combined surface UT-DSAEK MK values were significantly lower at 12 months post operation than before the operation by −1.42 ± 1.87 D. In contrast, after DMEK surgery, we found no significant differences in the anterior and combined surface MK values throughout the observation period compared to the baseline.

On the other hand, hyperopic outcomes tend to occur after posterior lamellar corneal transplantation. This hyperopic shift is very relevant after DSAEK and is described in the literature as ranging from 0.7 to 1.5 D [16]. Regarding UT-DSAEK, Busin et al. reported a significant hyperopic shift of 0.78 ± 0.59 D at the 1-year follow-up [3]. On the other hand, In their multicenter, prospective, double-masked, randomized, controlled clinical trial comparing DSAEK and UT-DSAEK, Dickman et al. observed a comparable hyperopic shift after both procedures [17]. Similarly, Dunker et al. showed no difference in hyperopic shift after the UT-DSAEK and DMEK surgery techniques [8].

In this study, we demonstrated a significant decrease in astigmatism power in the eyes after DMEK surgery that occurred from 3 months after surgery in the anterior, posterior and total corneas. In contrast, this effect was significantly prolonged in the anterior and total corneas and occurred only after 12 months post operation. We found no changes in posterior astigmatism throughout the observation period in the UT-DSAEK group. This allowed us to assume that the visual rehabilitation of patients after DMEK was shorter than that after UT-DSAEK. Indeed, data provided by Mencucci et al. lead to a similar assumption that postoperative recovery after DMEK might be quicker than that after UT-DSAEK [7]. Our results are also in line with those from the randomized controlled DETECT trial, which documented that DMEK was associated with a postoperative shift in posterior corneal astigmatism but not UT-DSAEK [18].

HOAs may increase after endothelial keratoplasty, which would significantly reduce visual acuity and influence vision quality. Throughout the observation period, we found no differences in the astigmatism asymmetry or HOA values for the anterior and total corneas between the DMEK and UT-DSAEK eyes. Importantly, the posterior absolute values of those parameters were significantly lower in the DMEK group than in the UT-DSAEK group at all follow-up time points. It is noteworthy that previous analyses that compared the changes in HOAs between DMEK and UT-DSAEK showed inconclusive results. In a recent study performed in 2020, Duggan et al. evaluated the outcomes of DMEK vs. UT-DSAEK patients and found that DMEK induced less posterior corneal HOAs than UT-DSAEK. The authors reported that posterior corneal HOA actually increased significantly in the UT-DSAEK group from the baseline to 3 months after surgery and remained significantly higher at 6 and 12 months. The HOAs of the anterior corneal surface in their sample did not differ significantly between DMEK and UT-DSAEK. These results are only partially in line with ours since we documented a similar pattern of decrease in the astigmatism asymmetry and the HOAs of the anterior, posterior and total corneas in both the DMEK and UT-DSAEK groups. Likewise, Mencucci et al. conducted a similar investigation and found that total and posterior corneal HOAs, posterior astigmatism and total coma were significantly lower after DMEK than after UT-DSAEK in both the 4 and 6 mm optical zones [7]. On the other hand, Torras-Sanvicens et al. did not observe statistically significant differences in total, anterior or posterior HOAs 12 months after surgery [6], which is in line with the results of other groups [19]. Altogether, it should be highlighted that the published data differ in terms of the operating techniques, corneal topographer device, definitions of UT-DSAEK grafts below 100 μm [8,9,20] or below 130 μm [3,7] and selection of study groups used, which makes it impossible to draw definite conclusions. It is worth mentioning that none of the previous studies compared the postoperative corneal curvature and topography parameters with their baseline values recorded preoperatively. To overcome this limitation, our study, for the first time, compared the changes in astigmatism asymmetry and HOAs compared to the baseline values between DMEK and UT-DSAEK eyes. We documented no significant differences between the two groups in the relative variations in any high-order aberration parameter at any follow-up time point. Our data seemed to represent an objective value in the comparative analysis between the UT-DSAEK and DMEK eyes. This approach eliminates the potential influence of the baseline corneal status on postoperative results between the study groups.

Bearing in mind that the presence of HOAs might affect the vision-related quality of life, several research groups have analyzed the objective and subjective visual quality and contrast sensitivity after both procedures. In their cross-sectional, comparative, and observational case series, Torras-Sanvicens et al. conducted an extended and comprehensive analysis that included objective visual quality variables, contrast sensitivity and subjective patient satisfaction, e.g., subjective quality of the surgical technique, level of comfort in the postoperative period, recovery time and preferred eye. The authors found no significant differences in any of the parameters studied between UT-DSAEK and DMEK eyes [6]. Accordingly, other research groups, e.g., Dukner et al., Ang et al. and Dunbar et al., reported no differences in vision-related quality of life between both procedures [10–12]. Interestingly, we observed that a decrease in the magnitudes of HOA values throughout the observation time was positively associated with a decrease in CCT. This strongly indicated that corneal thickness influenced the changes in corneal curvature and indicated a dynamic balance between corneal parameters due to the healing process within corneal tissue. Accordingly, postoperative visual acuity was significantly correlated with topographic characteristics of the cornea (the higher the aberrations, the lower the visual acuity was) in the UT-DSAEK eyes at subsequent postoperative visits. Similar observations were recorded by other study groups [7]. Importantly, our study seems to be the first to suggest that baseline vision acuity determines postoperative corneal thickness at the 12-month follow-up in both the DSAEK and DMEK groups. Further evidence is needed to establish causative links between changes in BCVA, central corneal thickness and corneal topographic outcomes after DMEK and UT-DSAEK surgery.

The results of our study clearly demonstrated that ECC loss after DMEK was less than that after UT-DSAEK. These results are comparable with those published by other research groups [6]. Conversely, Mencucci et al. [7] found no difference in ECC count between DMEK and UT-DSAEK eyes. Similar results were provided by Dunker et al. [8]. This observation is in line with those of several comparative DMEK and DSAEK studies that documented that endothelial cell loss was similar for both procedures [17,21,22]. The probable cause of such imbalances was, according to the authors, the increased handling of DMEK tissue during surgery. With regard to all the studies mentioned above, we can assume that endothelial cell loss after surgery is an individual quality that depends on the surgical technique, the experience of the operator and donor tissue preparatory procedures.

In conclusion, to the best of our knowledge, this is the first case series that compared changes in corneal topographic parameters with their baseline values between UT-DSAEK and DMEK groups at the 12-month follow-up. Accordingly, this might also be the first study in which the values of corneal topographic parameters in DMEK and UT-DSAEK eyes were studied using CASIA2 swept-source anterior segment OCT. Although DMEK showed a faster recovery during follow-up, along with lower pachymetry and a flatter posterior keratometry than UT DSAEK, UT-DSAEK seemed to be an easier and safer technique with similar outcomes regarding irregular corneal astigmatism with asymmetry of astigmatic components and HOAs.

Author Contributions: Conceptualization, A.M. and A.K.; methodology, A.M. and A.K.; software, n/a; validation, A.M., K.S. and A.K.; formal analysis, K.S.; investigation, A.K. and A.M.; resources, A.K. and A.M.; data curation, A.K., A.M., B.K. and K.S.; writing—original draft preparation, A.M. and A.K.; writing—review and editing, A.K. and A.M.; visualization, A.K., A.M. and B.K.; supervision, A.M.; project administration, A.M.; funding acquisition, n/a. All authors have read and agreed to the published version of the manuscript.

Funding: This research did not receive any specific grant from funding agencies in the public, commercial or not-for-profit sectors.

Institutional Review Board Statement: The study was conducted according to the guidelines of the Declaration of Helsinki. Ethical review and approval were waived due to the complete anonymization of the obtained data.

Informed Consent Statement: Informed consent was obtained from all subjects that were involved in the study.

Data Availability Statement: The data that were used to support the findings of this study are available from the corresponding author upon request.

Conflicts of Interest: The authors declare that there are no conflict of interest regarding the publication of this paper.

References

1. Dunker, S.L.; Armitage, W.J.; Armitage, M.; Brocato, L.; Figueiredo, F.C.; Heemskerk, M.B.; Hjortdal, J.; Jones, G.L.; Konijn, C.; Nuijts, R.M.; et al. Practice patterns of corneal transplantation in Europe: First report by the European Cornea and Cell Transplantation Registry (ECCTR). *J. Cataract. Refract. Surg.* 2021. [CrossRef]
2. Maier, P.; Reinhard, T.; Cursiefen, C. Descemet stripping endothelial keratoplasty–rapid recovery of visual acuity. *Dtsch. Aerzteblatt Online* 2013, *110*, 365–371. [CrossRef]
3. Busin, M.; Madi, S.; Santorum, P.; Scorcia, V.; Beltz, J. Ultrathin descemet's stripping automated endothelial keratoplasty with the microkeratome double-pass technique: Two-year outcomes. *Ophthalmology* 2013, *120*, 1186–1194. [CrossRef]
4. Kurji, K.H.; Cheung, A.Y.; Eslani, M.; Rolfes, E.J.; Chachare, D.Y.; Auteri, N.J.; Nordlund, M.L.; Holland, E.J. Comparison of Visual Acuity Outcomes Between Nanothin Descemet Stripping Automated Endothelial Keratoplasty and Descemet Membrane Endothelial Keratoplasty. *Cornea* 2018, *37*, 1226–1231. [CrossRef]
5. Tourabaly, M.; Chetrit, Y.; Provost, J.; Georgeon, C.; Kallel, S.; Temstet, C.; Bouheraoua, N.; Borderie, V. Influence of graft thickness and regularity on vision recovery after endothelial keratoplasty. *Br. J. Ophthalmol.* 2020, *104*, 1317–1323. [CrossRef] [PubMed]
6. Torras-Sanvicens, J.; Blanco-Domínguez, I.; Sánchez-González, J.-M.; Rachwani-Anil, R.; Spencer, J.-F.; Sabater-Cruz, N.; Peraza-Nieves, J.; Rocha-De-Lossada, C. Visual Quality and Subjective Satisfaction in Ultrathin Descemet Stripping Automated Endothelial Keratoplasty (UT-DSAEK) versus Descemet Membrane Endothelial Keratoplasty (DMEK): A Fellow-Eye Comparison. *J. Clin. Med.* 2021, *10*, 419. [CrossRef]
7. Mencucci, R.; Favuzza, E.; Marziali, E.; Cennamo, M.; Mazzotta, C.; Lucenteforte, E.; Virgili, G.; Rizzo, S. Ultrathin Descemet stripping automated endothelial keratoplasty versus Descemet membrane endothelial keratoplasty: A fellow-eye comparison. *Eye Vis.* 2020, *7*, 25–29. [CrossRef] [PubMed]
8. Dunker, S.L.; Dickman, M.M.; Wisse, R.P.; Nobacht, S.; Wijdh, R.H.; Bartels, M.C.; Tang, M.L.; Biggelaar, F.J.V.D.; Kruit, P.J.; Nuijts, R.M. Descemet Membrane Endothelial Keratoplasty versus Ultrathin Descemet Stripping Automated Endothelial Keratoplasty: A Multicenter Randomized Controlled Clinical Trial. *Ophthalmology* 2020, *127*, 1152–1159. [CrossRef]
9. Chamberlain, W.; Lin, C.C.; Austin, A.; Schubach, N.; Clover, J.; McLeod, S.D.; Porco, T.C.; Lietman, T.M.; Rose-Nussbaumer, J. Descemet Endothelial Thickness Comparison Trial: A Randomized Trial Comparing Ultrathin Descemet Stripping Automated Endothelial Keratoplasty with Descemet Membrane Endothelial Keratoplasty. *Ophthalmology* 2018, *126*, 19–26. [CrossRef] [PubMed]
10. Dunker, S.L.; Dickman, M.M.; Wisse, R.P.; Nobacht, S.; Wijdh, R.H.; Bartels, M.C.; Tang, N.M.; Biggelaar, F.J.V.D.; Kruit, P.J.; Winkens, B.; et al. Quality of vision and vision-related quality of life after Descemet membrane endothelial keratoplasty: A randomized clinical trial. *Acta Ophthalmol.* 2021, *99*, e1127–e1134. [CrossRef]
11. Dunbar, G.E.; Titus, M.; Stein, J.D.; Meijome, T.E.; Mian, S.I.; Woodward, M.A. Patient-Reported Outcomes After Corneal Transplantation. *Cornea* 2021, *40*, 1316–1321. [CrossRef] [PubMed]
12. Ang, M.J.; Chamberlain, W.; Lin, C.C.; Pickel, J.; Austin, A.; Rose-Nussbaumer, J. Effect of Unilateral Endothelial Keratoplasty on Vision-Related Quality-of-Life Outcomes in the Descemet Endothelial Thickness Comparison Trial (DETECT): A Secondary Analysis of a Randomized Clinical Trial. *JAMA Ophthalmol.* 2019, *137*, 747–754. [CrossRef]
13. Machalińska, A.; Kuligowska, A.; Kaleta, K.; Kuśmierz-Wojtasik, M.; Safranow, K. Changes in Corneal Parameters after DMEK Surgery: A Swept-Source Imaging Analysis at 12-Month Follow-Up Time. *J. Ophthalmol.* 2021, *2021*, 3055722. [CrossRef]
14. Pourhoseingholi, M.A.; Vahedi, M.; Rahimzadeh, M. Sample size calculation in medical studies. *Gastroenterol. Hepatol. Bed Bench* 2013, *6*, 14–17. [PubMed]
15. Goldich, Y.; Showail, M.; Avni-Zauberman, N.; Perez, M.; Ulate, R.; Elbaz, U.; Rootman, D.S. Contralateral eye comparison of descemet membrane endothelial keratoplasty and descemet stripping automated endothelial keratoplasty. *Am. J. Ophthalmol.* 2015, *159*, 155–159.e1. [CrossRef] [PubMed]
16. Lee, W.B.; Jacobs, D.; Musch, D.; Kaufman, S.C.; Reinhart, W.J.; Shtein, R. Descemet's stripping endothelial keratoplasty: Safety and outcomes: A report by the American Academy of Ophthalmology. *Ophthalmology* 2009, *116*, 1818–1830. [CrossRef] [PubMed]
17. Dickman, M.M.; Kruit, P.J.; Remeijer, L.; van Rooij, J.; Van der Lelij, A.; Wijdh, R.H.; Biggelaar, F.J.V.D.; Berendschot, T.T.; Nuijts, R.M. A Randomized Multicenter Clinical Trial of Ultrathin Descemet Stripping Automated Endothelial Keratoplasty (DSAEK) versus DSAEK. *Ophthalmology* 2016, *123*, 2276–2284. [CrossRef] [PubMed]
18. Werner, S.; Rose-Nussbaumer, J.; Lin, C.; Austin, A.; Chamberlain, W. Changes in Anterior and Posterior Corneal Astigmatism after Descemet Membrane Endothelial Keratoplasty versus Ultrathin Descemet Stripping Automated Endothelial Keratoplasty: Results from the Randomized Controlled DETECT Trial. *Investig. Ophthalmol. Vis. Sci.* 2019, *60*, 6294.
19. Maier, A.-K.B.; Gundlach, E.; Gonnermann, J.; Klamann, M.K.J.; Bertelmann, E.; Rieck, P.W.; Joussen, A.M.; Torun, N. Retrospective contralateral study comparing Descemet membrane endothelial keratoplasty with Descemet stripping automated endothelial keratoplasty. *Eye* 2014, *29*, 327–332. [CrossRef]
20. Hirabayashi, K.E.; Chamberlain, W.; Rose-Nussbaumer, J.; Austin, A.; Stell, L.; Lin, C.C. Corneal Light Scatter after Ultrathin Descemet Stripping Automated Endothelial Keratoplasty versus Descemet Membrane Endothelial Keratoplasty in Descemet Endothelial Thickness Comparison Trial: A Randomized Controlled Trial. *Cornea* 2020, *39*, 691–696. [CrossRef]

21. Guerra, F.P.; Anshu, A.; Price, M.; Price, F.W. Endothelial keratoplasty: Fellow eyes comparison of Descemet stripping automated endothelial keratoplasty and Descemet membrane endothelial keratoplasty. *Cornea* **2011**, *30*, 1382–1386. [CrossRef] [PubMed]
22. Li, S.; Liu, L.; Wang, W.; Huang, T.; Zhong, X.; Yuan, J.; Liang, L. Efficacy and safety of Descemet's membrane endothelial keratoplasty versus Descemet's stripping endothelial keratoplasty: A systematic review and meta-analysis. *PLoS ONE* **2017**, *12*, e0182275. [CrossRef] [PubMed]

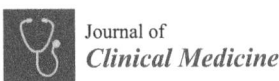

Article

Topo-Pachimetric Accelerated Epi-On Cross-Linking Compared to the Dresden Protocol Using Riboflavin with Vitamin E TPGS: Results of a 2-Year Randomized Study

Ciro Caruso [1,*], Robert Leonard Epstein [2], Pasquale Troiano [3], Francesco Napolitano [4], Fabio Scarinci [5] and Ciro Costagliola [6]

1. Corneal Transplant Center, Pellegrini Hospital, Via Portamedina alla Pignasecca, 41, 80127 Napoli, Italy
2. The Center for Corrective Eye Surgery, W. Elm Street, 5400, Mc Henry, IL 60050, USA; rlepstein@aol.com
3. Department of Ophthalmology Sacred Family, Fatebenefratelli Hospital, Via Fatebenefratelli, 20, 22036 Erba, Italy; ptroiano@fatebenefratelli.eu
4. Department of Ophthalmology, Pellegrini Hospital, Via Portamedina alla Pignasecca, 41, 80127 Napoli, Italy; eyenapoli@libero.it
5. Department of Ophthalmology, IRCCS Fondazione, Bietti, Via Livenza, 3, 00198 Roma, Italy; fabioscarinci@gmail.com
6. Eye Clinic, Department of Medicine and Health Sciences "V. Tiberio", University of Molise, Via Francesco De Sanctis, 1, 86100 Campobasso, Italy; ciro.costagliola@unimol.it
* Correspondence: cirocarusoeye@gmail.com; Tel.: +39-36-8772-5512

Abstract: In the present study (clinical trial registration number: NCT05019768), we compared the clinical outcome of corneal cross-linking with either the standard Dresden (sCXL) or the accelerated custom-fast (aCFXL) ultraviolet A irradiation protocol using riboflavin–D-α-tocopheryl poly(ethylene glycol)-1000 succinate for progressive keratoconus. Fifty-four eyes of forty-one patients were randomized to either of the two CXL protocols and checked before treatment and at the 2-year follow-up. The sCXL group was subjected to CXL with 30 min of pre-soaking and 3 mW/cm^2 UVA irradiation for 30 min. The aCFXL group was subjected to CXL with 10 min of pre-soaking and UVA irradiation of 1.8 ± 0.9 mW/cm^2 for 10 min ± 1.5 min. In both groups, a solution of riboflavin–vitamin E TPGS was used. Uncorrected distance visual acuity, corrected distance visual acuity, pachymetry, Scheimpflug tomography, and corneal hysteresis were performed at baseline and after 24 months. Both groups showed a statistically significant improvement in corrected distance visual acuity, and keratometric and corneal hysteresis compared to baseline conditions; no statistically significant differences in outcomes between the two groups were observed. Improvement in refractive, topographic, and biomechanical parameters were observed after sCXL and aCFXL, making the riboflavin–VE-TPGS solution an effective option as a permeation enhancer in CXL procedures. Deeper stromal penetration of riboflavin could be complemented by photo-protection against UVA and free radicals formed during photoinduced processes.

Keywords: riboflavin; vitamin E TPGS; aCFXL; sCXL

1. Introduction

Cross-linking (CXL) is a well-known treatment for keratoconus and ectatic cornea disorders, with various authors confirming its effectiveness in slowing or stopping the progression of the disease [1–3].

The induction of cross-links between corneal stromal fibrils by photosensitizing riboflavin and UV irradiation provides an increase in corneal stiffness and strength, thus stabilizing the ectatic process [4].

The results obtained with this treatment have shown a reduced need for keratoplasty in patients with keratoconus [5,6].

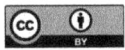

In recent years, the standard CXL (sCXL) Dresden protocol has been challenged by new therapeutic approaches, such as using higher UVA irradiation values (Table 1) [7].

Table 1. Different cross-linking protocols.

Differences among sCXL, aCXL, and aCFXL			
	sCXL	aCFXL	aCXL
Epithelium removal	Yes	No	Yes/No
Soaking time	30 min	10 min	Variable
Pre-soak eye drop frequency	Every 2 min	Every 15 s	Every 2 min
UVA fluence	3 mW/cm^2	1.8 ± 0.9 mW/cm^2	9 to 45 mW/cm^2
UVA fluence variation	Unchanging	Pachymetry and time dependent algorithm; fluence declining during treatment	Unchanging
Riboflavin during UVA	Yes; every 2 min	No; epithelial lavage before UVA	Yes; every 2 min
UVA irradiation time	30 min	10 ± 1.5 min	2 to 15 min
UVA irradiation method	Non-pulsed	Pulsed	Pulsed

Legend: sCXL, standard Dresden CXL; aCFXL, accelerated custom fast CXL; aCXL, accelerated CXL.

The rationale for the high-intensity approach is based on the Bunsen–Roscoe reciprocity law, which states that the time and intensity of irradiation can be varied without changing the total radiation energy of 5.4 J/cm^2 of the standard protocol of Dresden [8,9].

The intensity of 3 mW/cm^2 in the Dresden protocol was heuristically established; on the contrary, the accelerated custom fast CXL (aCFXL) protocol has been developed on a published mathematical model that takes into consideration objective variables such as the equation governing the UVA-induced riboflavin consumption rate and the corneal thickness at its thinnest point. By knowing both values, the mathematical model allows one to objectively calculate both the exact UVA irradiation value (intensity), expressed in mW/cm^2, and the irradiation time [10–12]. Furthermore, this procedure never exceeds the endothelial safety threshold of 0.35 mW/cm^2 [13,14]

Using this approach, it was possible to develop a customized, accelerated, pachymetry-dependent CXL protocol that has been named accelerated custom fast corneal cross-linking (aCFXL).

Reducing the UVA exposure time, and therefore the total time of the CXL procedure, can be beneficial for the patient.

So far, different CXL protocols have been proven effective in stopping the progression of keratoconus, with outcomes similar to standard CXL [1,15].

However, it is difficult to compare these studies, because different UVA irradiation profiles were applied [16].

In addition, there is no consensus among physicians about the clinical effectiveness of aCXL protocols in comparison with the sCXL protocol. Indeed, while some studies have found similar results [17–20], other studies have reported less topographical improvement after aCXL than sCXL [21–23].

So far, researchers have focused their attention on improving the clinical outcomes of the aCXL protocol only by modulating the intensity and time of UVA irradiation; conversely, little has been done in testing new and more effective solutions to improve riboflavin solution penetration. Indeed, in most of the studies performed so far, dextran was the only enhancer used. In a comparative study, in which dextran–riboflavin was used, a trend of increased corneal curvature was found in corneas that received aCXL with UVA irradiation at 9 mW/cm^2 for 10 min compared to standard sCXL. It was hypothesized that the lower clinical outcome after aCXL could be explained by a limited diffusion rate of dextran–riboflavin into the cornea when using a shorter treatment time.

In CXL based on accelerated but not customized UVA profiles, both the UVA irradiation and, therefore, the total soaking time are reduced. This can lead to a lower corneal concentration of riboflavin, which can result in less effective treatments.

In our previous comparative study, the time-dependent corneal accumulation of riboflavin–vitamin E TPGS or a control riboflavin solution was evaluated in both conditions: without epithelial debridement (epi-on) or after debridement (epi-off) [24]. No statistical differences were found between the solution containing the permeation enhancer (vitamin E TPGS (VE-TPGS)) and the control solution, thus demonstrating the efficacy of VE-TPGS–riboflavin solution in overcoming the resistance of the epithelium to corneal permeability.

To improve diffusion, in the present study, a VE-TPGS–riboflavin solution was used instead of the dextran–riboflavin solution.

D-α-tocopheryl poly(ethylene glycol)-1000 succinate (VE-TPGS) is a well-known non-ionic surfactant widely used as a solubilizer, emulsifier, and vehicle for lipid-based drug release formulations. VE-TPGS as a specific riboflavin transporter has been described in the rabbit corneal epithelium [25] and in human-derived retinoblastoma cells [26].

Furthermore, non-ionic surfactants have been widely described as enhancers of ocular permeation, with particular efficacy for the more hydrophilic molecules [27].

VE-TPGS has been proven effective in extinguishing potentially harmful oxidation-inducing substances, such as reactive oxygen species [28].

In recent years, we saw the introduction of VE-TPGS-enriched riboflavin solutions that showed enhanced stromal penetration during CXL's soaking phase. Riboflavin solution has also shown been to exert corneal endothelial layer protection during the irradiation step of CXL procedures. This feature has been exploited by physicians during the standard CXL procedure; indeed, continued riboflavin corneal wetting during UVA irradiation is mandatory in order to prevent UVA-induced corneal endothelium damage [14,24]. The epithelial layer is, in fact, the first corneal structure irradiated by UVA rays during CXL and consequently absorbs a large amount of radiation. Irradiation-induced damage to epithelial structures is well documented. Starting from this evidence, the aim of this comparative clinical study was to evaluate the safety and efficacy of the use of a riboflavin–VE-TPGS solution as an enhancer of the ocular permeation of the solution and as a photo-protective agent against UVA radiation in both procedures, sCXL and aCFXL UVA irradiation.

The study was a 2-year follow-up, evaluating clinical, visual, refractive, topographic, and biomechanical parameters.

To the best of our knowledge, there is no previous comparative CXL study between standard and different UVA irradiation protocols using riboflavin with VE-TPGS in both protocols.

2. Materials and Methods

2.1. Study Design and Patients

Based on the literature [29], the sample size was calculated to detect a difference of 0.95 D between the average Kmax changes in aCFXL and sCXL groups at 12 months, at a significance level of 5% and a power of 80%, assuming a standard deviation of 1.20 D. The sample size of the study was 54 observation (t-test for independent groups, two tails, using G*Power software version 3.1.9.7).

We randomized 54 eyes of 41 patients with keratoconus to either sCXL or aCFXL protocols and checked them before treatment and at the 2-year follow-up in this prospective, randomized controlled study. The randomization process was performed by using a cell phone app that was able to generate computerized random numbers. The allocation to either group was performed 1 week before the treatment when the patient was identified as eligible for the study.

This clinical study was conducted according to the ethical standards of the Declaration of Helsinki (revised in 2000). Patients were informed about the nature and purpose of the trial, and they provided informed consent. The approval of the institutional review/ethics committee (IRB) of the Corneal Transplant Center, Pellegrini Hospital, Napoli, Italy, was obtained (authorization 1269/2017). It was not appropriate or possible to involve patients or the public in the design, conduct, reporting, or dissemination plans of our research.

The patients were randomized (1:1) to receive either the standard or the customized protocol. In particular, 29 eyes were allocated to the sCXL group and 25 to the aCFXL group.

The mean age (±SD) of the patients in the sCXL and aCFXL groups was 28 ± 7.5 years and 26.3 ± 8.3 years, respectively. The mean follow-up period was 24.10 ± 3.30 months in the sCXL group and 25.20 ± 2.60 months in the aCFXL group.

The sCXL group underwent conventional UVA of 3 mW/cm^2 for 30 min, while the aCFXL group underwent the accelerated customized procedure (1.8 ± 0.9 mW/cm^2 for 10 min ± 1.5 min). The differences in CXL UVA irradiation treatment between the Dresden sCXL group and the aCFXL group are shown in Table 1. The Amsler–Krumeich classification system was used to define inclusion criteria. Furthermore, the treated eyes' distribution among the different keratoconus stages was as follows: sCXL stage 1 = 4, stage 2 = 16, and stage 3 = 9; aCFXL stage 1 = 3, stage 2 = 14, and stage 3 = 8.

The patients' eligibility was based on documented progressive keratoconus evaluated on corneal topography with Scheimpflug imaging (Pentacam HR; Oculus, Wetzlar Inc., Wetzlar, Germany) (increase of 1.0 D or more in the steepest keratometry), minimum corneal thickness reduction (thinnest point) of 5% or more on corneal pachymetry values, and changes in uncorrected distance visual acuity (UDVA) and corrected distance visual acuity (BCVA) (cylinder increase above 1.00 D or spherical equivalent greater than 0.50 D). To improve the reliability of topography measurements, a minimum of 3 acquisitions were obtained for each eye at each time interval. Topography evaluation was performed by only one trained operator to reduce inter-observer variation. If the value varied by more than 10% between the scans, then another scan was obtained. The best scan was then selected for analysis.

Visual acuity was measured with a logarithm of the minimum angle of resolution (logMAR) using the Early Treatment Diabetic Retinopathy Study chart at 4 m, and corneal hysteresis (CH) was measured using an Ocular Response Analyzer (ORA, Reichert, Depew, NY, USA). These parameters were evaluated for at least 6 months and up to 1 week before treatment. Patient demographic data with the mean clinical parameters for comparison of baseline characteristics between the Dresden sCXL group and the aCFXL group are shown in Table 2.

We excluded eyes with corneal pachymetry of less than 400 μm at the thinnest point, endothelial cell density (using a Tomey EM-3000 (Tomey Corp, Nagoya, Japan)) of less than 2000 cells/cm^2, corneal scarring, nystagmus or any motility disorder that prevented a fixed gaze during examination, and other significant pathologies. All patients discontinued contact lens use for at least 3 days prior to the screening visit.

The clinical observations were reported at 6 months and 1 week before treatment and at 1, 3, 6, 12, and 24 months after treatment. A complete ophthalmic examination was performed, including the best-corrected visual acuity (BCVA) with glasses based on the logMAR graph, manifest refraction, slit lamp, and dilated fundoscopy for all patients. Central minimum pachymetry was also measured using the Pentacam system.

The endothelial cell density was assessed using a non-contact specular microscope (Tomey EM-3000, Tomey Corp, Nagoya, Japan).

Table 2. Comparison of baseline parameters in the sCXL and aCFXL groups.

	sCXL (n = 29)	aCFXL (n = 25)	p-Value
Age years	28 ± 7.5	26.3 ± 8.3	0.432
Male/female eyes	18:11	15:10	0.194
Refractive parameters			
Corrected distance acuity (logMAR) (BCVA)	0.12 ± 0.12	0.10 ± 0.13	0.504
Spherical equivalent (D)	−4.11 ± 3.07	−4.70 ± 3.38	0.172
Refractive cylinder (D)	3.47 ± 1.35	3.25 ± 1.58	0.323
Topographical parameters			
Maximum keratometry (D) (6 months preoperative)	47.92 ± 5.22	47.65 ± 5.22	0.902
Maximum keratometry (D) (1 week preoperative)	49.93 ± 5.20	49.64 ± 5.20	0.326
Mean K (D) (6 months preoperative)	48.52 ± 4.17	46.82 ± 4.67	0.336
Mean K(D) (1 week preoperative)	49.48 ± 4.02	47.83 ± 4.66	0.184
Minimum corneal thickness (μm) (6 months preoperative)	435.0 ±54.8	461.0 ±56.3	1.000
Minimum corneal thickness (μm) (1 week preoperative)	449.0 ± 51.9	456.0 ± 56.6	0.582
Biomechanical parameters			
Corneal hysteresis (mmHg) (1 week preoperative)	7.91 ± 1.1	8.32 ± 1.7	0.676
Corneal resistance factor (mmHg) (1 week preoperative)	6.42 ± 1.3	6.58 ± 1.5	0.595
Endothelial cell density (cells/mm^2) (1 week preoperative)	2586 ± 246	2549 ± 263	0.184
Follow-up (months)	24.10 ± 3.30	25.20 ± 2.60	0.432

Legend: BCVA, best-corrected visual acuity; D, diopter; logMAR, logarithm of the minimum angle of resolution.

2.2. Surgical Technique

Both CXL procedures were performed under topical anesthesia and in the operating room. In the Dresden sCXL group, corneal pachymetry was performed before the procedure. The corneal epithelium was then partially removed from a treatment area of 9.0 mm using a smooth spatula after applying 10% diluted ethyl alcohol. A drop of 0.1% riboflavin–0.5% VE-TPGS solution (Ribocross, Iromed Group s.r.l., Rome, Italy) was instilled every 2 min for 30 min (15 drops).

Subsequently, the corneal thickness measurement was repeated and, if less than 400 μm, two drops of 0.1% hypotonic riboflavin solution (Ribofast, Iromed Group S.r.l., Rome, Italy) were instilled every 10–15 s until the corneal thickness was at least 400 μm. In this phase, we performed ultrasound thickness measurement with a 5 μ resolution pachymeter (Quantel Medical™, Cournon-d'Auvergne, France). The UV lighting device (CF-X LINKER, Iromed Group S.r.l., Rome, Italy) was the same for both protocols, positioned 5 cm away from the patient's eye. The riboflavin–vitamin E TPGS solution was then instilled every 2 min during the exposure, with a UV power of 3 mW/cm^2 for 30 min (total energy: 5.4 J/cm^2).

In the aCFXL group, a drop of 0.1% riboflavin–0.5% VE-TPGS solution (Ribocross, Iromed Group S.r.l., Rome, Italy) was instilled every 15 s for 10 min without removing the corneal epithelium. The eye was then rinsed thoroughly with a balanced salt solution and aligned under the UV lighting system (CF-X LINKER, Iromed Group S.r.l., Rome, Italy). Before starting the treatment, the corneal thinnest point value was entered into the device, which automatically calculated the treatment time and UV power for each patient. The modulated irradiation thus obtained was carried out at an average intensity of 1.8 ± 0.9 mW/cm^2 for 10 ± 1.5 min (total energy: 1.08 ± 0.6 J/cm^2). The main differences between the two protocols are summarized in Table 1. Briefly, in the sCXL protocol, continuous riboflavin–VE-TPGS solution administration on an epithelium-deprived cornea is necessary to better protect the endothelium, as demonstrated by Wallensak et al. [13,14]. Conversely, in the aCFXL protocol, riboflavin–VE-TPGS solution is applied once before UVA radiation without removing the epithelium. In addition, in the aCFXL protocol, the UVA fluency modulation is automatically modulated (using the published algorithm [10–12]) by the UV lighting system (CF-X LINKER, Iromed Group S.r.l., Rome, Italy).

In the Dresden sCXL group, a contact lens with a bandage was applied after the procedure; this was not necessary for the accelerated aCFXL group. In both protocols, patients took topical antibiotics (0.5% moxifloxacin hydrochloride) and steroids (0.12% prednisolone acetate); in the standard protocol, the therapy was gradually reduced during the first month after complete epithelial healing, while it only took 3 days for the customized protocol. All patients were examined after the procedure at 1 day, 1 week, and 1, 3, 6, 12, and 24 months.

2.3. Statistical Analysis

The normal data distribution was tested using the one-sample Kolomogorov–Smirnov test. Data were analyzed by one-way ANOVA for repeated measures, while Bonferroni correction was used to adjust for multiple comparisons. A probability of less than 5% ($p < 0.05$) was considered statistically significant. SPSS was the software used.

3. Results

Baseline characteristics showed no significant differences between the two groups (Table 2); furthermore, eye distribution among the different stages was non-statistically significant.

3.1. Refractive Parameters

Compared to baseline conditions, the BCVA improved significantly in both groups at the 12- and 24-month follow-up (one-way ANOVA for repeated measures: $f = 16.36$; $p < 0.0001$; sCXL group: 12 months, $p = 0.04$; 24 months, $p = 0.02$; aCFXL group: 12 months, $p = 0.05$; 24 months, $p = 0.012$; Table 3).

Table 3. Mean changes (postoperative values–preoperative values) of clinical outcomes in sCXL and aCFXL groups (n = studied eyes).

	sCXL (n = 29)				aCFXL (n = 25)			
	Mean ± SD		p-Value vs. Baseline		Mean ± SD		p-Value vs. Baseline	
Follow-up (months)	12 months	24 months	12 months	24 months	12 months	24 months	12 months	24 months
Refractive parameters								
Corrected distance acuity (logMAR)	−0.03 ± 0.013	−0.04 ± 0.015	0.04	0.02	−0.009 ± 0.004	−0.015 ± 0.005	0.05	0.012
Spherical equivalent (D)	0.38 ± 0.20	1.36 ± 0.53	0.12	0.02	0.6 ± 0.2	1.21 ± 0.37	0.012	0.006
Refractive cylinder magnitude (D)	0.36 ± 0.24	1.39 ± 0.53	0.28	0.02	0.95 ± 0.38	1.35 ± 0.46	0.02	0.014
Topographical parameters								
Maximum keratometry (D)	−0.78 ± 0.31	−0.97 ± 0.35	0.034	0.018	−0.99 ± 0.34	−1.1 ± 0.38	0.014	0.014
Mean K (D)	0.49 ± 0.2	0.49 ± 0.23	0.04	0.08	−0.58 ± 0.25	−0.59 ± 0.23	0.04	0.02
Minimum corneal thickness (μm)	−5.8 ± 4.1	−1.0 ± 3.5	0.2	1.0	−6.0 ± 5.5	−1.6 ± 2.9	0.4	1.0
Biomechanical parameters								
Corneal hysteresis (mmHg)	1.63 ± 0.5	1.09 ± 0.3	0.004	0.002	2.03 ± 0.78	1.94 ± 0.61	0.002	0.008

Similarly, the spherical equivalent improved at the 12- and 24-month follow-up in both groups (one-way ANOVA for repeated measures: $f = 110.56$; $p < 0.0001$). In particular, in the aCFXL group, the spherical equivalent had a p-value of 0.0012 at 12 months and $p = 0.006$ at 24 moths; the sCXL group showed a p-value of 0.02 at 24 months.

In contrast, while a significant decrease in cylinder correction was observed at both 12 and 24 months in the aCFXL group (one-way ANOVA for repeated measures: f = 96.22; $p < 0.0001$; $p = 0.02$ and $p = 0.014$, respectively), in the sCXL group, significant cylinder correction occurred only after 24 months ($p = 0.02$).

No significant difference was found for the analyzed parameter between 12 months and 24 months.

Intergroup analysis showed no statistically significant differences.

3.2. Topographic Parameters

Both Kmax and Kmean significantly improved in both groups at 12 and 24 months (one-way ANOVA for repeated measures: f = 86.31 and $p < 0.0001$ for Kmax and f = 61.05 and $p < 0.0001$ for Kmean; Table 3). For both groups, no statistical difference was observed in the minimum corneal thickness.

Intragroup comparison at 12 and 24 months showed no statistically significant differences.
Intergroup analysis showed no statistically significant differences.

3.3. Corneal Biomechanical Parameters

The CH significantly decreased in both groups at both 12 and 24 months (one-way ANOVA for repeated measures: f = 106.43; $p < 0.0001$; aCFXL: $p = 0.002$ at 12 months and $p = 0.008$ at 24 months; sCXL: $p = 0.004$ at 12 months and $p = 0.021$ at 24 months).

No significant differences were found between 12 and 24 months in both groups.
Intergroup analysis showed no statistically significant differences between groups.

3.4. Complications

Two patients in the sCXL group developed late-onset deep stromal scarring. In both cases, the stromal scar formation was located far from the visual axis and did not affect the final best spectacle-corrected visual acuity. There were no long-term complications in the aCFXL group.

4. Discussion

The results of this 2-year follow-up study of CXL treatment demonstrated that by using VE-TPGS-enriched riboflavin, it is possible to obtain overlapping clinical results using both surgical techniques: aCFXL and sCXL. Indeed, both groups showed statistically significant improvements in BCVA, Kmax, and CH parameters, and there were no significant differences in the observed changes between the two groups.

Currently, there is no agreement on the safety and effectiveness of aCFXL compared with the standard Dresden protocol. In this study, both groups showed improvement in the BCVA (logMAR) at 12 and 24 months after treatment.

An in vitro CXL study showed a lower biomechanical stiffening effect in high-UV-power accelerated protocols in porcine corneas [30].

The group that received the highest UV intensity (18 mW/cm^2 for 5 min) had the same stiffness values as the control group after the treatment. Since oxygen is required for covalent bond formation through a photo-oxidative reaction, this study hypothesized that oxygen depletion is the reason behind the subsidiary effect of accelerated CXL [31,32].

Oxygen depletion could be caused by the disparity between its diffusion capacity and its consumption in the corneal stroma with greater irradiation.

Using customized accelerated UVA irradiation profiles with the same riboflavin–vitamin E TPGS solution led to a significant improvement in keratometric outcomes after both aCFXL and sCXL treatments [33,34].

The results described in our study further highlight the ability of CXL (both sCXL and aCFXL) to improve the CH, an effect that remains constant till after 24 months.

The CH is a biomechanical parameter together with the corneal resistance factor (CRF). The CH is an indicator of corneal viscosity, while the CRF represents the cornea's ability to counteract deformation [35,36].

The ORA system is a non-contact applanation tonometer that assesses the corneal response to indentation (change in shape) induced by an air pulse.

CXL-induced CH variation has been studied by several authors, with conflicting results. While Sedaghat et al. [37], Goldich et al. [35], and Spoerl et al. [38] reported little to no variation in both the CH and the CRF, authors such as Lanchares et al. and Wollensak et al. [39,40] highlighted an increased corneal rigidity following CXL. These conflicting results can be explained by taking into consideration two main factors: one methodological and one pathology linked. Regarding the methodological factor, Sedaghat et al. [37], Goldich et al. [35], and Spoerl et al. [38] used the ORA in vivo system; on the contrary, Lanchares et al. and Wollensak et al. [39,40] used the strip extensometry in vitro system.

The pathology-related factor is the non-homogeneous corneal curvature. This implies that taking the mean of the variable measurements may lead to neglect the subtle changes in the CH and CRF [8]. Regarding this, it is worth noting that Spoerl and coworkers reported conflicting results in the same study by measuring the CH and CRF at different points on the cornea [38].

This suggests that the ORA is not able to measure the cross-linking-induced changes in the CH and CRF. Indeed, the ORA measures the biomechanics of collagen fibers and the viscous ground substance (proteoglycans and glycosaminoglycans), while CXL changes only collagen fibers. Therefore, using a static method may provide a better evaluation of the CXL effects on the cornea [9,10]. Despite the abovementioned limitations, we collected and reported the ORA CH data for two main reasons: First, we aimed to provide a complete picture of the differences we identified; second, the ORA is the only system able to provide such data in vivo. However, the validation of such procedure is out of the scope of this study.

Our findings, together with the already published ones, become even more relevant if we consider that sCXL and non-customized aCXL procedures usually involve removal of the corneal epithelium. Indeed, the epithelium prevents the passage of riboflavin, limiting the concentration of the molecule in the corneal stroma and, therefore, the effectiveness of the treatment. At the same time, low concentrations of stromal riboflavin increase the risk of tissue photodamage after UVA irradiation [14].

Removal of the corneal epithelium causes pain, ocular photophobia, and transient blurring. These symptoms persist until the corneal epithelium has been restored. In addition, the use of lubricating eye drops and antibiotics, analgesic oral therapy, and therapeutic contact lenses is necessary for healing. Occasionally, complications such as infections, keratitis, edema, and corneal scarring may arise, potentially leading to further loss of vision. Corneal thickness is also an essential parameter in CXL treatments. UV damage to deeper structures, especially the endothelial layer, is even more likely in thin corneas. It is known that the minimum safe corneal thickness to protect against endothelial damage is 400 µm [41].

Unfortunately, many patients with progressive keratoconus have corneas thinner than this threshold and, therefore, are excluded from treatment. Since the thickness of the human corneal epithelium is reported to be around 50 µm [42], avoiding the removal of the epithelium can allow for more patients to be treated. Several approaches have been described so far to overcome these problems. Hyposmolar riboflavin solutions have been used to swell the corneal stroma by more than 400 µm to treat thinner corneas, but without consistent evidence. Other procedures have been described as treatment of thin corneas, such as the accelerated cross-linking nomograms, the sub-400 protocol, the M nomogram for standardized treatment of thin corneas, contact-lens-assisted treatments, and the smile-lenticule-assisted epi-off CXL [43–45].

The introduction of the aCFXL protocol avoids debridement of the corneal epithelium, while increasing the corneal concentration of riboflavin by using corneal permeation stimulators such as VE-TPGS.

Since data from the present study were collected using only one type of equipment, different type of cameras might provide different results; therefore, the date described in the present manuscript might be not translated on different equipment [46].

5. Conclusions

In conclusion, this is the first study comparing 2-year outcomes after standard sCXL and aCFXL protocols customized using riboflavin–VE-TPGS in both irradiation profiles.

Since both study groups achieved similar clinical results, we can conclude that using riboflavin–VE-TPGS solution during both sCXL or aCFXL is a safe and effective approach. Furthermore, since it has been already shown that vitamin E is an effective candidate as a permeation enhancer in CXL procedures, we can also speculate that riboflavin–VE-TPGS solution might also positively impact the CXL procedure. Indeed, due to a deeper stromal penetration of riboflavin, more efficient photo-protection against UVA rays and free radicals formed during photoinduced processes can be achieved. Larger, prospective, randomized controlled trials with longer follow-ups are now necessary to confirm the long-term safety and efficacy of riboflavin–VE-TPGS solution in CXL with different irradiation profiles.

Author Contributions: Conceptualization, C.C. (Ciro Caruso) and C.C. (Ciro Costagliola); investigation, R.L.E., F.N., and P.T.; writing—original draft preparation, C.C. (Ciro Caruso), R.L.E., and P.T.; writing—review and editing, F.S.; supervision, C.C. (Ciro Caruso). All authors have read and agreed to the published version of the manuscript.

Funding: This research received no external funding.

Institutional Review Board Statement: The approval of the institutional review/ethics committee (IRB) of the Corneal Transplant Center, Pellegrini Hospital, Napoli, Italy, was obtained (authorization 1269/2017).

Informed Consent Statement: Informed consent was obtained from all subjects involved in the study.

Data Availability Statement: The data presented in this study are available on request from the corresponding author. The data are not publicly available due to privacy and ethical reasons.

Conflicts of Interest: The authors declare no conflict of interest.

References

1. Sorkin, N.; Varssano, D. Corneal collagen crosslinking: A systematic review. *Ophthalmologica* **2014**, *232*, 10–27. [CrossRef] [PubMed]
2. Shetty, R.; Pahuja, N.K.; Nuijts, R.M.; Ajani, A.; Jayadev, C.; Sharma, C.; Nagaraja, H. Current protocols of corneal collagen cross-linking: Visual, refractive, and tomographic outcomes. *Am. J. Ophthalmol.* **2015**, *160*, 243–249. [CrossRef]
3. Meiri, Z.; Keren, S.; Rosenblatt, A.; Sarig, T.; Shenhav, L.; Varssano, D. Efficacy of corneal collagen cross-linking for the treatment of keratoconus: A systematic review and meta-analysis. *Cornea* **2016**, *35*, 417–428. [CrossRef] [PubMed]
4. Schumacher, S.; Oeftiger, L.; Mrochen, M. Equivalence of biomechanical changes induced by rapid and standard corneal cross-linking, using riboflavin and ultraviolet radiation. *Investig. Opthalmol. Vis. Sci.* **2011**, *52*, 9048–9052. [CrossRef]
5. Sandvik, G.F.; Thorsrud, A.; Råen, M.; Østern, A.E.; Sæthre, M.; Drolsum, L. Does corneal collagen cross-linking reduce the need for keratoplasties in patients with keratoconus? *Cornea* **2015**, *34*, 991–995. [CrossRef]
6. Godefrooij, D.A.; Gans, R.; Imhof, S.M.; Wisse, R.P. Nationwide reduction in the number of corneal transplantations for keratoconus following the implementation of cross-linking. *Acta Ophthalmol.* **2016**, *94*, 675–678. [CrossRef]
7. Beckman, K.A.; Gupta, P.K.; Farid, M.; Berdahl, J.P.; Yeu, E.; Ayres, B.; Chan, C.C.; Gomes, J.A.; Holland, E.J.; Kim, T.; et al. Corneal crosslinking: Current protocols and clinical approach. *J. Cataract Refract. Surg.* **2019**, *45*, 1670–1679. [CrossRef]
8. Rubinfeld, R.S.; Caruso, C.; Ostacolo, C. Corneal cross-linking: The science beyond the myths and misconceptions. *Cornea* **2019**, *38*, 780–790. [CrossRef]
9. Brindley, G.S. The Bunsen-Roscoe law for the human eye at very short durations. *J. Physiol.* **1952**, *118*, 135–139. [CrossRef] [PubMed]
10. Caruso, C.; Barbaro, G.; Epstein, R.L.; Tronino, D.; Ostacolo, C.; Sacchi, A.; Pacente, L.; Del Prete, A.; Sala, M.; Troisi, S.; et al. Corneal Cross-Linking: Evaluating the Potential for a Lower Power, Shorter Duration Treatment. *Cornea* **2016**, *35*, 659–662. [CrossRef] [PubMed]
11. Caruso, C.; Epstein, R.L.; Ostacolo, C.; Pacente, L.; Troisi, S.; Barbaro, G. Customized corneal cross-linking-a mathematical model. *Cornea* **2017**, *36*, 600–604. [CrossRef]

12. Kling, S.; Hafezi, F. Biomechanical stiffening: Slow low-irradiance corneal crosslinking versus the standard Dresden protocol. *J. Cataract Refract. Surg.* **2017**, *43*, 975–979. [CrossRef] [PubMed]
13. Wollensak, G.; Spoerl, E.; Wilsch, M.; Seiler, T. Endothelial cell damage after riboflavin-ultraviolet-A treatment in the rabbit. *J. Cataract Refract. Surg.* **2003**, *29*, 1786–1790. [CrossRef]
14. Wollensak, G.; Aurich, H.; Wirbelauer, C.; Sel, S. Significance of the riboflavin film in corneal collagen crosslinking. *J. Cataract Refract. Surg.* **2010**, *36*, 114–120. [CrossRef] [PubMed]
15. Lim, L.; Lim, E.W.L. A review of corneal collagen cross-linking—Current trends in practice applications. *Open Ophthalmol. J.* **2018**, *12*, 181–213. [CrossRef] [PubMed]
16. Kobashi, H.; Tsubota, K. Accelerated versus standard corneal cross-linking for progressive keratoconus: A meta-analysis of randomized controlled trials. *Cornea* **2020**, *39*, 172–180. [CrossRef]
17. Kanellopoulos, A.J. Long term results of a prospective randomized bilateral eye comparison trial of higher fluence, shorter duration ultraviolet A radiation, and riboflavin collagen cross linking for progressive keratoconus. *Clin. Ophthalmol.* **2012**, *6*, 97–101. [CrossRef] [PubMed]
18. Çinar, Y.; Cingü, A.K.; Türkcü, F.M.; Çınar, T.; Yuksel, H.; Özkurt, Z.G.; Çaça, I. Comparison of accelerated and conventional corneal collagen cross-linking for progressive keratoconus. *Cutan. Ocul. Toxicol.* **2014**, *33*, 218–222. [CrossRef]
19. Hashemian, H.; Jabbarvand, M.; Khodaparast, M.; Ameli, K. Evaluation of corneal changes after conventional versus accelerated corneal cross-linking: A randomized controlled trial. *J. Refract. Surg.* **2014**, *30*, 837–842. [CrossRef] [PubMed]
20. Jiang, L.; Jiang, W.; Qiu, S. Conventional vs. pulsed-light accelerated corneal collagen cross-linking for the treatment of progressive keratoconus: 12-month results from a prospective study. *Exp. Ther. Med.* **2017**, *14*, 4238–4244. [CrossRef] [PubMed]
21. Brittingham, S.; Tappeiner, C.; Frueh, B.E. Corneal cross-linking in keratoconus using the standard and rapid treatment protocol: Differences in demarcation line and 12-month outcomes. *Investig. Opthalmol. Vis. Sci.* **2014**, *55*, 8371–8376. [CrossRef]
22. Ng, A.L.; Chan, T.C.; Cheng, A.C. Conventional versus accelerated corneal collagen cross-linking in the treatment of keratoconus. *Clin. Exp. Ophthalmol.* **2016**, *44*, 8–14. [CrossRef] [PubMed]
23. Chow, V.W.; Chan, T.C.Y.; Yu, M.; Wong, V.W.Y.; Jhanji, V. One-year outcomes of conventional and accelerated collagen crosslinking in progressive keratoconus. *Sci. Rep.* **2015**, *5*, 14425. [CrossRef] [PubMed]
24. Ostacolo, C.; Caruso, C.; Tronino, D.; Troisi, S.; Laneri, S.; Pacente, L.; Del Prete, A.; Sacchi, A. Enhancement of corneal permeation of riboflavin-5′-phosphate through vitamin E TPGS: A promising approach in corneal trans-epithelial cross linking treatment. *Int. J. Pharm.* **2013**, *440*, 148–153. [CrossRef]
25. Hariharan, S.; Janoria, K.G.; Gunda, S.; Zhu, X.; Pal, D.; Mitra, A.K. Identification and functional expression of a carrier-mediated riboflavin transport system on rabbit corneal epithelium. *Curr. Eye Res.* **2006**, *31*, 811–824. [CrossRef] [PubMed]
26. Kansara, V.; Pal, D.; Jain, R.; Mitra, A.K. Identification and functional characterization of riboflavin transporter in human-derived retinoblastoma cell line (Y-79): Mechanisms of cellular uptake and translocation. *J. Ocul. Pharmacol. Ther.* **2005**, *21*, 275–287. [CrossRef] [PubMed]
27. Saettone, M.; Chetoni, P.; Cerbai, R.; Mazzanti, G.; Braghiroli, L. Evaluation of ocular permeation enhancers: In vitro effects on corneal transport of four β-blockers, and in vitro/in vivo toxic activity. *Int. J. Pharm.* **1996**, *142*, 103–113. [CrossRef]
28. Constantinides, P.P.; Han, J.; Davis, S.S. Advances in the use of tocols as drug delivery vehicles. *Pharm. Res.* **2006**, *23*, 243–255. [CrossRef] [PubMed]
29. Lombardo, M.; Giannini, D.; Lombardo, G.; Serrao, S. Randomized controlled trial comparing transepithelial corneal cross-linking using iontophoresis with the dresden protocol in progressive keratoconus. *Ophthalmology* **2017**, *124*, 804–812. [CrossRef] [PubMed]
30. Hammer, A.; Richoz, O.; Mosquera, S.A.; Tabibian, D.; Hoogewoud, F.; Hafezi, F. Corneal biomechanical properties at different corneal cross-linking (CXL) irradiances. *Investig. Opthalmol. Vis. Sci.* **2014**, *55*, 2881–2884. [CrossRef]
31. Richoz, O.; Hammer, A.; Tabibian, D.; Gatzioufas, Z.; Hafezi, F. The biomechanical effect of corneal cross-linking (CXL) with riboflavin and UV-A is oxygen dependent. *Transl. Vis. Sci. Technol.* **2013**, *2*, 6. [CrossRef]
32. Kamaev, P.; Friedman, M.D.; Sherr, E.; Muller, D. Photochemical kinetics of corneal cross-linking with riboflavin. *Investig. Ophthalmol. Vis. Sci.* **2012**, *53*, 2360–2367. [CrossRef]
33. Caruso, C.; Epstein, R.L.; Troiano, P.; Ostacolo, C.; Barbaro, G.; Pacente, L.; Bartollino, S.; Costagliola, C. Topography and pachymetry guided, rapid Epi-on corneal cross-linking for keratoconus: 7-year study results. *Cornea* **2020**, *39*, 56–62. [CrossRef]
34. Caruso, C.; Ostacolo, C.; Epstein, R.L.; Barbaro, G.; Troisi, S.; Capobianco, D. Transepithelial corneal cross-linking with vitamin E-enhanced riboflavin solution and abbreviated, low-dose UV-A: 24-month clinical outcomes. *Cornea* **2016**, *35*, 145–150. [CrossRef] [PubMed]
35. Goldich, Y.; Barkana, Y.; Morad, Y.; Hartstein, M.; Avni, I.; Zadok, D. Can we measure corneal biomechanical changes after collagen cross-linking in eyes with keratoconus?—A pilot study. *Cornea* **2009**, *28*, 498–502. [CrossRef] [PubMed]
36. Luce, D.A. Determining in vivo biomechanical properties of the cornea with an ocular response analyzer. *J. Cataract Refract. Surg.* **2005**, *31*, 156–162. [CrossRef]
37. Sedaghat, M.; Naderi, M.; Zarei-Ghanavati, M. Biomechanical parameters of the cornea after collagen crosslinking measured by waveform analysis. *J. Cataract Refract. Surg.* **2010**, *36*, 1728–1731. [CrossRef] [PubMed]
38. Spoerl, E.; Terai, N.; Scholz, F.; Raiskup, F.; Pillunat, L.E. Detection of biomechanical changes after corneal cross-linking using Ocular Response Analyzer software. *J. Refract. Surg.* **2011**, *27*, 452–457. [CrossRef]

39. Lanchares, E.; Del Buey, M.A.; Cristóbal, J.A.; Lavilla, L.; Calvo, B. Biomechanical property analysis after corneal collagen cross-linking in relation to ultraviolet A irradiation time. *Graefes Arch. Clin. Exp. Ophthalmol.* **2011**, *249*, 1223–1227. [CrossRef]
40. Wollensak, G.; Iomdina, E. Long-term biomechanical properties of rabbit cornea after photodynamic collagen crosslinking. *Acta Ophthalmol.* **2009**, *87*, 48–51. [CrossRef]
41. Hafezi, F. Limitation of collagen cross-linking with hypoosmolar riboflavin solution: Failure in an extremely thin cornea. *Cornea* **2011**, *30*, 917–919. [CrossRef]
42. Reinstein, D.Z.; Gobbe, M.; Archer, T.J.; Silverman, R.H.; Coleman, D.J. Epithelial thickness in the normal cornea: Three-dimensional display with Artemis very high-frequency digital ultrasound. *J. Refract. Surg.* **2008**, *24*, 571–581. [CrossRef]
43. Hafezi, F.; Kling, S.; Gilardoni, F.; Hafezi, N.; Hillen, M.; Abrishamchi, R.; Gomes, J.A.P.; Mazzotta, C.; Randleman, J.B.; Toress-Netto, E.A. Individualized corneal cross-linking with riboflavin and UV-A in ultrathin corneas: The Sub400 protocol. *Am. J. Ophthalmol.* **2021**, *224*, 133–142. [CrossRef]
44. Cagini, C.; Riccitelli, F.; Messina, M.; Piccinelli, F.; Torroni, G.; Said, D.; Al Maazmi, A.; Dua, H.S. Epi-off-lenticule-on corneal collagen cross-linking in thin keratoconic corneas. *Int. Ophthalmol.* **2020**, *40*, 3403–3412. [CrossRef] [PubMed]
45. Jacob, S.; Srivatsa, S.; Agarwal, A. Contact lens assisted corneal cross linking in thin ectatic corneas—A review. *Indian J. Ophthalmol.* **2020**, *68*, 2773–2778. [CrossRef] [PubMed]
46. Brunner, M.; Czanner, G.; Vinciguerra, R.; Romano, V.; Ahmad, S.; Batterbury, M.; Britten, C.; Willoughby, C.; Kaye, S.B. Improving precision for detecting change in the shape of the cornea in patients with keratoconus. *Sci. Rep.* **2018**, *8*, 12345. [CrossRef] [PubMed]

Article

Establishment of a Robust and Simple Corneal Organ Culture Model to Monitor Wound Healing

Sandra Schumann [1,*], Eva Dietrich [2,3], Charli Kruse [1,2], Salvatore Grisanti [3] and Mahdy Ranjbar [3,4]

1. Institute for Medical and Marine Biotechnology, University of Luebeck, Moenkhofer Weg 239a, 23562 Luebeck, Germany; charli.kruse@uni-luebeck.de or charli.kruse@emb.fraunhofer.de
2. Fraunhofer Research Institution for Marine Biotechnology and Cell Technology, Moenkhofer Weg 239a, 23562 Luebeck, Germany; eva-dietrich@mail.de
3. Department of Ophthalmology, University of Luebeck, Ratzeburger Allee 160, 23538 Luebeck, Germany; Salvatore.Grisanti@uksh.de (S.G.); eye.research101@gmail.com (M.R.)
4. Laboratory for Angiogenesis & Ocular Cell Transplantation, University of Luebeck, Ratzeburger Allee 160, 23538 Luebeck, Germany
* Correspondence: s.schumann@uni-luebeck.de; Tel.: +49-451-38444814

Abstract: The use of in vitro systems to investigate the process of corneal wound healing offers the opportunity to reduce animal pain inflicted during in vivo experimentation. This study aimed to establish an easy-to-handle ex vivo organ culture model with porcine corneas for the evaluation and modulation of epithelial wound healing. Cultured free-floating cornea disks with a punch defect were observed by stereomicroscopic photo documentation. We analysed the effects of different cell culture media and investigated the impact of different wound sizes as well as the role of the limbus. Modulation of the wound healing process was carried out with the cytostatic agent Mitomycin C. The wound area calculation revealed that after three days over 90% of the lesion was healed. As analysed with TUNEL and lactate dehydrogenase assay, the culture conditions were cell protecting and preserved the viability of the corneal tissue. Wound healing rates differ dependent on the culture medium used. Mitomycin C hampered wound healing in a concentration-dependent manner. The porcine cornea ex vivo culture ideally mimics the in vivo situation and allows investigations of cellular behaviour in the course of wound healing. The effect of substances can be studied, as we have documented for a mitosis inhibitor. This model might aid in toxicological studies as well as in the evaluation of drug efficacy and could offer a platform for therapeutic approaches based on regenerative medicine.

Keywords: cornea; wound healing; epithelium; disease model; cell migration

1. Introduction

The cornea is a transparent, avascular tissue which forms an important barrier through tight junctions present at its superficial layer [1]. This highly specialized tissue has been used extensively as a model system to study wound healing in the human body as its anatomic location causes the cornea to be subject to abrasive forces and physical damage [2]. Corneal epithelial erosion and ulceration are common ocular injuries resulting from multiple causes such as trauma, chemical burns, infections and refractive surgery [3].

Wound healing of the cornea involves the removal of necrotic cells, infiltration of neutrophils, migration of cells from the wound edge covering the wound, mitosis as well as migration of limbal epithelial stem cells, and differentiation of newly formed epithelial cells to more mature, anterior, stratified epithelial cells to restore a smooth multilayered formation [4]. Epithelial lesions normally resolve within several days, without any fibrotic response. However, wound healing speed might be impacted by various diseases such as diabetes, autoimmune disorders or infection of the tissue. During this period, various eye drops are used to support healing and prevent infection. These agents should not adversely affect re-epithelization and reduce scar tissue formation [3].

Several animal models of corneal wound healing have been developed, which played a major role in understanding the regeneration process and helped in the assessment of potential therapeutic medications. Use of in vitro systems offer a great relief from in vivo experiments on animals, but are not able to mimic the complex interaction of different cell types in a vivid surrounding. Alternatives, such as ex vivo organ culture models, are in demand as they combine the advantages of both. However, most of these models are quite difficult to set up from a technical point of view and reproducibility is therefore also often not given, especially for less experienced experimenters [5].

Here, we report an easy-to-establish ex vivo organ culture model for the evaluation and modulation of corneal wound healing. This model has improved on the development of corneal edema with several modifications and as this model uses globes from porcine cadavers, it is closer to the in vivo condition than in vitro cell cultures. In addition, the tissue is regularly available and easy to obtain. As such, this model might aid in toxicological studies as well as in the evaluation of drug efficacy and could offer a platform for therapeutic approaches based on regenerative medicine.

2. Materials and Methods

2.1. Preparation and Cultivation of Porcine Corneas

Specimens were prepared as previously described [6]. In brief, the pig eyes used for tissue culture were obtained from a local abattoir. Shortly post mortem the eyes were removed and kept cool (4 °C) in phosphate buffered saline (PBS; Thermo Fisher Scientific GmbH, Waltham, MA, USA). The overall preparation of corneal tissue was performed within 6 h. The eyes were freed of excess muscle and connective tissue and placed in a disinfectant solution (penicillin/streptomycin with amphotericin B (Merck KGaA, Darmstadt, Germany) in PBS) for 10 min. The corneal wound was made by carefully pressing a biopsy punch (4 mm or 8 mm diameter; Kai Europe GmbH, Solingen, Germany) onto the middle of the eye while avoiding too much pressure. The epithelium within the resulting circle was then abraded using a hockey knife, so that a defined defect area (corneal erosion) was created. The corneal tissue with the wound was then cut out completely through a 10 mm biopsy punch (Acuderm, Lauderdale, FL, USA) and with the help of scissors. The specimens were then transferred to a 12-well plate with 1 mL of organ culture medium per well and cultivated in the incubator at 37 °C and 5% CO_2 for 72 h. The medium was changed daily.

Wound healing of the corneal lesions was observed with a Stemi 2000-C stereomicroscope (Carl Zeiss Microscopy GmbH, Oberkochen, Germany). Various culture media (Table 1) and conditions (Table 2) were evaluated.

2.2. Determination of Corneal Wound Area

To observe the epithelial wound area, images of the porcine corneas were taken at regular intervals over 72 h using the Stemi-2000C stereo microscope using the darkfield filter. The wound area was quantified using ImageJ (NIH, Version 1.48b, Bethesda, Rockville, MD, USA). For this purpose, the wound margin was outlined with the mouse (polygon tool) and the size of this area was determined in pixels (measure). The number of pixels was converted to mm^2 using an internal standard.

2.3. Lactate Dehydrogenase Assay for Cytotoxicity Estimation

In order to estimate the tissue integrity and viability of the corneal disks during ex vivo culture the Cytotoxicity Detection Kit PLUS LDH (Roche, Basel, Switzerland) was used. This colorimetric assay quantified cell death and cell lysis, based on the measurement of lactate dehydrogenase (LDH) activity released from the cytosol of damaged cells into the medium. The cell culture supernatants from the organ culture were collected and stored at −20 °C until further use. After thawing the supernatants were centrifuged by $250\times g$ and 4 °C for 5 min followed by the transfer of a 100 µL volume per sample in a well of a 96 well plate. The test was subsequently carried out according to the manufacturer's instructions.

The formed red formazan was detected spectroscopically. The absorption of the samples was measured at 492 nm and 690 nm in a microplate reader (CLARIOstar, BMG Labtech GmbH, Ortenberg, Germany). Media samples cultivated without cornea tissues served as controls. The values measured at an absorption of 690 nm represented the background and were subtracted from the measured values at 490 nm. Finally, the mean values of the media controls were subtracted from the difference values of $[A_{492}-A_{690}]$. The amount of formazan is proportional to the amount of LDH and thus a measure of cytotoxicity.

Table 1. Composition of culture media for corneal ex vivo cultivation.

Medium	Ingredients	Distributor
DMEM	Dulbeccos Modified Eagle Medium, high Glucose, w/L-Glutamin	Thermo Fisher Scientific GmbH, Waltham, MA, USA
	Penicillin/Streptomycin solution 1×	Merck KGaA, Darmstadt, Germany
	2.5 µg/mL Amphotericin B	Merck KGaA, Darmstadt, Germany
	6% Dextran-500	Carl Roth GmbH + Co. KG, Karlsruhe, Germany
KGM2	Keratinocyte Growth Medium 2	PromoCell, Heidelberg, Germany
	Supplement Mix including Bovine Pituitary Extract, Epidermal Growth Factor, Insulin, Hydrocortisone, Epinephrine, Transferrin, CaCl$_2$	PromoCell, Heidelberg, Germany
	Penicillin/Streptomycin solution 1×	Merck KGaA, Darmstadt, Germany
	2.5 µg/mL Amphotericin B	Merck KGaA, Darmstadt, Germany
	6% Dextran-500	Carl Roth GmbH + Co. KG, Karlsruhe, Germany
OcuLife	OcuLife ™ Epithelial Basal Medium	CellSystems GmbH, Troisdorf, Germany
	OcuLife Supplements ("Life Factors") including Insulin, Glutamin, Epinephrin, Apo-Transferrin, Extract P^{TM}, Hydrocortisone, OcuFactor^{TM}	CellSystems GmbH, Troisdorf, Germany
	Penicillin/Streptomycin solution 1×	Merck KGaA, Darmstadt, Germany
	2.5 µg/mL Amphotericin B	Merck KGaA, Darmstadt, Germany
	6% Dextran-500	Carl Roth GmbH + Co. KG, Karlsruhe, Germany
WEM	William's Medium E	Merck KGaA, Darmstadt, Germany
	10 µg/mL Insulin	Sigma-Aldrich Chemie GmbH, Taufkirchen, Germany
	0.1 µg/mL Hydrocortisone	Sigma-Aldrich Chemie GmbH, Taufkirchen, Germany
	2 mM L-Glutamine	PAA Laboratories GmbH, Cölbe, Germany
	Penicillin/Streptomycin solution 1×	Merck KGaA, Darmstadt, Germany
	2.5 µg/mL Amphotericin B	Merck KGaA, Darmstadt, Germany
	6% Dextran-500	Carl Roth GmbH + Co. KG, Karlsruhe, Germany

Table 2. Summary of parameters for optimization and evaluation of corneal organ culture.

Influence on Test Model	Parameters
Defect size	4 mm vs. 8 mm
Role of limbus	With vs. without limbus
Organ culture medium	DMEM vs. KGM2 vs. Oculife vs. WEM
Mitomycin C as cytostatic, antiproliferative agent	50 µg/mL vs. 100 µg/mL vs. 200 µg/mL

2.4. Tissue Processing for Paraffin Sections

The porcine corneas were initially placed in embedding cassettes (VWR International GmbH, Darmstadt, Germany). They were fixed in formalin, dehydrated through a series of graded ethanol baths and finally embedded in paraffin (Sigma-Aldrich, Taufkirchen, Germany). Paraffin wax blocks with embedded tissue were created and stored at 4 °C until further processing. The paraffin sections were cut with a thickness of 4 µm using a microtome. The sections were initially stored overnight at 37 °C and until further use at room temperature. Before usage for further analysis (e.g., HE staining) the tissue sections had to be dewaxed. Therefore, the sections were dipped three times for 7 min each in xylene, twice for 3 min each in 100% ethanol and then they were hydrated for 2 min each in a descending alcohol series. Until further use, the sections were placed in distilled water (dH$_2$O) for at least 5 min.

2.5. Haematoxylin and Eosin Staining of Corneal Sections

After an initial brief rinse in dH$_2$O, the corneal paraffin sections were stained for 3 min with Mayer's hemalum solution (Carl Roth, GmbH + Co. KG, Karlsruhe, Germany). The sections were then briefly washed again in dH$_2$O and then blued for 20 min under running tap water. After another washing step in dH$_2$O, the samples were stained with eosin solution (Carl Roth, GmbH + Co. KG, Karlsruhe, Germany) for 30 s, washed in dH$_2$O and immersed for a short time in solutions of ascending alcohol series (70, 80, 90, 96%). Finally, the sections were covered with Euparal (Carl Roth, GmbH + Co. KG, Karlsruhe, Germany) and left to dry for at least 1 h. Tissue sections were analysed with the Discovery.V8 stereomicroscope (Carl Zeiss Microscopy GmbH, Oberkochen, Germany) and histological overviews were created using the mosaic tool.

2.6. Evaluation of Apoptosis with TUNEL Assay

To detect apoptosis in the corneal tissue sections the "In situ Cell Death Detection Kit, TMR red" (Roche, Basel, Switzerland) was used according to the manufacturer's instructions. This TUNEL (Terminal deoxynucleotidyl transferase dUTP nick end labeling)-Assay is based on the detection of single and double strand breaks in the DNA that occur during early apoptosis. For this method, the paraffin tissue sections were first dewaxed for 30 min in xylene, 5 min in isopropanol and were then rehydrated for 5 min in 70% ethanol and for a short time in PBS. The sections were permeabilized for 8 min with the TUNEL permeabilization solution and then washed twice with PBS. The samples were then incubated for 1 h at 37 °C using the reaction mix containing terminal deoxynucleotidyl transferase (TdT) and tetramethylrhodamine (TMR)-dUTP. The negative control was incubated without a reaction mix, whereas the positive control was incubated with deoxyribonuclease (DNase) I beforehand for 30 min. The samples were then washed three times with PBS following a nuclear staining using 4′,6-diamidino-2-phenylindole (DAPI; Roche, Basel, Switzerland) for 10 min. Finally, sections were covered with Vectashield (Vector Laboratories, Burlingame, CA, USA) and were analysed using the Axio Observer Z.1 fluorescence microscope (Carl Zeiss Microscopy GmbH, Oberkochen, Germany). The left edge area of the defect, the middle area and the right edge area of the defect were recorded.

2.7. Statistical Analysis

For each experiment at least 3 biological replicates were studied. The data were tested for normality using the Shapiro–Wilk test. Values are expressed as median (min–max). Statistical analyses were performed by Mann–Whitney test or Kruskall–Wallis test followed by Dunn post-test correction. For evaluation of two factors a mixed-model analysis was done. Differences were considered statistically significant at $p < 0.05$. Analyses were performed with Prism (GraphPad Prism version 9.0).

3. Results

3.1. Tissue Preparation for Corneal Ex Vivo Culture

Pig eyes were easily obtained at scheduled time points and in great numbers from the abattoir, so that several experiments could be performed in parallel. The experimental procedure for wound setting and preparation of corneal tissue was simple and robust. For one wounded cornea it took less than 5 min from the first step of tissue preparation until the start of ex vivo culture in a multiwell plate. Every process step could be followed with a stereomicroscope (Figure 1). For the handling it was an advantage to set the wound area with the smaller punch first and then cutting out the whole area with the 10 mm punch: (I) The scratching with a hockey knife could be carried out more precisely and reproducible, because the eyeball served as robust and stable support and (II) when positioning the 10 mm punch for cutting out, the wound was exactly placed in the middle. The excised corneal tissue sheets were cultivated free floating in a multiwell plate with the wound upward. During the culture period a swell-up of the tissue specimens was noticeable and the previously translucent corneal tissue became opaque. This effect is also known for human corneal transplants, which are often stored in a medium with dextran as deswelling agent until keratoplasty. While we used 6% dextran-500 as dehydrating additive in our media, the swelling could not be completely prevented.

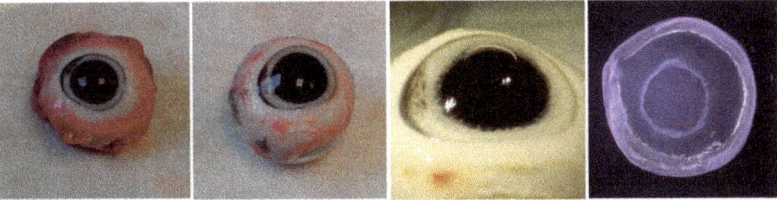

Figure 1. Preparation of pig eyes, wounding and corneal tissue isolation for organ culture photo documentation of the corneal preparation to start cornea organ culture. After removal of muscle and connective tissue the wound was prepared using a small biopsy punch (here 4 mm diameter) and a hockey knife. The resulting epithelial defect was visible with optimized illumination. The whole corneal tissue is excised from the eye with a 10 mm biopsy punch and was cultivated free floating in a microplate well.

3.2. Optical Documentation of the Corneal Defect for 72 h

To establish the corneal ex vivo culture initial experiments were conducted with Dulbecco's Modified Eagle's Medium (DMEM), which is used for a wide range of cells or tissues. The corneal tissues were analysed by a stereomicroscope and pictures were taken every day. New epithelial tissue at the wound margin was detectable after a few hours and the area of newly formed cells enlarged with progressed cultivation period (Figure 2). The wound edges of the regenerating epithelium were clearly visible, so that the wound size was calculated at every time point. Wound size decreased significantly over 72 h from 9.94 (9.29–10.71) mm^2 to 0.89 (0.87–2.02) mm^2 (Figure 2B). Whether the newly formed epithelium was a result of cell divisions or cell migration had to be discussed. In this regard, a statistically significant decline of the wound healing rate over time could be seen. Initially the gap closed at a speed of 0.196 (0.180–0.201) mm^2/h, but slowed down significantly to 0.022 (0.018–0.045) mm^2/h during the final 24 h (Figure 2C). Correspondingly, LDH concentration in the supernatant decreased with increasing closure of the gap (Figure 2D). Following an initial peak right after inducing the trauma through trepanation LDH was reduced by almost 50% at final follow-up.

3.3. Histological Analysis of Corneal Wound Healing

To get more insight into the structure and behaviour of corneal regeneration, paraffin sections were stained with haematoxylin and eosin and analysed with a stereomicroscope. The histological analysis confirmed the visually determined observations: The regeneration of the epithelial defect started at the first day with cells that migrated from the wound edge to close the gap (Figure 3). The newly formed epithelium was just 1–2 cell layers thin. The closure of the wound progressed over the cultivation period as the epithelial cells pushed themselves further and further over the corneal stroma. After 72 h a thin epithelium closed the wound.

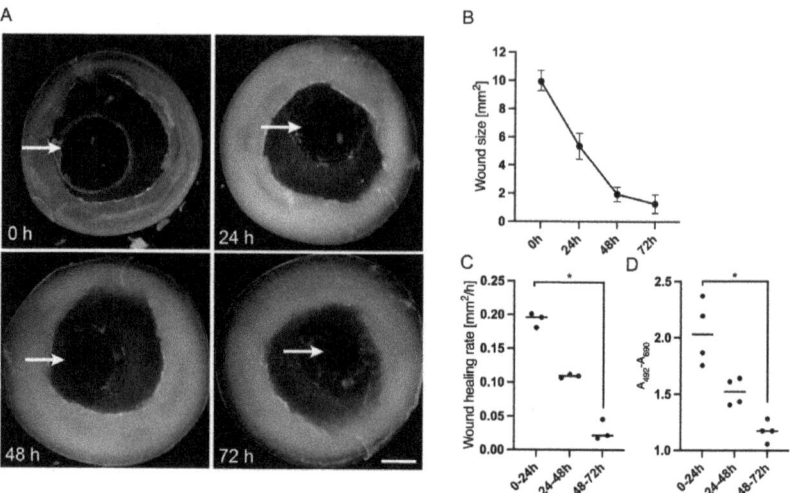

Figure 2. Optical documentation and analysis of wound healing in corneal organ culture model for 72 h. The wound healing process of corneas during ex vivo culture was monitored with a stereomicroscope. The specimens were cultivated in DMEM (see Table 2) for up to 72 h. (**A**) The epithelial wound margin after using a 4 mm punch could be identified at the start of the experiment (arrow, 0 h). During wound healing the margins of the newly formed epithelium could be followed visually (arrows at 24, 48 and 72 h). (**B**) The wound area was calculated at 0 h, 24 h, 48 h and 72 h and the median (range) was calculated from three specimens. (**C**) The wound healing rate was calculated for every 24 h from the start as mm^2 per hour. D: Vitality of the corneal tissue was evaluated by measuring release of lactate dehydrogenase (LDH). The absorbance of organ culture supernatant was evaluated after 24 h, 48 h and 72 h. Scale bar measures 2 mm. Sample size $n = 3$ for (**B**,**C**), $n = 4$ for (**D**). Statistically significant differences are indicated as *: $p < 0.05$.

3.4. Evaluation of Apoptotic Cells in the Wound Area in the Course of Cornea Ex Vivo Cultivation

To detect apoptosis in the wound area of the corneas, paraffin sections were prepared at the beginning of the experiment and after one, two and three days of organ culture. The sections were examined using a TUNEL staining via the "In Situ Cell Death Detection Kit". Cells with single- and double-stranded DNA breaks that occur at the early stages of apoptosis were labelled with TMR, a red fluorescent dye. At the start of the experiment (d 0), no red-coloured and thus apoptotic cells were visible (Figure 4). On day 1, apoptotic cells were detectable at the epithelial wound margin and in the upper area of the stroma. In the stroma area beneath the defect apoptotic keratocytes were particularly numerous. On day 2, apoptotic cells were mainly detectable in the stroma. After three days only a few apoptotic cells were visible in the stroma, but none in the epithelium.

3.5. Influence of Defect Size and Presence of Limbus on Corneal Wound Healing

Organ culture with living tissues is being influenced by several factors. With increasing culture time, negative effects from dying cells increase. Nevertheless, a sufficient period of time should be available to observe all cellular processes during wound healing. Here we will investigate whether the dynamics of wound healing change with epithelial erosions of different sizes. In addition to the defect of 4 mm in diameter, a defect of 8 mm was caused. Moreover, it was analysed whether the presence or absence of the limbus has an impact on corneal wound healing. Since the limbus is a reservoir for limbal stem cells, which can divide quickly in case of injury and replace the defective epithelium, the influence of this stem cell niche should be investigated. All different corneal specimens were cultured after wounding for three days and the wound size was calculated at the start of the experiment and then after 24 h, 48 h and 72 h (Figure 5A). Furthermore, the speed of wound healing was calculated by determination of the wound healing rate (mm^2/h). First, the influence of different defect sizes with 4 and 8 mm was analysed in ex vivo cultivated corneas with limbus. Both the 4 mm and the 8 mm defects showed a significant decrease in wound sizes over 72 h. The former started at a median of 9.11 (8.86–10.35) mm^2 and ended at 3.25 (1.81–3.87) mm^2 (p = 0.014), while the latter had a median of 40.17 (39.79–43.71) mm^2 initially and 29.68 (28.87–30.42) mm^2 (p = 0.048) at final follow-up (Figure 5B). In both setups, the most dynamic passage of wound healing was seen within the first 48 h. However, during this phase healing speed was not significantly different (0.14 vs. 0.19, p = 0.10) between the two wound sizes (Figure 5D). As reproducibility of initial lesion area was slightly higher with the 4 mm trephine, we decided to continue the following experiments with this size. Following that, the presence of limbal stem cells and their influence on corneal wound healing was checked. The wound closure of a 4 mm defect in a cornea with limbus was compared to a cornea without limbus (Figure 5C). Even without the limbal support the wound closed significantly from 9.94 (9.29–10.71) mm^2 at baseline to 0.89 (0.87–2.02) mm^2 after 72 h (p = 0.011). After three days over 90% of the lesion was healed, but there were no statistically significant differences compared to corneas with limbus (p = 0.308). Since the curves nearly ran parallel the presence of the limbus seemingly did not have any significant effect at a lesion size of 4 mm. There were also no significant differences in the wound healing rate (0.14 vs. 0.16, p = 0.10) during the first 48 h. With the aim of establishing a robust and easy to use ex vivo model, only corneas without limbus were cultivated in the following.

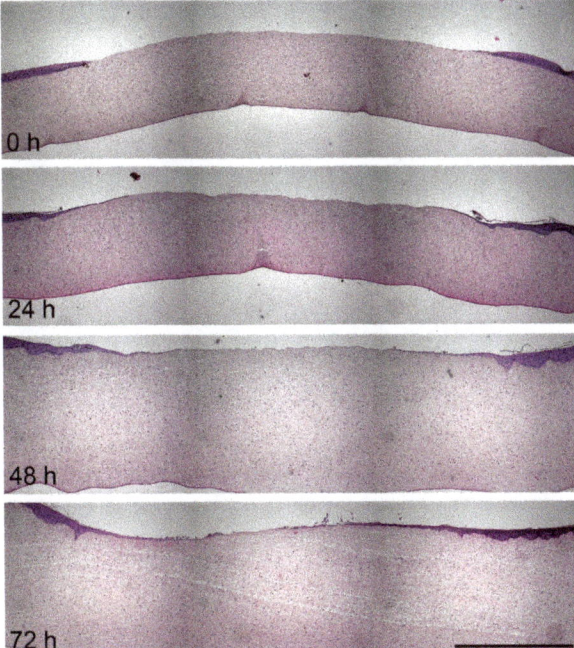

Figure 3. Histological documentation of the corneal wound healing process in HE-stained paraffin sections. HE-stained paraffin sections of the cornea were analysed with a stereomicroscope to follow wound healing of a 4 mm defect at day 1, 2 and 3. Thickening of the corneal stroma due to swelling processes is evident. Several single images were taken in a good magnification and via mosaic tool combined to a cornea overview. Scale bar represents 1 mm.

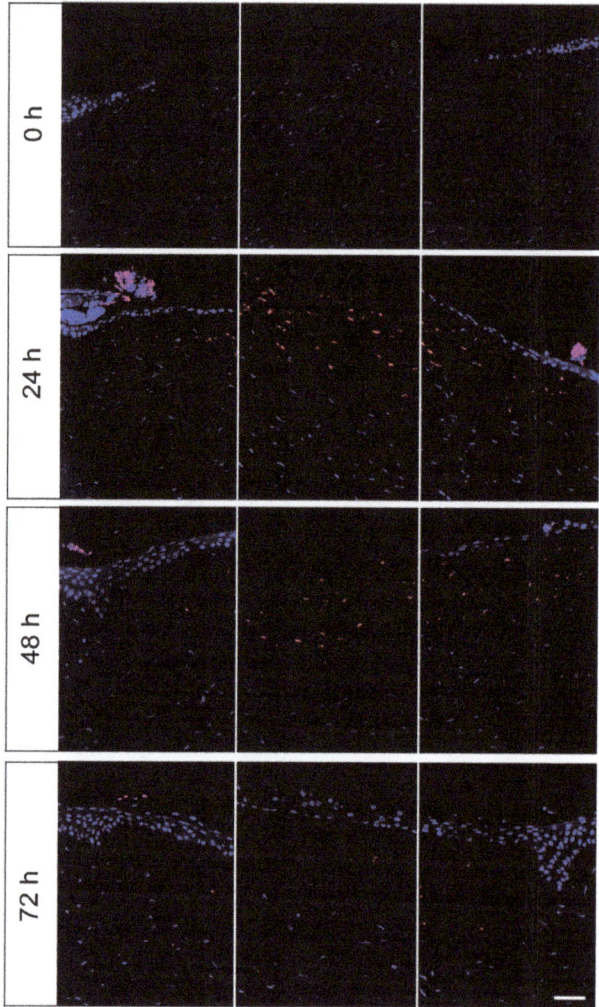

Figure 4. TUNEL-Assay on paraffin sections of the organ culture model after 0 h, 24 h, 48 h and 72 h. Apoptotic cells in cornea paraffin sections were determined at the start of the culture (0 h) and during ex vivo cultivation on days 1–3. Specimens had been cultured in DMEM and the lesion had a diameter of 4 mm. Images present the left wound margin (left panels), the centre of the defect (middle panels) and the right wound margin (right panels). Apoptotic cells were stained with TMR (red) and all cell nuclei were stained with DAPI (blue). Scale bar represents 50 µm.

3.6. Influence of Culture Medium on Corneal Wound Healing

During the organ culture optimization phase, a classic serum-containing medium based on DMEM was initially used. For the in vitro culture of epithelia such as skin, there are also other special media that are considered to be beneficial for keratinocytes. Therefore, the wound healing in the cornea model was analysed in various media in order to find the optimal medium composition. During culture the wound size was determined at the start of the experiment and then 24 h, 48 h and 72 h after the lesion was generated. As shown in Figure 6, the following media were compared: William's E Medium (WEM; purple line), a medium which is often used for skin organ culture, Keratinocyte Growth Medium 2 (KGM2; green line), which is designed for in vitro culture of epidermal keratinocytes and

OcuLife (yellow line), which is optimized for the culture of human corneal epithelial cells. The application of all media resulted in a statistically significant wound size reduction. The results indicated that DMEM was superior compared to each of the other media at any time point. At final follow-up after 72 h the median lesion was 0.96 (0.14–2.52) mm^2 for DMEM, 9.44 (8.06–9.44) mm^2 for KGM2, 9.38 (9.35–10.19) mm^2 for OcuLife and 6.85 (6.38–6.85) mm^2 for WEM. However, during the dynamic phase (0–48 h) the wound healing rate of DMEM was significantly higher compared to OcuLife ($p = 0.036$) and KGM2 ($p = 0.014$), but not to WEM ($p = 0.78$).

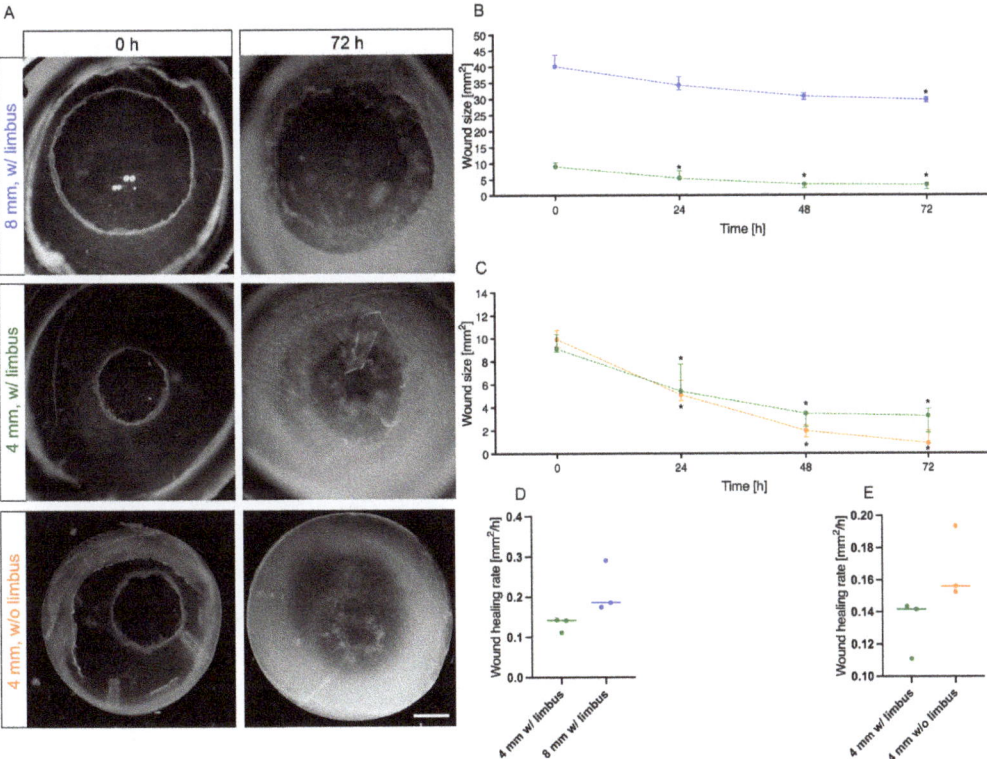

Figure 5. Influence of defect size and presence of limbus. For optimizing the organ culture model parameters like wound size and the presence of limbal stem cells in the limbus were evaluated. (**A**) Images were taken at 0 h and 72 h to monitor wound closure during different experimental settings. First panel (blue): Wound size 8 mm with limbus; second panel (green): Wound size 4 mm with limbus; third panel (orange): Wound size 4 mm without limbus. (**B**) Comparison of the wound closure progression of corneas with limbus for wound sizes of 4 mm (green line) and 8 mm (blue line). (**C**) Comparison of the wound closure progression of 4 mm diameter wounds of corneas with limbus (green line) and without limbus (orange line). (**D**) Wound healing rates of corneas with limbus calculated between 0 h and 48 h for wound sizes of 4 mm (green) and 8 mm (blue). (**E**) Wound healing rates of 4 mm diameter wounds calculated between 0 h and 48 h of corneas with limbus (green) and without limbus (orange). Scale bar measures 2 mm. Sample size $n = 3$. Statistically significant differences are indicated as *: $p < 0.05$.

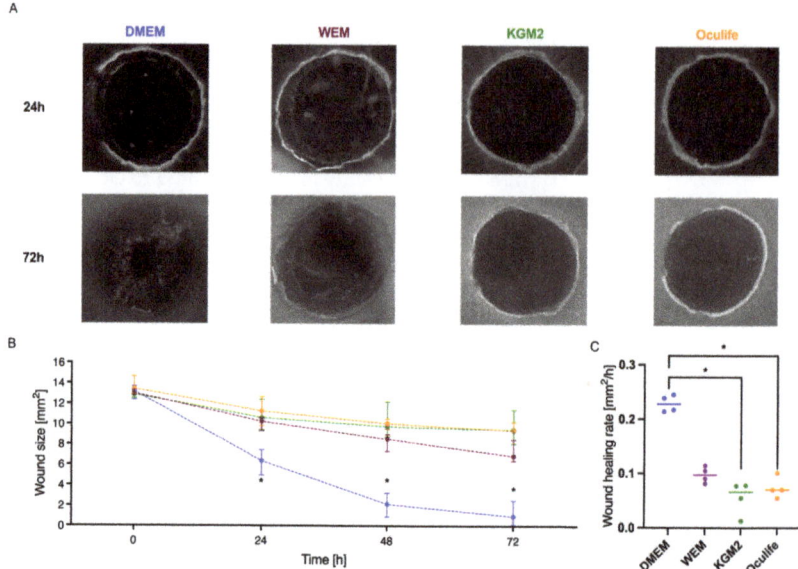

Figure 6. Comparison of wound healing rates in different cell culture media. The wound healing of ex vivo cultured corneas was determined evaluating the effect of different culture media. The corneal lesion was generated with a 4 mm biopsy punch. After 24 h, 48 h and 72 h of culture the wound size was calculated. (**A**) Images, which illustrate the wound healing performance were shown for 24 h and 72 h. (**B**) The tested media were Dulbecco's modified eagle medium (DMEM, blue line), Williams E Medium (WEM, purple line), Keratinocyte Growth Medium 2 (KGM2, green line) and OcuLife (yellow line). (**C**) The wound healing rates were also calculated for the period from 0 h to 48 h. Sample size n = 4. Statistically significant differences are indicated as *: $p < 0.05$.

3.7. Modulation of the Cornea Model with the Wound Healing Inhibitor Mitomycin

For the aim to use a tissue or organ model for test purposes, it must be sensitive, so that differences in wound healing performance can be measured. Since biologic specimens are always heterogenous, standard deviations should be small to see the effects of the analysed substances. Here we analysed the influence of increasing concentrations of mitomycin C (MMC), an antimetabolite which induces cell cycle arrest, on corneal wound healing, a process were cell division and cell migration are essential. Figure 7 shows the harmful effect of MMC, which negatively affected wound healing. Nevertheless, in all specimens the wound size showed a significant decrease over 72 h regardless of the MMC concentration. Yet, comparing the MMC setups to the DMEM control a significant, slightly delayed, dose-dependent impact was evident. At final follow-up, median wound size was 4.82 (4.74–6.69) mm^2 for MMC 50 µg/mL, 7.11 (5.74–7.33) mm^2 for MMC 100 µg/mL and 8.30 (7.72–9.79) mm^2 for 200 µg/mL, which were significantly larger compared to DMEM. While the wound healing rate of the samples incubated with 200 µg/mL MMC (0.11 mm^2/h, p = 0.019) was significantly decreased compared to the culture in DMEM (0.22 mm^2/h), the lower concentrations showed no significant effect on the wound healing rate.

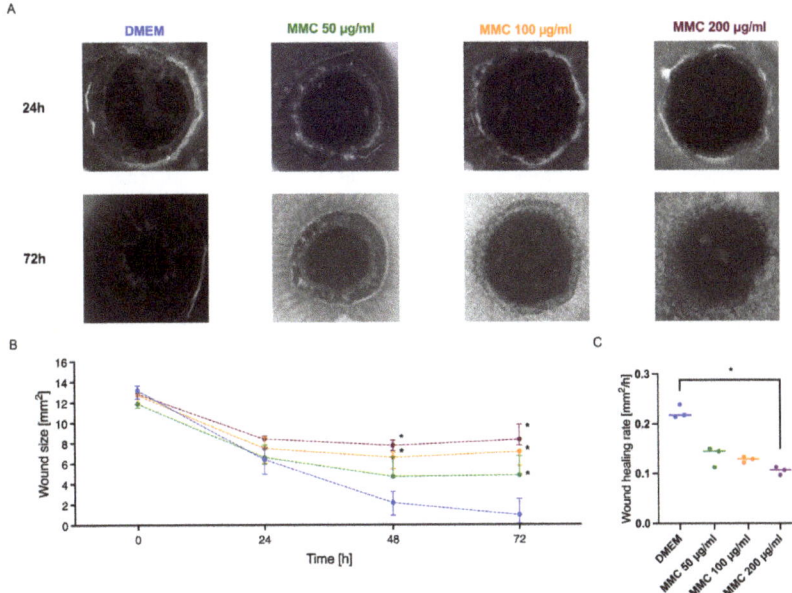

Figure 7. Effect of mitomycin C on corneal wound healing. The regeneration capacity of ex vivo cultured corneas was determined under the influence of the cytostatic agent mitomycin C. (**A**) Images, which illustrate the wound healing performance were shown for 24 h and 72 h. (**B**) The corneal lesion was generated with a 4 mm biopsy punch. After 24 h, 48 h and 72 h of culture the wound size was calculated. Different concentrations of mitomycin were tested: 0 µg/mL (DMEM, blue line), 50 µg/mL (green line), 100 µg/mL (orange line) and 200 µg/mL (purple line). (**C**) The wound healing rates were also calculated for the different mitomycin c concentrations evaluating the period from 0 to 48 h. Sample size n = 3. Statistically significant differences are indicated as *: $p < 0.05$.

4. Discussion

The use of organ culture models has several advantages and will often provide results that correspond better to the situation in vivo than in vitro models with primary cells or immortalized cell lines. Since human tissue is not regularly available and animal in vivo experiments have several ethical issues next to experimental challenges, the established organ culture model with porcine corneas appears to be the optimal alternative. First of all, the corneal architecture is maintained in those 3D models and the cells crosstalk, i.e., between keratocytes and epithelial cells remains possible. Furthermore, there is no need for elaborate equipment and since pig eyes are regularly available from the abattoir even larger experimental approaches are cost effective. In addition, this ex vivo tissue models allow the simple and easy testing of admitted exogenous factors like drugs, cytokines or even transplanted cells. Moreover, evaluation and analysis of the results is possible with quite a few procedures: Optical real time imaging of wound closure, histology of embedded cornea tissue, protein analysis of culture media, etc.

In the last few years, many research groups have already established ex vivo cornea models with animal tissues and optimized them for certain applications. Since they follow different key objectives, there are many different experimental approaches and care should be taken when comparing the results obtained.

With our model we had the aim to establish a robust and easy-to-handle ex vivo organ culture model, which allows us to study early wound healing effects, so that influences of media compositions, drugs or cell-based transplantation strategies can be analysed. Many researchers put a lot of effort into adapting the cornea culture to the in vivo situation in the best possible way. Some debate exists about the type of tissue culture: Submerged or at an air–liquid interface [7–13]. Richard et al. compared the ex vivo air-interface organ culture with submerged, epithelial side down cultured human corneas [7]. Together with rocking the culture plates to irrigate cornea tissues they can show a better epithelial integrity for the corneas cultured at the air–liquid interface. This approach seems to decrease intracellular edema, preserve stromal keratocytes and improve epithelial cell morphology. The system permits a long-term culture of human corneas for up to three weeks. A more recent work from Janin-Magnificat et al. followed a similar approach with air/liquid interface as well as immersed organ cultures with the difference of cultivating the submerged human corneas with the epithelial side up [14]. For laser-caused wounds they found almost no differences when comparing the expression of epithelial and wound healing specific proteins. Only the epithelial thickness was reduced to one cell layer in the submerged culture conditions compared to the air–liquid equivalents.

In the last years several groups adapt these culture systems to enable a more standardized handling and the maintenance of corneal curvature by using support structures for the cultured tissue specimens. Some groups sought to stabilize the tissue explants with the use of plastic domes from falcon tubes [9,11] or Luer Lock syringe covers [3]. Other groups use agar and collagen to fill up the corneal half shells with a gelatinous material [8,12,13,15]. Zhao and co-workers established even a sophisticated chamber system with perfusion and drop wise irrigation of rabbit corneas [10].

Our cornea 3D culture of epithelial side up, free floating cornea disks followed the approach from Janin-Magnificat et al. and is a submerged organ culture with a minimum of processing and the advantages of optimal nutritional supply and better perfusion with soluble factors [14].

The results from the lactate dehydrogenase assay, which measured cell viability, corroborate the presumption that our culture conditions were cell-protecting and preserved the viability of the corneal tissue. The initially high LDH values at the start of the culture are due to the inevitable trauma of punching out the wound and the corneal disk, but over the culture period of 72 h the LDH values and therefore cytotoxicity declined. Moreover, the results from the TUNEL assay indicate that the cultivation procedure was tissue-conserving. The apoptotic cells were mainly located in the stroma beneath the defect. The early disappearance of keratocytes after epithelial injury had been reported from others and is called "phenomenon of disappearing keratocytes". The effect is caused by crosstalk of epithelial cells and stromal cells [16].

In addition, there was no need of adhesives to fix the tissues, i.e., with acrylate glue, which has been used by other groups to immobilize corneas and may be toxic [3,11]. Free floating corneal disks have furthermore the advantage that opacity of the cornea could be avoided, as it was observed when the tissue rests on blotting paper, agar or acrylic surfaces [9,14,17,18].

Problems like opacity and swelling of cornea tissue were also addressed in our organ culture model through addition of dextran. Dextran, a polysaccharide, increases the osmolarity of the culture medium. Such compounds are essential parts of classic ocular storage media, when tissues should be preserved for transplantation (i.e., Optisol-GS). In our ex vivo model, the addition of dextran was mandatory, because without it the corneal defect could not be located anymore due to swelling and opacification (data not shown). In the literature there is some debate about cytotoxicity of dextran, since it accumulates within the cornea [19–21]. However, the ex vivo culture of the cornea in dextran-containing medium for a maximum of four days is considered to be unproblematic [19].

Aiming to analyse early wound healing effects in a model, which therefore did not need to be long-term viable, we examined the effects of the presence or absence of the limbus. As the limbus is a reservoir for stem cells, this tissue between cornea and sclera has a central role in cornea regeneration. Epithelial lesions normally resolve within a couple of days in a concentric fashion due to the proliferation and migration of stem cells from the limbus or from other parts of the epithelium [14]. Comparing the corneas cultured with and without limbus there were no statistically significant differences in the general wound healing performance or the wound healing rate. These findings are in line with the work of Chang and co-workers, as they demonstrated that early re-epithelialisation after wounding is due to proliferation and migration of cells from the basal and suprabasal layers of the epithelium [22]. Corneal epithelial recovery seems to be independent of limbal epithelial stem cells at least in the first 12 h after injury as migration dominates proliferation. This suggestion is also underlined by the observation that MMC in each concentration did not change the wound healing rate within the first 24 h. Either most of the cells passed the vulnerable S and G2/M phase of the cell cycle and were at G1 stage, which is quite unlikely as cells usually are quite heterogenous in their mitosis rhythm, or migration is the major force during this initial wound healing period. We decided to use limbal-free corneal disks for further experiments, since they were easier to handle. It must be pointed out, however, that in our ex vivo model the reconstruction of a multi-layered corneal epithelium will not be possible, as no cell replenishment from the limbus is available. In fact, this is also confirmed by the histological analyses in which the regenerated epithelium remains in a single layer even three days after injury.

Regarding the defect area, no difference in the rate of wound healing could be determined between the lesion of 4 mm and 8 mm in diameter. The observation confirms studies on cultured rabbit corneas, in which the defect size also had no influence on the average rate of cellular migration during the linear healing phase. It is postulated that the epithelial cells move at a constant rate until coverage was complete and that cellular migration is the limiting step during wound healing [23]. Since the wound was closed within three days in the case of the 4 mm injuries, which was rated as a well observable healing dynamic, this defect size was used in all further investigations.

When comparing different serum-free cell culture media for the pig organ culture, the classic DMEM promoted the healing of the corneas best. Since DMEM is used for many different cell types and organisms, it seems reasonable to assume that it is generally useful in an organ culture model with different cell types, like keratinocytes, keratocytes and endothelial cells. Indeed, serum-free Minimum Essential Medium had been already used for the organ culture of human corneas, which retain vitality and remain suitable for transplantation [24]. KGM2 and OcuLife are normally used for the in vitro culture of human corneal epithelial cells or cell lines [25,26]. Their poorer performance in the wound healing model could be due to the fact that they are supportive for only one cell type. Interestingly, the WEM which was successfully established for wound healing studies in frog and human skin organ cultures [27,28] supported corneal wound healing of the pig cornea punches slightly better than KGM2 and OcuLife. In addition, it also cannot be ruled out that there are species-specific effects, so that media for human cells are not optimal suitable for pig cells. If there a specific wound healing promoting factors in DMEM or inhibitors of healing in the other media had to be analyzed in further studies.

The wound healing rates determined for the cultured pig corneas are slightly lower, but still comparable to ex vivo cultured corneas from other experimenters. Foreman et al. determined a wound healing rate for ex vivo cultured bovine corneas of 0.75 mm^2/h for excisional wounds with a diameter of 5 mm [8]. Zhao et al. used also bovine corneas, which were cultivated in a chamber system with perfusion and irrigation [10]. They discovered different wound healing rates for their 7 mm defects according to their culture media: 0.78 mm^2/h in serum containing media and 1.29 mm^2/h in serum free media.

The transferability of the data gained from an animal model to humans is often a critical issue. For the selection of a suitable model, which is as close as possible to the human eye, several parameters should be considered. Among the classically used experimental animals such as rats, mice, rabbits, pigs or cattle, the eye size of pigs is closest to the human eye. In addition, the corneal thickness of pig eyes (0.68 mm) is better comparable to human eyes (0.5 mm), as other species like bovine (0.8 mm) or rabbit (0.37 mm) [15]. There are also differences in the corneal anatomical structure between the species [29]. While human and porcine corneas contain a Bowman's layer, this layer is missing in rabbit corneas [15].

A limitation of our model is that the use of a manual trephine results in uneven wounds and cannot be reproduced identically from cornea to cornea. This can be avoided by using an excimer laser [30]. However, naturally occurring wounds are not all equivalent in depth and perfectly round. Therefore, using a trephine does actually mimic the situation in real-life more realistically. Moreover, swelling of the corneal stroma may limit the cultural duration of our model. Yet, evaluations up to five days were easily achievable, which is within the critical time frame for corneal epithelial regeneration processes. Yet, this might also vary from specimen to specimen due to baseline properties (e.g., size, thickness, endothelial cell count, stromal composition, post-mortem changes). Therefore, heterogenicity of samples could be a downside [31]. Nevertheless, the primary outcome parameter of our study (wound size) demonstrated a quite narrow range between replicates, which indicates a certain reproducibility.

In conclusion, this easy-to-handle organ culture model of pig corneas is suitable for analysing early wound healing effects. It facilitates observation of the time course and dynamic of wound closure by the use of non-invasive optical documentation with a simple stereomicroscope. The effect of substances can be studied, as we have documented for MMC, which stopped cell division and therefore hampered wound closure. Further experiments need to be performed, so that other factors like wound healing inducers or the effect of transplanted stem cells can be assessed.

Author Contributions: Conceptualization, S.S. and M.R.; Data curation, S.S., E.D. and M.R.; Formal analysis, E.D.; Investigation, S.S. and E.D.; Methodology, S.S., E.D. and M.R.; Supervision, S.S. and M.R.; Validation, S.S., E.D. and M.R.; Visualization, S.S. and M.R.; Writing—original draft, S.S.; Writing—review & editing, S.S., E.D., C.K., S.G. and M.R. All authors have read and agreed to the published version of the manuscript.

Funding: This research received no external funding.

Institutional Review Board Statement: The study was conducted according to the guidelines of the Declaration of Helsinki, and approved by the Ethics Committee of the University of Lübeck (protocol code 18-102, date of approval 27 June 2018).

Informed Consent Statement: Informed consent was obtained from all subjects involved in the study.

Data Availability Statement: The data that support the findings of this study are available from the authors, S.S. and M.R., upon reasonable request.

Conflicts of Interest: The authors declare no conflict of interest.

References

1. Kinoshita, S.; Adachi, W.; Sotozono, C.; Nishida, K.; Yokoi, N.; Quantock, A.J.; Okubo, K. Characteristics of the Human Ocular Surface Epithelium. *Prog. Retin. Eye Res.* **2001**, *20*, 639–673. [CrossRef]
2. Carrier, P.; Deschambeault, A.; Talbot, M.; Giasson, C.J.; Auger, F.A.; Guérin, S.L.; Germain, L. Characterization of Wound Reepithelialization Using a New Human Tissue-Engineered Corneal Wound Healing Model. *Investig. Ophthalmol. Vis. Sci.* **2008**, *49*, 1376–1385. [CrossRef] [PubMed]
3. Proietto, L.R.; Whitley, R.D.; Brooks, D.E.; Schultz, G.E.; Gibson, D.J.; Berkowski, W.M., Jr.; Salute, M.E.; Plummer, C.E. Development and Assessment of a Novel Canine Ex Vivo Corneal Model. *Curr. Eye Res.* **2017**, *42*, 813–821. [CrossRef] [PubMed]
4. Dua, H.S.; Gomes, J.A.; Singh, A. Corneal Epithelial Wound Healing. *Br. J. Ophthalmol.* **1994**, *78*, 401–408. [CrossRef] [PubMed]
5. Bukowiecki, A.; Hos, D.; Cursiefen, C.; Eming, S.A. Wound-Healing Studies in Cornea and Skin: Parallels, Differences and Opportunities. *Int. J. Mol. Sci.* **2017**, *18*, 1257. [CrossRef] [PubMed]
6. Holzhey, A.; Sonntag, S.; Rendenbach, J.; Ernesti, J.S.; Kakkassery, V.; Grisanti, S.; Reinholz, F.; Freidank, S.; Vogel, A.; Ranjbar, M. Development of a Noninvasive, Laser-Assisted Experimental Model of Corneal Endothelial Cell Loss. *J. Vis. Exp. JoVE* **2020**, *158*, e60542. [CrossRef]
7. Richard, N.R.; Anderson, J.A.; Weiss, J.L.; Binder, P.S. Air/Liquid Corneal Organ Culture: A Light Microscopic Study. *Curr. Eye Res.* **1991**, *10*, 739–749. [CrossRef]
8. Foreman, D.M.; Pancholi, S.; Jarvis-Evans, J.; McLeod, D.; Boulton, M.E. A Simple Organ Culture Model for Assessing the Effects of Growth Factors on Corneal Re-Epithelialization. *Exp. Eye Res.* **1996**, *62*, 555–564. [CrossRef] [PubMed]
9. Chuck, R.S.; Behrens, A.; Wellik, S.; Liaw, L.L.; Dolorico, A.M.; Sweet, P.; Chao, L.C.; Osann, K.E.; McDonnell, P.J.; Berns, M.W. Re-Epithelialization in Cornea Organ Culture after Chemical Burns and Excimer Laser Treatment. *Arch. Ophthalmol.* **2001**, *119*, 1637–1642. [CrossRef] [PubMed]

10. Zhao, B.; Cooper, L.J.; Brahma, A.; MacNeil, S.; Rimmer, S.; Fullwood, N.J. Development of a Three-Dimensional Organ Culture Model for Corneal Wound Healing and Corneal Transplantation. *Investig. Ophthalmol. Vis. Sci.* **2006**, *47*, 2840–2846. [CrossRef]
11. Castro-Combs, J.; Noguera, G.; Cano, M.; Yew, M.; Gehlbach, P.L.; Palmer, J.; Behrens, A. Corneal Wound Healing Is Modulated by Topical Application of Amniotic Fluid in an Ex Vivo Organ Culture Model. *Exp. Eye Res.* **2008**, *87*, 56–63. [CrossRef] [PubMed]
12. Deshpande, P.; Ortega, Í.; Sefat, F.; Sangwan, V.S.; Green, N.; Claeyssens, F.; MacNeil, S. Rocking Media over Ex Vivo Corneas Improves This Model and Allows the Study of the Effect of Proinflammatory Cytokines on Wound Healing. *Investig. Ophthalmol. Vis. Sci.* **2015**, *56*, 1553–1561. [CrossRef]
13. Castro, N.; Gillespie, S.R.; Bernstein, A.M. Ex Vivo Corneal Organ Culture Model for Wound Healing Studies. *J. Vis. Exp. JoVE* **2019**, *144*, e58562. [CrossRef]
14. Janin-Manificat, H.; Rovère, M.-R.; Galiacy, S.D.; Malecaze, F.; Hulmes, D.J.S.; Moali, C.; Damour, O. Development of Ex Vivo Organ Culture Models to Mimic Human Corneal Scarring. *Mol. Vis.* **2012**, *18*, 2896–2908.
15. Piehl, M.; Gilotti, A.; Donovan, A.; DeGeorge, G.; Cerven, D. Novel Cultured Porcine Corneal Irritancy Assay with Reversibility Endpoint. *Toxicol. Vitr.* **2010**, *24*, 231–239. [CrossRef] [PubMed]
16. Dohlman, C.H.; Gasset, A.R.; Rose, J. The Effect of the Absence of Corneal Epithelium or Endothelium on the Stromal Keratocytes. *Investig. Ophthalmol.* **1968**, *7*, 520–534.
17. Xu, K.P.; Li, X.F.; Yu, F.S. Corneal Organ Culture Model for Assessing Epithelial Responses to Surfactants. *Toxicol. Sci. Off. J. Soc. Toxicol.* **2000**, *58*, 306–314. [CrossRef]
18. Sriram, S.; Gibson, D.J.; Robinson, P.; Pi, L.; Tuli, S.; Lewin, A.S.; Schultz, G. Assessment of Anti-Scarring Therapies in Ex Vivo Organ Cultured Rabbit Corneas. *Exp. Eye Res.* **2014**, *125*, 173–182. [CrossRef] [PubMed]
19. Redbrake, C.; Salla, S.; Nilius, R.; Becker, J.; Reim, M. A Histochemical Study of the Distribution of Dextran 500 in Human Corneas during Organ Culture. *Curr. Eye Res.* **1997**, *16*, 405–411. [CrossRef]
20. Borderie, V.M.; Baudrimont, M.; Lopez, M.; Carvajal, S.; Laroche, L. Evaluation of the Deswelling Period in Dextran-Containing Medium after Corneal Organ Culture. *Cornea* **1997**, *16*, 215–223. [CrossRef]
21. Thuret, G.; Manissolle, C.; Campos-Guyotat, L.; Guyotat, D.; Gain, P. Animal Compound-Free Medium and Poloxamer for Human Corneal Organ Culture and Deswelling. *Investig. Ophthalmol. Vis. Sci.* **2005**, *46*, 816–822. [CrossRef] [PubMed]
22. Chang, C.-Y.; Green, C.R.; McGhee, C.N.J.; Sherwin, T. Acute Wound Healing in the Human Central Corneal Epithelium Appears to Be Independent of Limbal Stem Cell Influence. *Investig. Ophthalmol. Vis. Sci.* **2008**, *49*, 5279–5286. [CrossRef] [PubMed]
23. Crosson, C.E.; Klyce, S.D.; Beuerman, R.W. Epithelial Wound Closure in the Rabbit Cornea. A Biphasic Process. *Investig. Ophthalmol. Vis. Sci.* **1986**, *27*, 464–473.
24. Müller, L.J.; Pels, E.; Vrensen, G.F. The effects of organ-culture on the density of keratocytes and collagen fibers in human corneas. *Cornea* **2001**, *20*, 86–95. [CrossRef]
25. Robertson, D.M.; Li, L.; Fisher, S.; Pearce, V.P.; Shay, J.W.; Wright, W.E.; Cavanagh, H.D.; Jester, J.V. Characterization of growth and differentiation in a telomerase-immortalized human corneal epithelial cell line. *Investig. Ophthalmol. Vis. Sci.* **2005**, *46*, 470–478. [CrossRef]
26. Fukuda, T.; Gouko, R.; Eitsuka, T.; Suzuki, R.; Takahashi, K.; Nakagawa, K.; Sugano, E.; Tomita, H.; Kiyono, T. Human-Derived Corneal Epithelial Cells Expressing Cell Cycle Regulators as a New Resource for in vitro Ocular Toxicity Testing. *Front. Genet.* **2019**, *10*, 587. [CrossRef]
27. Meier, N.T.; Haslam, I.S.; Pattwell, D.M.; Zhang, G.-Y.; Emelianov, V.; Paredes, R.; Debus, S.; Augustin, M.; Funk, W.; Amaya, E.; et al. Thyrotropin-releasing hormone (TRH) promotes wound re-epithelialisation in frog and human skin. *PLoS ONE* **2013**, *8*, e73596. [CrossRef]
28. Liao, T.; Lehmann, J.; Sternstein, S.; Yay, A.; Zhang, G.; Matthießen, A.E.; Schumann, S.; Siemers, F.; Kruse, C.; Hundt, J.E.; et al. Nestin+ progenitor cells isolated from adult human sweat gland stroma promote reepithelialisation and may stimulate angiogenesis in wounded human skin ex vivo. *Arch Dermatol. Res.* **2019**, *311*, 325–330. [CrossRef] [PubMed]
29. Van den Berghe, C.; Guillet, M.C.; Compan, D. Performance of Porcine Corneal Opacity and Permeability Assay to Predict Eye Irritation for Water-Soluble Cosmetic Ingredients. *Toxicol. Vitr.* **2005**, *19*, 823–830. [CrossRef]
30. Hafezi, F.; Gatzioufas, Z.; Angunawela, R.; Ittner, L.M. Absence of IL-6 Prevents Corneal Wound Healing after Deep Excimer Laser Ablation in Vivo. *Eye* **2018**, *32*, 156–157. [CrossRef] [PubMed]
31. Napoli, P.E.; Nioi, M.; Gabiati, L.; Laurenzo, M.; De-Giorgio, F.; Scorcia, V.; Grassi, S.; d'Aloja, E.; Fossarello, M. Repeatability and Reproducibility of Post-Mortem Central Corneal Thickness Measurements Using a Portable Optical Coherence Tomography System in Humans: A Prospective Multicenter Study. *Sci. Rep.* **2020**, *10*, 14508. [CrossRef] [PubMed]

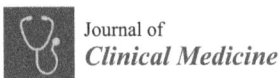

Article

Visual Acuity and Number of Amniotic Membrane Layers as Indicators of Efficacy in Amniotic Membrane Transplantation for Corneal Ulcers: A Multicenter Study

Javier Lacorzana [1,2,*], Antonio Campos [3,4], Marina Brocal-Sánchez [5], Juan Marín-Nieto [6], Oswaldo Durán-Carrasco [7], Esly C. Fernández-Núñez [7], Andrés López-Jiménez [8], Jose L. González-Gutiérrez [9], Constantinos Petsoglou [10] and Jose L. García Serrano [11]

1. Department of Ophthalmology, Virgen de las Nieves University Hospital, 18006 Granada, Spain
2. Doctoral Program in Clinical Medicine and Public Health, University of Granada, 18006 Granada, Spain
3. Tissue Engineering Group, Department of Histology, University of Granada, 18006 Granada, Spain; acampos@ugr.es
4. Institute of Biosanitary Research ibs. Granada, University of Granada, 18006 Granada, Spain
5. Department of Ophthalmology, Son Espases University Hospital, 07120 Palma de Mallorca, Spain; mabroc2@hotmail.com
6. Department of Ophthalmology, Virgen de la Victoria University Hospital, 29010 Malaga, Spain; juan7_m@hotmail.com
7. Department of Ophthalmology, Nuestra Señora de la Candelaria University Hospital, 38010 Santa Cruz de Tenerife, Spain; oswaldurancarrasco@gmail.com (O.D.-C.); fernandez_729@hotmail.com (E.C.F.-N.)
8. Department of Ophthalmology, Reina Sofía University Hospital, 30003 Murcia, Spain; andreslj_2005@hotmail.com
9. Department of Ophthalmology, Juan Ramón Jimenez, University Hospital, 21005 Huelva, Spain; joselgogu@hotmail.com
10. Department of Ophthalmology, Sydney Eye Hospital, Sydney 2100, Australia; conpetsoglou@hotmail.com
11. Department of Ophthalmology, San Cecilio University Hospital, 18006 Granada, Spain; jopalace@hotmail.com
* Correspondence: javilacor@gmail.com

Abstract: Background: To evaluate new indicators in the efficacy of amniotic membrane transplantation (AMT) for non-healing corneal ulcers (NHCUs). Methods: Retrospective, multicenter study. In total, 223 AMTs for NHCU in 191 patients were assessed. The main outcomes studied were the success rate of AMT (complete re-epithelization), postoperative visual acuity (VA) gain, and number of AM layers transplanted. Results: The overall AMT success rate was 74.4%. In 92% of our patients VA stability or improvement. Postoperative VA was significantly higher than preoperative VA in the entire cohort ($p < 0.001$) and in all etiological groups of ulcers (post-bacterial, $p \leq 0.001$; post-herpetic, $p \leq 0.0038$; neurotrophic ulcers, $p \leq 0.014$; non-rheumatic peripheral, $p \leq 0.001$; and ulcers secondary to lagophthalmos and eyelid malposition or trauma, $p \leq 0.004$). Most participants (56.5%) presented a preoperative VA equal to or less than counting fingers (≤ 0.01). Of these, 13.5% reached a postoperative VA equal to or better than legal blindness (≥ 0.05) after AMT. A higher success rate was observed in the monolayer than in the multilayer AMT (79.5% and 64.9%, respectively; $p = 0.018$). No statistically significant values were found between the number of layers transplanted and VA gain ($p = 0.509$). Conclusion: AMT is not only beneficial in achieving complete re-epithelialization in NHCUs but also in improving postoperative VA; these improvements are independent of etiologies of ulcers. Furthermore, the use of monolayer AMT seems to be a more appropriate option than multilayer AMT for NHCU since the multilayer AMT did not present better outcomes (success rate and VA gain) compared to monolayer AMT in the different types of ulcers studied.

Keywords: amniotic membrane; amniotic membrane transplantation; cornea; corneal ulcer; corneal ulceration; non healing corneal ulcer; visual acuity; persistent epithelial defects

---

Citation: Lacorzana, J.; Campos, A.; Brocal-Sánchez, M.; Marín-Nieto, J.; Durán-Carrasco, O.; Fernández-Núñez, E.C.; López-Jiménez, A.; González-Gutiérrez, J.L.; Petsoglou, C.; Serrano, J.L.G. Visual Acuity and Number of Amniotic Membrane Layers as Indicators of Efficacy in Amniotic Membrane Transplantation for Corneal Ulcers: A Multicenter Study. *J. Clin. Med.* **2021**, *10*, 3234. https://doi.org/10.3390/jcm10153234

Academic Editor: Vincenzo Scorcia

Received: 31 May 2021
Accepted: 13 July 2021
Published: 22 July 2021

Publisher's Note: MDPI stays neutral with regard to jurisdictional claims in published maps and institutional affiliations.

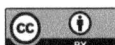

Copyright: © 2021 by the authors. Licensee MDPI, Basel, Switzerland. This article is an open access article distributed under the terms and conditions of the Creative Commons Attribution (CC BY) license (https://creativecommons.org/licenses/by/4.0/).

1. Introduction

The cornea is a body surface exposed to the external environment. The protective factors of the cornea include the eyelids and the tear film among others. The latter is responsible for nourishing the avascular cornea while providing a stable refractive surface.

A stable tear film and an integrated corneal surface are of great importance for good visual acuity (VA) [1,2]. Different authors [2–4] have studied the histological and immunohistochemical methods for the alterations of the tear film and the cornea and their implication in VA.

A non-healing corneal ulcer (NHCU) is defined as an ulcer that does not show any indication of complete corneal epithelialization within two weeks despite the administration of proper medical treatment [5]. It can be caused by multiple conditions such as neurotrophic keratitis, infection, rheumatic disease, eyelid malposition, trauma, and corneal dystrophy [5,6]. NHCUs can progress to descemetoceles or perforations, which is why their rapid treatment is highly recommended. In this regard, amniotic membrane transplantation (AMT) has been suggested as an excellent therapeutic option [5,6].

The amniotic membrane (AM) is the innermost layer of the placenta. It is a thin (20–500 μm), semi-transparent membrane. Histologically, the AM comprises three layers: epithelium, basement membrane, and avascular stroma [7–13].

This tissue has multiple biological properties, including the induction of cell proliferation, reduction of neovascularization, anti-scarring properties, increasing migration of cells such as keratinocytes, pool corneal regeneration, and little or no immunogenicity [7,14–20]. Heavy chain hyaluronan/pentraxin 3 (HC-HA/PTX3), a matrix component of AM, is a key factor responsible for the aforementioned AM's properties [16,17,21]. These properties favor its use in ophthalmological pathologies, such as persistent corneal ulcers (neurotrophic, post-herpetic) [7,22–28], descemetoceles [29], perforations [7,14,26,30–32], and chemical burns [7,14,33–39].

Although the usefulness of AMT in treating NHCU has previously been investigated, several questions remain unanswered, especially with regard to VA gain and the number of layers used [6,31,40–42]. The current uncertainties may be due to the differences in the etiology of ulcers, insufficient statistical approach, or indicators evaluated [5,6,31,40,42,43]. In order to address these limitations, the present multicenter study sought to assess the efficacy of AMT in a large sample of patients with NHCUs while considering the VA gain and number of layers used. In addition, we aimed to explore these effects on different etiological groups and the possible influence of numbers of layers used in VA gain, a novel approach to be considered [6,40].

2. Materials and Methods

2.1. Patients

This retrospective multicenter study was conducted to evaluate the efficacy of AMT in treating NHCUs at Spanish National Healthcare hospitals. Patient records from January 2012 to June 2018 were obtained. Our study covered 17 participating hospitals throughout Spain. The patient population from these hospitals represents 13.78% (6,436,043/46,720,000) of the Spanish population. Written informed consent was obtained from all patients prior to the transplantation. This study was approved by the local Ethics Committee (Study code: 1272-N-18) and adhered to the tenets of the Declaration of Helsinki.

We analyzed data from 223 AMT cases in 191 patients with NHCUs of different etiologies. In all cases, cryopreserved AMs were used as they contain high concentrations of growth factors [7,44] and lubricin, a boundary lubricant (Figure 1) [17,45]. Cryopreserved AMs are most widely used because of their biosafety [43] The protocols of provincial and regional biobanks established by the National Health System were followed, with sterility controls and serological studies of donors and recipients [15].

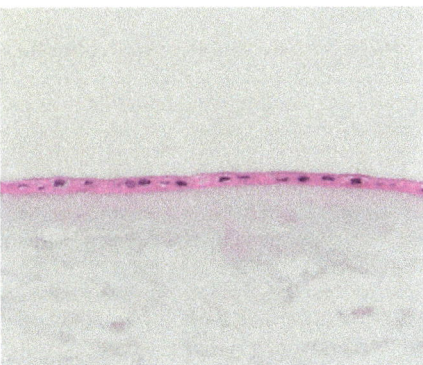

Figure 1. Amniotic membrane (×20) stained with *hematoxylin and eosin* provided by Biobank. Epithelium and avascular stroma.

Patients with corneal ulcers refractory to medical treatment, surgically treated with cryopreserved AM, were included. Only patients with a minimum follow-up of 18 months post-surgery were included in accordance with the inclusion criteria. The ulcers were categorized as post-bacterial ulcers, post-herpetic ulcers, neurotrophic ulcers, peripheral corneal ulcers not associated with a rheumatic disease, and ulcers caused by lagophthalmos, eyelid malposition, or trauma [6,40,43]. The exclusion criteria were as follows: inability to follow-up, incomplete records, and coadjutant surgery (e.g., conjunctival flap, tarsorrhaphy, or lamellar keratoplasty). Incomplete or unclear records were evaluated by two investigators with expertise (LJ and GSJL). In cases of disparity, the patient was excluded. NHCUs with an active infection, descemetocele, or perforation were excluded. Furthermore, patients with ulcers due to bullous keratopathy, post-keratoplasty ulcers, rheumatic corneal ulcers, stem cell deficiencies (requiring different surgical techniques), or chemical burns (requiring AMT within two weeks, thus not qualified as an NHCU) were excluded [5,46]. The measurement of ulcers' width was not standardized at all centers, which is why this parameter was excluded from our study. An identity document (ID) was assigned to each center, and each AMT used for treatments received an individualized ID. The outcome variable was the success or failure of the surgery.

Success was defined as the complete epithelialization of the refractory corneal ulcer eight weeks after surgery (lack of fluorescein staining at the slit lamp examination). Confocal microscopy studies have shown that AM may be present up to six weeks, and it might not be detectable eight weeks after surgery [47] AMT failure was defined as incomplete corneal epithelization within eight weeks after intervention. If two or more AMTs were performed, the results were analyzed. If other types of reconstructive surgery were performed post-AMT, the results were censored at this time [40].

The independent variables collected in each case included the following: sex, age, number of AMTs performed in each patient, number of AM layers used in each AMT, etiology of the ulcers, whether AMT was the primary surgical option or not, VA before transplantation, VA after the last follow-up, and corneal transparency after AMT. The corneal opacification was based on the Sotozono classification [48]: transparent (grade 0), partially opaque (grades 1 and 2), and opaque (grade 3) corneas.

VA was evaluated in all patients using the Snellen's original test with conversions to decimal and logMAR scales [49,50] for statistical analyses. Lower VAs were calculated as follows: counting fingers, 1/100 (logMAR 2); hand motions, 1/200 (logMAR 2.3); light perception, 1/666 (logMAR 2.8) [51], and amaurosis, 0 (logMAR 3).

2.2. Surgery and Follow-Up

All surgeries were performed by consultant ophthalmologists (n = 21). To homogenize their results, the following quality criteria were required: fill in a single and unified questionnaire, clearly defined ulcer type, definition of success or failure of AMT, performed in public hospitals with training program in ophthalmology, and surgery performed by ocular surface specialists with more than five years of experience.

The cryopreserved AMs were prepared according to the Tseng method [15]. The surgeons obtained the AMs from the regional tissue banks maintained by the Spanish government. All patients underwent a thorough preoperative examination. Surgery was performed under topical, peribulbar, or general anesthesia, as determined by the surgeon. Prior to the AMT, necrotic edges of the ulcer were debrided. Depending on the severity, the AMs were applied as a monolayer or as multilayers (≥ 2), fixed with interrupted or uninterrupted 10-0 nylon sutures or fibrin sealants. The AMs could be transplanted using different techniques: (1) inlay—it was placed over the ocular defect without extending beyond its edges; (2) overlay—it was used as a patch suturing it beyond the edges of the ocular defect; and (3) a combination of both methods, known as the "sandwich" technique [7,40].

Postoperatively, the patients received treatment with antibiotics and topical corticosteroids, in addition to the etiological treatment for the ulcer. Follow-up examinations were performed the day after, and approximately one, two, four, and eight weeks after the operation. The patients were treated in the emergency department in case of any complications. Subsequent follow-ups were performed at the discretion of the physician for at least 18 months. When AMT was not the primary surgical option, the alternative options were conjunctival flap, tarsorrhaphy, and lamellar or penetrating keratoplasty [23,52].

2.3. Statistical Analysis

Statistical analysis was performed using the SPSS Statistics 19 software (IBM Corp., Armonk, NY, USA). The numerical variables are expressed as means ± standard deviations. The categorical variables are described as absolute (n) and relative (%) frequencies. For nonparametric data distribution, a Mann-Whitney test was used. Odds ratios (ORs) were calculated for variables related to success, along with their 95% confidence intervals (CIs). For differences between the types of ulcers, a Kruskal-Wallis test was applied. VA data were normalized to the logMAR scale, and a Wilcoxon signed-rank test was applied to analyze the relationship between the VAs before and after the intervention. These values were also expressed on the Snellen optotype scale. A p-value < 0.05 was considered statistically significant.

For the determination of the sample size, 34 AMTs would be needed in each of the 5 subgroups (n = 170); accepting an alpha risk of 0.005 and beta risk of 0.2 in a two-sided test, and estimating the significant post-AMT VA gain at 0.3 logMAR and the variance at 0.8. Furthermore, an exhaustive review of the literature on this subject was carried out. It was found that the studies with the largest sample size and best design were those of Schuerch et al. [6] and Uhlig et al. [40] (149 and 108 patients, respectively). In our article, we analyzed data from 191 patients (223 AMT cases).

3. Results

In our study, we analyzed 223 AMTs that were used in 191 patients (94 male and 97 female patients) with NHCUs of different etiologies (Figure 2).

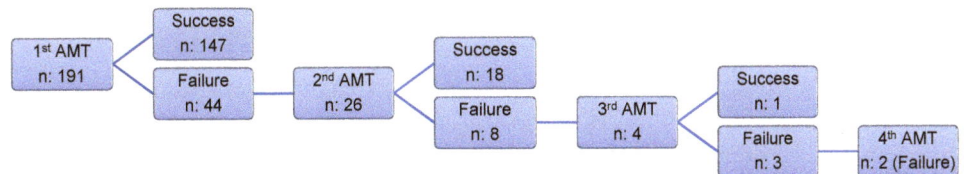

Figure 2. Flowchart of success and failure after amniotic membrane transplantation.

3.1. Sex and Age

Sex distribution analysis revealed that 46.6% (n = 104) of the 223 AMTs were performed in male patients and 53.4% (n = 119) in female patients (Table 1). The mean age of patients receiving an AMT was 65 ± 18.3 years (range 11–102 years) (Table 1).

Table 1. Amniotic membrane transplantation for each type of ulcer.

	BACT	HERP	NEUROT	PERIPH	LAGOPH
	N = 39	N = 31	N = 87	N = 18	N = 48
	−17.50%	−13.90%	−39.00%	−8.10%	−21.50%
Sex					
Male	21 (53.8%)	16 (51.6%)	36 (41.4%)	9 (50%)	22 (45.8%)
Female	18 (46.2%)	15 (48.4%)	51 (58.6%)	9 (50%)	26 (54.2%)
Age (mean ± SD)	66.4 ± 16.9	63.6 ± 15.5	66.4 ± 17.8	65.4 ± 16.9	61.9 ± 22.4
1ª surgical option	32 (82.1%)	24 (77.4%)	73 (83.9%)	14 (77.8%)	42 (87.5%)
Corneal opacification					
Grade 0	9 (23.1%)	1 (3.2%)	17 (19.5%)	12 (66.7%)	12 (25%)
Grade 1–2	6 (15.4%)	1 (3.2%)	24 (27.6%)	2 (11.1%)	9 (18.8%)
Grade 3	24 (61.5%)	29 (93.5%)	46 (52.9%)	4 (22,2%)	27 (56.2%)

BACT, post-bacterial ulcers; HERP, post-herpetic ulcers; NEUROT, neurotrophic ulcers; PERIPH, non-rheumatic peripheral ulcers; LAGOPH, ulcers secondary to lagophthalmos and eyelid malposition or trauma; SD, standard deviation; 1ª surgical option, primary surgical option.

3.2. Success and Failure

Of all the AMTs, 74.4% (166/223) were successful, and there were no statistically significant differences among the NHCU cases of various etiologies ($p = 0.755$) (Figure 3).

3.3. Corneal Opacification

Since these were refractory ulcers secondary to a serious corneal pathology, transparency was reduced at the beginning. The cornea was transparent after AMT (grade 0 classification Sotozone) in 22.4% (51/223), partially opaque (grades 1 and 2) in 18.8% (42/223), and opaque (grade 3) in 58.3% (130/223) (Table 1).

3.4. Visual Acuity

Preoperative VA was significantly different in each type of ulcer ($p = 0.001$). Preoperative VA was significantly worse in post-herpetic ulcers compared to those in neurotrophic ulcers ($p = 0.03$), and non-rheumatic peripheral ulcers ($p = 0.003$) (Figure 4).

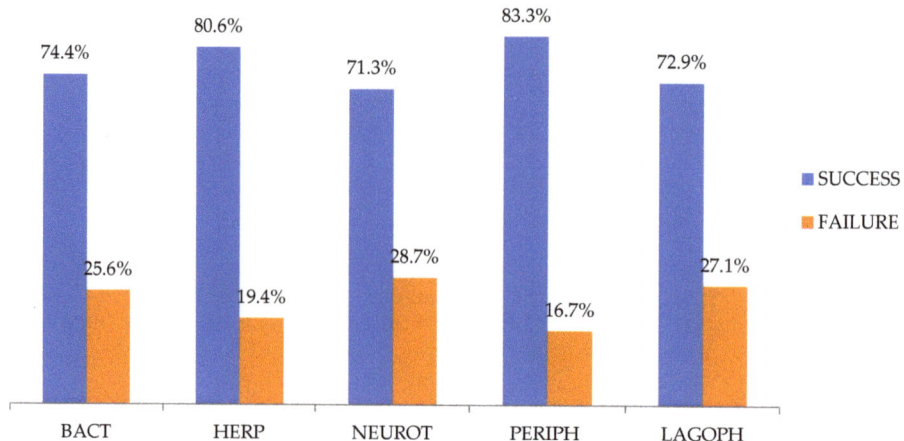

Figure 3. Amniotic membrane transplantation success and failure rates for each group of corneal ulcers. BACT, post-bacterial ulcers; HERP, post-herpetic ulcers; NEUROT, neurotrophic ulcers; PERIPH, non-rheumatic peripheral ulcers; LAGOPH, ulcers secondary to lagophthalmos and eyelid malposition or trauma.

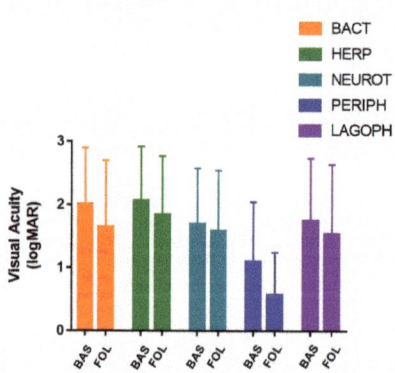

Figure 4. Bar chart representing visual acuity (VA) in logMAR at baseline and at the last follow-up. VA, visual acuity; BACT, post-bacterial ulcers; HERP, post-herpetic ulcers; NEUROT, neurotrophic ulcers; PERIPH, non-rheumatic peripheral ulcers; LAGOPH, ulcers secondary to lagophthalmos and eyelid malposition or trauma; BAS, at baseline; FOL, at the last follow-up.

In the entire study population, the VA significantly improved from 1.77 ± 0.93 to 1.54 ± 1.02 logMAR ($p < 0.001$). Postoperative VA was significantly higher than preoperative VA in all etiological groups of ulcers: post-bacterial ulcers ($p \leq 0.001$), post-herpetic ulcers ($p \leq 0.0038$), neurotrophic ulcers ($p \leq 0.014$), non-rheumatic peripheral corneal ulcers ($p \leq 0.001$) and in ulcers secondary to lagophthalmos and eyelid malposition or trauma ($p \leq 0.004$) (Figure 4).

VA stability or improvement was seen in 92% (205/223) of the cases (Table 2). The participants presented a preoperative VA equal to or less than counting fingers (≤ 0.01) in 56.5% of the study population (126/223). Of those, 13.5% (17/126) reached a postoperative VA equal to or better than legal blindness (≥ 0.05) due to AMT [53,54].

Table 2. Functional results (visual acuity) of amniotic membrane transplantation for each type of ulcer. The minimum last follow-up was 18 months.

	BACT	HERP	NEUROT	PERIPH	LAGOPH
VA at baseline					
- Amaurosis	6 (15.4%)	1 (3.2%)	3 (3.4%)	1 (5.6%)	2 (4.2%)
- LP	7 (17.9%)	12 (38.8%)	13 (14.9%)	2 (11.1%)	16 (33.3%)
- HM	10 (25.6%)	5 (16.1%)	22 (25.3%)	1 (5.6%)	6 (12.5%)
- CF	4 (10.3%)	5 (16.1%)	10 (11.5%)	0 (0%)	0 (0%)
- ≥0.05 a 1 Snellen	12 (30.8%)	8 (25.8%)	39 (44.8%)	14 (77.8%)	24 (50%)
VA at last follow-up					
- Amaurosis	6 (15.4%)	1 (3.2%)	4 (4.6%)	1 (5.5%)	2 (4.2%)
- LP	5 (12.8%)	8 (25.8%)	11 (12.6%)	0 (0%)	14 (29.2%)
- HM	7 (17.9%)	5 (16.1%)	19 (21.9%)	0 (0%)	5 (10.4%)
- CF	1 (2.6%)	7 (22.7%)	13 (14.9%)	0 (0%)	1 (2.1%)
- ≥0.05 a 1	20 (51.3%)	10 (32.3%)	40 (46%)	17 (94.5%)	26 (54.2%)
Changes in VA					
Worsening	1 (2.6%)	5 (16.1%)	8 (9.2%)	1 (5.6%)	3 (6.3%)
Equal	22 (56.4%)	15 (48.4%)	54 (62.1%)	2 (11.1%)	30 (62.5%)
Improvement	16 (41%)	11 (35.5%)	25 (28.7%)	15 (83.3%)	15 (31.3%)

VA, visual acuity; BACT, post-bacterial ulcers; HERP, post-herpetic ulcers; NEUROT, neurotrophic ulcers; PERIPH, non-rheumatic peripheral ulcers; LAGOPH, ulcers secondary to lagophthalmos and eyelid malposition or trauma; CF, counting fingers; HM, hand motions; LP; light perception.

3.5. Efficacy of Monolayer Versus Multilayer AMT

Monolayer and multilayer AMTs were performed in 65.5% (146/223) and 34.5% (77/223) of the cases, respectively. The success rate was higher in the monolayer (79.5%) than in the multilayer AMTs (64.9%) ($p = 0.018$) (Table 3).

Table 3. Relationship between the number of AM layers and success rate according to ulcer etiology.

	BACT	HERP	NEUROT	PERIPH	LAGOPH
MON	88.9%	90.9%	75.0%	77.8%	75.7%
MUL	61.9%	55.6%	63.0%	88.9%	63.6%
TOTAL	74.4%	80.6%	71.3%	85.3%	72.9%
p	$p = 0.058$	$p = 0.043$	$p = 0.186$	$p = 0.500$	$p = 0.334$

MON, monolayer; MUL, multilayer; BACT, post-bacterial ulcers; HERP, post-herpetic ulcers; NEUROT, neurotrophic ulcers; PERIPH, non-rheumatic peripheral ulcers; LAGOPH, ulcers secondary to lagophthalmos and eyelid malposition or trauma.

3.6. Correlation of Monolayer/Multilayer AMT and VA Gain

In the monolayer and multilayer AMT, the VA improved from 2.04 ± 0.88 to 1.80 ± 1.01 logMAR ($p = 0.093$) and 1.49 ± 0.91 to 1.28 ± 0.97 logMAR ($p = 0.056$), respectively. Table 4 shows the relationship between the number of amniotic membrane layers and VA gain according to ulcer etiology (Table 4).

There were no statistically significant differences in VA gain between the monolayer and multilayer AMT in the entire cohort ($p = 0.509$) or in all etiological groups (post-bacterial ulcers, $p = 0.208$; post-herpetic ulcers, $p = 0.338$; neurotrophic ulcers, $p = 0.737$; non-rheumatic peripheral ulcers, $p = 0.054$; ulcers secondary to lagophthalmos and eyelid malposition or trauma, $p = 0.371$).

Table 4. Relationship between the number of amniotic membrane layers and visual acuity gain according to ulcer etiology.

		BACT	HERP	NEUROT	PERIPH	LAGOPH
MON	logMAR VA at baseline (mean ± SD)	2.19 ± 0.93	2.20 ± 0.79	1.89 ± 0.87	1.56 ± 1.05	2.21 ± 0.86
	logMAR VA last follow-up (mean ± SD)	1.88 ± 1.14	1.84 ± 0.97	1.82 ± 0.94	0.61 ± 0.33	2.11 ± 0.97
MUL	logMAR VA at baseline (mean ± SD)	1.69 ± 0.79	1.81 ± 0.94	1.48 ± 0.85	0.81 ± 0.80	1.52 ± 0.98
	logMAR VA last follow-up (mean ± SD)	1.28 ± 0.79	1.84 ± 0.89	1.35 ± 0.93	0.55 ± 0.85	1.25 ± 1.05

VA, visual acuity; MON, monolayer; MUL, multilayer; BACT, post-bacterial ulcers; HERP, post-herpetic ulcers; NEUROT, neurotrophic ulcers; PERIPH, non-rheumatic peripheral ulcers; LAGOPH, ulcers secondary to lagophthalmos and eyelid malposition or trauma; SD, standard deviation.

4. Discussion

Several studies have described the benefits of AMTs as a treatment for various ocular surface pathologies [14,34,35,55], including NHCUs [56–58]. However, the diverse etiologies of the ulcers, the small sample sizes, and the adjuvant treatments used or the analysis of the different variables make direct comparisons difficult [5,6,31,40,42,43]. Our multicenter study aimed to study a series of indicators in a large sample size, with a special emphasis on VA gain and number of layers. Thus, we sought to assess and confirm ideas related to the effectiveness of the use of AMT, all the while suggesting new ones to reinforce its use.

The mean age of the participants in our study and other studies were between 64 and 68 years [6,40,51,59]. We found that AMT was a safe and non-aggressive technique and so can be used in a wide range of ages, a fact that was also supported by other studies [6,40,59]. Therefore, in the absence of a response to pharmacological treatment, AMT became the first surgical option for NHCU in the hospitals enrolled in our study. This idea was also supported by a recently published article that revealed that corneal ulcers are the first indications for AMTs [60].

Our overall percentage of success was 74.4% (166/223). Success rates of AMT on the ocular surface are highly variable, ranging from 49% to 97–100% [6,40,43,57]. Success rates as high as 49% (66/135) and 70% (105/149) have been reported by Uhlig et al. [40] and Schuerch et al. [6], respectively. The success rate in our study is consistent with that observed in these studies, with a comparatively larger sample size. Nevertheless, when comparing the results of these studies, the fact that the NHCU cases treated with AMT did not have a homogeneous etiological classification should be considered. Schuerch et al. [6] studied the same etiologies as the ones studied here. Moreover, they focused on other etiologies, such as post-keratoplasty associated with rheumatic disease, secondary to bullous keratopathy, and ulcers due to chemical burns. Uhlig et al. [40] divided NHCU cases into four groups (neurotrophic, post-herpetic, post-bacterial, and rheumatologic). Among their examined groups, there were no significant differences in the epithelization percentages. Liu et al. [43] also reported no significant differences between their infectious and non-infectious ulcer groups. In line with the results reported above, no significant differences were observed in the percentages of AMT success (71.3% to 83.3%) among our five groups of corneal ulcers.

Preoperative VA was very low throughout the cohort. Schuerch et al. [6] observed no difference in the preoperative VA between different etiological groups. However, we found that preoperative VA was significantly worse in the group with post-herpetic ulcers compared to the other NHCU etiological groups. Post-herpetic ulcers presented a high percentage of opacification, even though they were well re-epithelialized. Although AMT is an effective technique for the closure of these ulcers in many cases, the initial treatment of the post-herpetic ulcers should be faster since the loss of transparency was more frequent than in other ulcers. Therefore, despite the healing that was achieved, the VA at the last follow-up was low in most cases.

In contrast to our postoperative VA findings, Uhlig et al. [40], Letko et al. [41], Prabhasawat et al. [31], and Brocks et al. [61] did not find significant improvements in postoperative VA compared to the baseline values despite reporting high percentages of re-epithelization. Schuerch et al. [6] observed significant improvements in VA in the entire cohort but not in the etiological groups. In our study, we found significant improvements in VA across the entire cohort and also in all the etiological groups. Thus, since all groups improved, the etiology of ulcers does not seem to be a decisive factor in the VA improvements. Although, these improvements were small in some cases, even these small VA gains are relevant in the daily lives of patients with such low VA. Moreover, this gain may allow some of them to stop being blind (13.5%, 17/126), with all that this visual improvement entails clinically, as we have been able to observe in our results. HC-HA/PTX3's anti-scarring and anti-angiogenic effects of AM could help explain the VA improvements [16,21,62].

A recent study using self-retained cryopreserved AMs (Prokera®; Bio-Tissue, Inc., Miami, FL, USA) has shown significant VA gain in a limited number of cases (n = 24); however, this study only analyzed Prokera® in infectious ulcers but not in NHCUs. Others studies on Prokera® did not find this significant VA gain [61].

A total of 92% (205/223) of our patients maintained or improved their VA scores. This result made us consider several ideas. First, vascular progression and persistent inflammation often facilitate the closure of ulcers, with secondary consequence being the loss of corneal transparency and reduction in VA. AMTs could help avoid this by self-integration into the host corneal tissue in different patterns (subepithelial, intraepithelial, or intrastromal) [63,64]. However, if we use it later, there may already be a certain component of fibrotic stroma that reduces corneal transparency in a pronounced way. The initial treatment of these chronic ulcers must be aggressive and rapid to prevent the loss of initial VA; otherwise, only a low percentage of patients will have moderate vision restored. Hence, we strongly recommend that AMT should be used as soon as possible. Second, AMTs can improve VA by regularizing the corneal surface and improving the transparency of the cornea [41,65]; this may delay the employment of more aggressive surgical options. In the future, many of these patients could receive a corneal transplant since their cornea will have been epithelialized and will be less inflamed [23,26,43].

With regard to AM layers and the success rate, there are two previous studies that included a relatively low number of cases (n = 28 in each study) and reported that the success rate of monolayer AMT ranged from 64% to 80% and that of multilayer AMT ranged from 72% to 84.6% [31,42]. In our multicenter study, the success rate was significantly higher with the monolayer AMT than with the multilayer AMT (79.5% and 64.9%, respectively). This result must be cautiously interpreted as the ulcers' depth could be analyzed (descemetoceles were discarded) but not the ulcers' width. Perhaps, larger ulcers lead surgeons to apply more layers in order to try achieving greater success or this may depend on the surgeons' preferences. Another possible hypothesis is that AM does not integrate well when used as a multilayer. This hypothesis could be evaluated at the level of optical microscopy in future studies.

Regarding the influence of the number of AM layers on VA gain, our results showed that there were no significant differences between monolayer and multilayer AMT in all etiological groups.

Thus, since the success rate and VA gain were not better in multilayer AMT than in monolayer AMT, the use of multilayer AMT could not be justified in NHCU. Nonetheless, the use of multilayer AMT could be indicated in specific cases such as descemetoceles and perforations [19,26,27,63,64].

A limitation to our study could be its retrospective and multicenter nature. AM availability, surgeons' therapeutic preferences, and prevalence of ulcers could have conditioned the selection of the different cases in our studied hospitals. Possibly, the assessment of the ulcers' width would have helped to better explain our results; however, these data were not consistent and, thus, were excluded from our study.

In conclusion, this multicenter study has assessed VA gain and the number of AM layers transplanted as new indicators in the evaluation of NHCUs. Our results revealed not only that the use of AMT is beneficial in achieving complete re-epithelialization in NHCUs but also that it improves the postoperative VA independent of the etiology of the ulcers. Moreover, we demonstrated that the use of multilayer AMT in NHCUs does not improve the outcomes (success rate and VA gain) in comparison to monolayer AMT in the different types of ulcers studied. In addition, to the best of our knowledge, this is the largest sample size included in a study evaluating the efficacy of AMT as a treatment for patients with NHCUs [6,40].

Author Contributions: Conceptualization, J.L., J.L.G.S. and A.C.; methodology, J.L. and J.L.G.S.; data curation, all authors; writing—original draft preparation, J.L.; writing—review and editing, all authors; visualization, all authors; supervision, all authors. All authors have read and agreed to the published version of the manuscript.

Funding: This research received a grant from the Andalusian Society of Ophthalmology. The funding source had no role in the study design, data collection and analysis, decision to publish, or preparation of the manuscript.

Institutional Review Board Statement: This study was approved by the local Ethics Committee (*Cómité Ético de Investigación Médica Provincial de Granada*) (Study code: 1272-N-18) and adhered to the tenets of the Declaration of Helsinki.

Informed Consent Statement: Written informed consent was not necessary because no patient data has been included in the manuscript. Informed consent was not requested for the present study because of its retrospective nature, the large number of patients, the non-exposure of personal data, and the acceptance by the ethics committee of the total anonymity of the study population. The data collection and analysis were carried out completely anonymized.

Data Availability Statement: The data presented in this study are available on request from the corresponding author. The data are not publicly available due to restrictions of privacy.

Acknowledgments: The authors are grateful to the Andalusian Society of Ophthalmology for their support of our project, to Manuela Expósito Ruiz, statistician at the Bio-health Research Institute (FIBAO), for statistical analysis, and to Biobank for its excellent work in preparing the AMs. This study forms part of the Doctoral Thesis of Javier Lacorzana Rodríguez.

Conflicts of Interest: The authors have no conflict of interest to declare.

References

1. Mead, O.; Tighe, S.; Tseng, S.C.G. Amniotic membrane transplantation for managing dry eye and neurotrophic keratitis. *Taiwan J. Ophthalmol.* **2020**, *10*, 13–21. [CrossRef]
2. Napoli, P.E.; Nioi, M.; D'Aloja, E.; Loy, F.; Fossarello, M. The architecture of corneal stromal striae on optical coherence Tomography and histology in an animal model and in humans. *Sci. Rep.* **2020**, *10*, 19861. [CrossRef] [PubMed]
3. Napoli, P.E.; Nioi, M.; D'Aloja, E.; Fossarello, M. The bull's eye pattern of the tear film in humans during visual fixation on en-face optical coherence tomography. *Sci. Rep.* **2019**, *9*, 1413. [CrossRef]
4. Nioi, M.; Napoli, P.E.; Demontis, R.; Locci, E.; Fossarello, M.; D'Aloja, E. Morphological analysis of corneal findings modifications after death: A preliminary OCT study on an animal model. *Exp. Eye Res.* **2018**, *169*, 20–27. [CrossRef]
5. Zhang, T.; Wang, Y.; Jia, Y.; Liu, D.; Li, S.; Shi, W.; Gao, H. Active pedicle epithelial flap transposition combined with amniotic membrane transplantation for treatment of nonhealing corneal ulcers. *J. Ophthalmol.* **2016**, *2016*, 5742346. [CrossRef] [PubMed]
6. Schuerch, K.; Baeriswyl, A.; Frueh, B.E.; Tappeiner, C. Efficacy of amniotic membrane transplantation for the treatment of corneal ulcers. *Cornea* **2020**, *39*, 479–483. [CrossRef] [PubMed]
7. Lacorzana, J. Amniotic membrane, clinical applications and tissue engineering. Review of its ophthalmic use. *Arch. Soc. Esp. Oftalmol.* **2020**, *95*, 15–23. [CrossRef] [PubMed]
8. Meller, D.; Pauklin, M.; Thomasen, H.; Westekemper, H.; Steuhl, K.-P. Amniotic membrane transplantation in the human eye. *Dtsch. Aerztebl. Int.* **2011**, *108*, 243–248. [CrossRef]
9. Alemañy González, J.; Camacho Ruaigip, F. Usos de la membrana amniótica humana en oftalmología. *Rev. Cuba Oftalmol.* **2006**, *19*, 1–7.

10. Kobayashi, M.; Yakuwa, T.; Sasaki, K.; Sato, K.; Kikuchi, A.; Kamo, I.; Yokoyama, Y.; Sakuragawa, N. Multilineage potential of side population cells from human amnion mesenchymal layer. *Cell Transplant.* **2008**, *17*, 291–301. [CrossRef]
11. Hasegawa, M.; Fujisawa, H.; Hayashi, Y.; Yamashita, J. Autologous amnion graft for repair of myelomeningocele: Technical note and clinical implication. *J. Clin. Neurosci.* **2004**, *11*, 408–411. [CrossRef]
12. Favaron, P.; Carvalho, R.C.; Borghesi, J.; Anunciação, A.; Miglino, M. The amniotic membrane: Development and potential applications—A review. *Reprod. Domest. Anim.* **2015**, *50*, 881–892. [CrossRef] [PubMed]
13. van Herendael, B.; Oberti, C.; Brosens, I. Microanatomy of the human amniotic membranes. *Am. J. Obstet. Gynecol.* **1978**, *131*, 872–880. [CrossRef]
14. Lacorzana, J.; García-Serrano, J.; Prieto-Moreno, C.G.; Castillo-Rodríguez, S.; Lucena-Martín, J.; Pozo-Jiménez, I. Amniotic membrane, review of its ophthalmic use and results in the last five years (2013–2017) in Granada. Preliminary study. *Actual Med.* **2018**, *103*, 82–86. [CrossRef]
15. Tseng, S.C.; Espana, E.M.; Kawakita, T.; Di Pascuale, M.A.; Li, W.; He, H.; Liu, T.-S.; Cho, T.-H.; Gao, Y.-Y.; Yeh, L.-K.; et al. How does amniotic membrane work? *Ocul. Surf.* **2004**, *2*, 177–187. [CrossRef]
16. Tseng, S.C.G. HC-HA/PTX3 purified from amniotic membrane as novel regenerative matrix: Insight into relationship between inflammation and regeneration. *Investig. Opthalmol. Vis. Sci.* **2016**, *57*, ORSFh1–ORSFh8. [CrossRef]
17. Wang, J.; Chen, D.; A Sullivan, D.; Xie, H.; Li, Y.; Liu, Y. Expression of lubricin in the human amniotic membrane. *Cornea* **2020**, *39*, 118–121. [CrossRef]
18. Sabater, A.L.; Perez, V.L. Amniotic membrane use for management of corneal limbal stem cell deficiency. *Curr. Opin. Ophthalmol.* **2017**, *28*, 363–369. [CrossRef]
19. Murri, M.S.; Moshirfar, M.; Birdsong, O.C.; Ronquillo, Y.C.; Ding, Y.; Hoopes, P.C. Amniotic membrane extract and eye drops: A review of literature and clinical application. *Clin. Ophthalmol.* **2018**, *12*, 1105–1112. [CrossRef]
20. Utheim, T.P.; Utheim, A.; Salvanos, P.; Jackson, C.; Schrader, S.; Geerling, G.; Sehic, A. concise review: Altered versus unaltered amniotic membrane as a substrate for limbal epithelial cells. *Stem Cells Transl. Med.* **2018**, *7*, 415–427. [CrossRef]
21. Zhu, Y.-T.; Li, F.; Zhang, Y.; Chen, S.-Y.; Tighe, S.; Lin, S.-Y.; Tseng, S.C.G. HC-HA/PTX3 purified from human amniotic membrane reverts human corneal fibroblasts and myofibroblasts to keratocytes by activating BMP signaling. *Investig. Opthalmol. Vis. Sci.* **2020**, *61*, 62. [CrossRef]
22. Kruse, F.E.; Rohrschneider, K.; Völcker, H.E. Multilayer amniotic membrane transplantation for reconstruction of deep corneal ulcers. *Ophthalmology* **1999**, *106*, 1504–1511. [CrossRef]
23. Lambiase, A.; Sacchetti, M. Diagnosis and management of neurotrophic keratitis. *Clin. Ophthalmol.* **2014**, *8*, 571–579. [CrossRef]
24. Saad, S.; Abdelmassih, Y.; Saad, R.; Guindolet, D.; El-Khoury, S.; Doan, S.; Cochereau, I.; Gabison, E.E.; El Khoury, S. Neurotrophic keratitis: Frequency, etiologies, clinical management and outcomes. *Ocul. Surf.* **2020**, *18*, 231–236. [CrossRef] [PubMed]
25. Di Zazzo, A.; Coassin, M.; Varacalli, G.; Galvagno, E.; De Vincentis, A.; Bonini, S. Neurotrophic keratopathy: Pros and cons of current treatments. *Ocul. Surf.* **2019**, *17*, 619–623. [CrossRef]
26. Singhal, D.; Nagpal, R.; Maharana, P.K.; Sinha, R.; Agarwal, T.; Sharma, N.; Titiyal, J.S. Surgical alternatives to keratoplasty in microbial keratitis. *Surv. Ophthalmol.* **2020**, *66*. [CrossRef] [PubMed]
27. Chen, H.-J.; Pires, R.T.F.; Tseng, S.C.G. Amniotic membrane transplantation for severe neurotrophic corneal ulcers. *Br. J. Ophthalmol.* **2000**, *84*, 826–833. [CrossRef] [PubMed]
28. Dua, H.S.; Said, D.G.; Messmer, E.M.; Rolando, M.; Benitez-Del-Castillo, J.M.; Hossain, P.N.; Shortt, A.J.; Geerling, G.; Nubile, M.; Figueiredo, F.C.; et al. Neurotrophic keratopathy. *Prog. Retin. Eye Res.* **2018**, *66*, 107–131. [CrossRef]
29. Agarwal, R.; Nagpal, R.; Todi, V.; Sharma, N. Descemetocele. *Surv. Ophthalmol.* **2020**, *66*, 2–19. [CrossRef] [PubMed]
30. Rodríguez-Ares, M.T.; Touriño, R.; López-Valladares, M.J.; Gude, F. Multilayer amniotic membrane transplantation in the treatment of corneal perforations. *Cornea* **2004**, *23*, 577–583. [CrossRef]
31. Prabhasawat, P.; Smith, G.T.; Liu, C.S.C. Single and multilayer amniotic membrane transplantation for persistent corneal epithelial defect with and without stromal thinning and perforation. *Br. J. Ophthalmol.* **2001**, *85*, 1455–1463. [CrossRef]
32. Fan, J.; Wang, M.; Zhong, F. Improvement of amniotic membrane method for the treatment of corneal perforation. *BioMed Res. Int.* **2016**, *2016*, 1693815. [CrossRef]
33. Joseph, A.; Dua, H.S.; King, A. Failure of amniotic membrane transplantation in the treatment of acute ocular burns. *Br. J. Ophthalmol.* **2001**, *85*, 1065–1069. [CrossRef]
34. Navas, A.; Guerrero, F.S.M.; López, A.D.; Chávez-García, C.; Partido, G.; Graue-Hernández, E.O.; Sánchez-García, F.J.; Garfias, Y. Anti-inflammatory and anti-fibrotic effects of human amniotic membrane mesenchymal stem cells and their potential in corneal repair. *Stem Cells Transl. Med.* **2018**, *7*, 906–917. [CrossRef] [PubMed]
35. Sharma, N.; Kaur, M.; Agarwal, T.; Sangwan, V.S.; Vajpayee, R.B. Treatment of acute ocular chemical burns. *Surv. Ophthalmol.* **2018**, *63*, 214–235. [CrossRef] [PubMed]
36. Sharma, N.; Singh, D.; Maharana, P.K.; Kriplani, A.; Velpandian, T.; Pandey, R.M.; Vajpayee, R.B. Comparison of amniotic membrane transplantation and umbilical cord serum in acute ocular chemical burns: A randomized controlled trial. *Am. J. Ophthalmol.* **2016**, *168*, 157–163. [CrossRef] [PubMed]
37. Chen, Y.; Yan, X.-M.; Wu, H.-R.; Rong, B. An experimental study on the fate of the amniotic membrane after amniotic membrane transplantation for acute alkaline burn of rat cornea. *Zhonghua Yan Ke Za Zhi* **2012**, *48*, 27–32.

38. Eslani, M.; Baradaran-Rafii, A.; Cheung, A.Y.; Kurji, K.H.; Hasani, H.; Djalilian, A.R.; Holland, E.J. Amniotic membrane transplantation in acute severe ocular chemical injury: A randomized clinical trial. *Am. J. Ophthalmol.* **2019**, *199*, 209–215. [CrossRef]
39. Sahay, P.; Goel, S.; Maharana, P.K.; Sharma, N. Amniotic membrane transplantation in acute severe ocular chemical injury: A randomized clinical trial. *Am. J. Ophthalmol.* **2019**, *205*, 202–203. [CrossRef] [PubMed]
40. Uhlig, C.E.; Frings, C.; Rohloff, N.; Harmsen-Aasman, C.; Schmitz, R.; Kiesel, L.; Eter, N.; Busse, H.; Alex, A.F. Long-term efficacy of glycerine-processed amniotic membrane transplantation in patients with corneal ulcer. *Acta Ophthalmol.* **2015**, *93*, e481–e487. [CrossRef]
41. Letko, E.; Stechschulte, S.U.; Kenyon, K.R.; Sadeq, N.; Romero, T.R.; Samson, C.M.; Nguyen, Q.D.; Harper, S.L.; Primack, J.D.; Azar, D.T.; et al. Amniotic membrane inlay and overlay grafting for corneal epithelial defects and stromal ulcers. *Arch. Ophthalmol.* **2001**, *119*, 659. [CrossRef]
42. Dekaris, I.; Gabrić, N.; Mravicić, I.; Karaman, Z.; Katusić, J.; Lazić, R.; Spoljarić, N. Multilayer vs. monolayer amniotic membrane transplantation for deep corneal ulcer treatment. *Coll. Antropol.* **2001**, *25*, 23–28.
43. Liu, J.; Li, L.; Li, X. Effectiveness of cryopreserved amniotic membrane transplantation in corneal ulceration: A meta-analysis. *Cornea* **2019**, *38*, 454–462. [CrossRef]
44. Rodríguez-Ares, M.T.; López-Valladares, M.J.; Touriño, R.; Vieites, B.; Gude, F.; Silva, M.T.; Couceiro, J. Effects of lyophilization on human amniotic membrane. *Acta Ophthalmol.* **2009**, *87*, 396–403. [CrossRef]
45. Samsom, M.; Iwabuchi, Y.; Sheardown, H.; Schmidt, T.A. Proteoglycan 4 and hyaluronan as boundary lubricants for model contact lens hydrogels. *J. Biomed. Mater. Res. Part B Appl. Biomater.* **2017**, *106*, 1329–1338. [CrossRef]
46. Ghosh, S.; Salvador-Culla, B.; Kotagiri, A.; Pushpoth, S.; Tey, A.; Johnson, Z.K.; Figueiredo, F. Acute chemical eye injury and limbal stem cell deficiency—A prospective study in the United Kingdom. *Cornea* **2019**, *38*, 8–12. [CrossRef]
47. Nubile, M.; Dua, H.S.; Lanzini, T.E.-M.; Carpineto, P.; Ciancaglini, M.; Toto, L.; Mastropasqua, L. Amniotic membrane transplantation for the management of corneal epithelial defects: An in vivo confocal microscopic study. *Br. J. Ophthalmol.* **2007**, *92*, 54–60. [CrossRef] [PubMed]
48. Sotozono, C.; Ang, L.P.; Koizumi, N.; Higashihara, H.; Ueta, M.; Inatomi, T.; Yokoi, N.; Kaido, M.; Dogru, M.; Shimazaki, J.; et al. New grading system for the evaluation of chronic ocular manifestations in patients with Stevens–Johnson syndrome. *Ophthalmology* **2007**, *114*, 1294–1302. [CrossRef]
49. Rabbettts RB: Visual acuity and contrast sensitivity. In *Clinical Visual Optics*; Rabbetts, R.B. (Ed.) Buttwerworth Heineman: Oxford, UK, 1998; pp. 19–61.
50. Risse, J.F. Acuité visuelle. In *Exploration de la Fonction Visuelle*; Risse, J.F., Ed.; Masson: Paris, France, 1999; pp. 99–128.
51. Yokogawa, H.; Kobayashi, A.; Yamazaki, N.; Masaki, T.; Sugiyama, K. Surgical therapies for corneal perforations: 10 years of cases in a tertiary referral hospital. *Clin. Ophthalmol.* **2014**, *8*, 2165–2170. [CrossRef] [PubMed]
52. Abdulhalim, B.-E.H.; Wagih, M.M.; Gad, A.A.M.; Boghdadi, G.; Nagy, R.R.S. Amniotic membrane graft to conjunctival flap in treatment of non-viral resistant infectious keratitis: A randomised clinical study. *Br. J. Ophthalmol.* **2015**, *99*, 59–63. [CrossRef] [PubMed]
53. Rim, T.H.; Kim, D.W.; Chung, E.J.; Kim, S.S. Nationwide incidence of blindness in South Korea: A 12-year study from 2002 to 2013. *Clin. Exp. Ophthalmol.* **2017**, *45*, 773–778. [CrossRef]
54. Lee, C.M.; Afshari, N.A. The global state of cataract blindness. *Curr. Opin. Ophthalmol.* **2017**, *28*, 98–103. [CrossRef]
55. Chirapapaisan, C.; Prabhasawat, P.; Srivannaboon, S.; Roongpoovapatr, V.; Chitsuthipakorn, P. Ocular injury due to potassium permanganate granules. *Case Rep. Ophthalmol.* **2018**, *9*, 132–137. [CrossRef] [PubMed]
56. Westekemper, H.; Figueiredo, F.; Siah, W.F.; Wagner, N.; Steuhl, K.-P.; Meller, D. Clinical outcomes of amniotic membrane transplantation in the management of acute ocular chemical injury. *Br. J. Ophthalmol.* **2017**, *101*, 103–107. [CrossRef] [PubMed]
57. Paolin, A.; Cogliati, E.; Trojan, D.; Griffoni, C.; Grassetto, A.; Elbadawy, H.; Ponzin, D. Amniotic membranes in ophthalmology: Long term data on transplantation outcomes. *Cell Tissue Bank.* **2016**, *17*, 51–58. [CrossRef] [PubMed]
58. Bouchard, C.S.; John, T. Amniotic membrane transplantation in the management of severe ocular surface disease: Indications and outcomes. *Ocul. Surf.* **2004**, *2*, 201–211. [CrossRef]
59. Röck, T.; Bartz-Schmidt, K.U.; Landenberger, J.; Bramkamp, M.; Röck, D. Amniotic membrane transplantation in reconstructive and regenerative ophthalmology. *Ann. Transplant.* **2018**, *23*, 160–165. [CrossRef]
60. Sabater-Cruz, N.; Figueras-Roca, M.; Ventosa, A.G.; Padró-Pitarch, L.; Tort, J.; Casaroli-Marano, R.P. Current clinical application of sclera and amniotic membrane for ocular tissue bio-replacement. *Cell Tissue Bank.* **2020**, *21*, 597–603. [CrossRef]
61. Brocks, D.; Mead, O.G.; Tighe, S.; Tseng, S.C.G. Self-retained cryopreserved amniotic membrane for the management of corneal ulcers. *Clin. Ophthalmol.* **2020**, *14*, 1437–1443. [CrossRef]
62. Yin, H.Y.; Cheng, A.M.S.; Tighe, S.; Kurochkin, P.; Nord, J.; Dhanireddy, S.; Swan, R.; Alpert, S. Self-retained cryopreserved amniotic membrane for treating severe corneal ulcers: A comparative, retrospective control study. *Sci. Rep.* **2020**, *10*, 17008. [CrossRef] [PubMed]
63. Resch, M.D.; Schlötzer-Schrehardt, U.; Hofmann-Rummelt, C.; Sauer, R.; Kruse, F.E.; Beckmann, M.W.; Seitz, B. Integration patterns of cryopreserved amniotic membranes into the human cornea. *Ophthalmology* **2006**, *113*, 1927–1935. [CrossRef] [PubMed]

64. Resch, M.D.; Schlötzer-Schrehardt, U.; Hofmann-Rummelt, C.; Sauer, R.; Cursiefen, C.; Kruse, F.E.; Beckmann, M.W.; Seitz, B. Adhesion structures of amniotic membranes integrated into human corneas. *Investig. Opthalmol. Vis. Sci.* **2006**, *47*, 1853–1861. [CrossRef] [PubMed]
65. Lee, S.-H.; Tseng, S.C. Amniotic membrane transplantation for persistent epithelial defects with ulceration. *Am. J. Ophthalmol.* **1997**, *123*, 303–312. [CrossRef]

MDPI
St. Alban-Anlage 66
4052 Basel
Switzerland
www.mdpi.com

Journal of Clinical Medicine Editorial Office
E-mail: jcm@mdpi.com
www.mdpi.com/journal/jcm

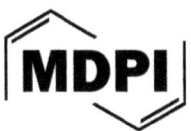

Disclaimer/Publisher's Note: The statements, opinions and data contained in all publications are solely those of the individual author(s) and contributor(s) and not of MDPI and/or the editor(s). MDPI and/or the editor(s) disclaim responsibility for any injury to people or property resulting from any ideas, methods, instructions or products referred to in the content.

www.ingramcontent.com/pod-product-compliance
Lightning Source LLC
LaVergne TN
LVHW070616100526
838202LV00012B/659